W9-BQX-555

Cod, cool Book.

The
Complete Book of
MINERALS
for
HEALTH

ALL-NEW EDITION

The Complete Book of MINERALS *for* HEALTH

ALL-NEW EDITION

BY
SHARON FAELTEN
AND THE EDITORS OF
Prevention®
MAGAZINE

RODALE PRESS EMMAUS, PA

Copyright © 1981 by Rodale Press, Inc.

All rights reserved. No part of this publication may be reproduced or transmitted in any form or by any means, electronic or mechanical, including photocopy, recording, or any information storage and retrieval system, without the written permission of the publisher.

Book Design by Jerry O'Brien   Illustrations by Jeanne Stock

Printed in the United States of America on recycled paper, containing a high percentage of de-inked fiber.

Library of Congress Cataloging in Publication Data

Faelten, Sharon.
    The complete book of minerals for health.

    Previous ed. by: J.I. Rodale. 1972.
    Includes bibliographical references and
index.
    1. Minerals in the body. 2. Health.
I. Rodale, J. I. (Jerome Irving),
1898-1971. Complete book of minerals for
health. II. Prevention (Emmaus, Pa.)
III. Title.
QP533.F23   1981   613.2'8   81-8684
ISBN 0-87857-360-7   hardcover   AACR2
    6   8   10   9   7   hardcover

Address all inquiries to: Rodale Books
                            Rodale Press, Inc.
                            33 East Minor Street
                            Emmaus, Pennsylvania 18049

Notice

This book is intended as a reference volume only, not as a medical manual or guide to self-treatment. If you suspect that you have a medical problem, we urge you to seek competent medical help. Keep in mind that nutritional needs vary from person to person, depending on age, sex, health status and total diet. Information here is intended to help you make informed decisions about your diet, not to substitute for any treatment that may have been prescribed by your doctor.

Editors: Mark Bricklin
Emrika Padus

Contributions by: Carol Baldwin
Dominick Bosco
John Feltman
William Gottlieb
Carol Keough
Laurie Lucas
Eileen Mazer
Kerry Pechter
Linda Shaw
Carl Sherman
Larry Stains
Jonathan Uhlaner
John Yates

Research Chief: Carol Baldwin

Assistant Research Chief: Carol Matthews

Research Associates: Martha Capwell
Holly Clemson
Takla Gardey
Sue Ann Gursky
Christy Kohler
Carol Munson
Susan Nastasee
Susan Rosenkrantz
Joann Williams

Copy Editor: Marian Wolbers

Supervisor of Publication
Recipe Testing: Anita Hirsch

Test Kitchen Personnel: JoAnn Benedick
Rhonda Diehl
Janice Kay
Irene Nicholson
Gretel Rupert

Office Personnel: Carol Petrakovich
Barbara Hill
Brenda Peluso

CONTENTS

List of Tables and Charts

Acknowledgments

Special thanks go out to the many physicians and researchers who shared their thoughts and experiences with us and shed light on new developments in their field of mineral nutrition. Among those who were especially helpful are: Anthony Albanese, Ph.D., Burke Rehabilitation Center, White Plains, New York; Joseph Boone, Ph.D., Centers for Disease Control, Atlanta, Georgia; Richard Jacobs, Ph.D., acting chief of nutrient toxicity—Division of Nutrition, Food and Drug Administration; Sheldon V. Pollack, M.D., Duke University Medical Center, Durham, North Carolina; Leslie M. Klevay, M.D., USDA Human Nutrition Laboratory, Grand Forks, North Dakota; Pekko Koivistoinen, Ph.D., University of Helsinki, Finland; Gerhard N. Schrauzer, Ph.D., University of California, La Jolla, California.

Thanks, too, to Anne C. Marsh, Consumer Nutrition Center, U.S. Department of Agriculture, Washington, D.C., who answered countless questions and provided a wealth of information concerning the nutrient value of foods, and to Carol Matthews for her invaluable advice and recommendations in preparing the recipe section of the book.

And finally, I'd like to offer my personal thanks to Emrika and Mark for their confidence and guidance, and to my husband John for his encouragement while work was in progress.

FOREWORD

Most of us have been hearing about vitamins since we were children. All the vitamins in the world do us little good without minerals, though. In fact, minerals are not only as important as vitamins, but in many cases they may be *more* important. Since the first edition of this book was printed, a surge of new research on minerals has spurred medical progress in almost every area of health. Consider:

• Twenty or 30 years ago, the notion that something as time-honored as salt—sodium chloride—could be to blame for an insidious killer disease was not taken very seriously. Now, most doctors urge people with high blood pressure to cut down on sodium, possibly saving millions from stroke, heart attack or kidney failure.

• In the past 15 years or so, insulin has come a long way as the one and only way to control the erratic blood sugar levels of diabetes. But research now indicates that the trace mineral chromium helps the body use insulin much more efficiently, thereby helping to save diabetics from the long-term and sometimes fatal effects of the disease.

• Ten years ago, cutting cholesterol intake was touted as the single most important way to escape heart disease. Low-fat diets took center stage. Now, a defense line of minerals is stepping forward as the guardians of our hearts and arteries.

• In the past few years, doctors have turned serious attention to nutrition as a possible means of fighting cancer. Selenium, one of the newest trace minerals on the scene, has begun to show promise not only as an effective aid to cancer therapy, but as a preventative as well.

Progress hasn't been limited to the life-threatening diseases, either. The thin, crumbly bones of osteoporosis—the bane of five million older women a year—appears to be the upshot of long-term embezzlement of calcium from bones. Reducing diets, childbearing, breastfeeding, lack of exercise, emotional stress and hormonal changes all foster calcium losses. Fragile bones need not team up with gray hair and wrinkles as a by-product of age, though. A high-calcium diet not only fends off those antibone factors, but bone losses can even be reversed in some cases. There's no reason why we all can't have the same strong bones at age 70 that we do at 25.

Aside from great strides toward mastering the more disabling health problems, other research has pointed out that minerals are responsible for helping us feel our best *every* day.

• Chronic fatigue drags more people to their doctors than any other problem. Faulty nutrition may often be the hidden cause. Certain minerals—magnesium, potassium and iron—are particularly important. Those minerals were used in actual studies in which people who had been tired for more than two years felt terrific again after minerals were added to their diet.

• Dips in sexual vigor in men—or even actual impotence—may improve with zinc therapy. Zinc supplementation dramatically reversed the sexual woes of kidney dialysis patients in one study. And it just might do the same for "ordinary" impotence, say researchers.

• If you should find yourself laid up in bed with a broken bone or surgical incision, zinc can get you out of bed in record time. Whether you gash your foot or have your gallbladder out, healing is improved if zinc is in good supply. Doctors have found that zinc levels—before *and* after surgery—are a good barometer of how well patients heal after surgery. Without enough zinc, incisions refuse to close up and infections set in. Healing becomes a long, drawn-out—and frustrating—affair. With plenty of zinc, though, wounds heal up tight, smooth and clean.

Those are just a handful of many similar discoveries. So far, 28 conditions—from body odor and migraine headaches to arthritis and prostate trouble—seem to be related to mineral imbalance in some way. In fact, we now know of 21 minerals that exhibit critical roles in health.

When you think about it, minerals are bound to be important. After all, rocks are the parent material for soil—which is the main source of nutrition for plants, animals and us, ultimately. While single, stark deficiencies of any one mineral are rare, what happens if we're marginally low in several minerals? The effects are often very subtle. To top it off, absorption of minerals such as iron and chromium declines with age.

Stress and exposure to environmental pollution raises our requirements for zinc, calcium, iron and others.

Then there's the case against harmful minerals—notably lead, cadmium and mercury—from industrial pollution. Even casually accepted elements like chlorine are coming under close scrutiny.

Clearly, minerals can no longer be taken for granted. This all-new version of *The Complete Book of Minerals for Health,* completely rewritten from start to finish, not only brings you up to date on the many important developments, but shows how you can use that information to build good health into your diet as well.

Mark Bricklin
Executive Editor, *Prevention®* magazine

PART
I

INTRODUCTION

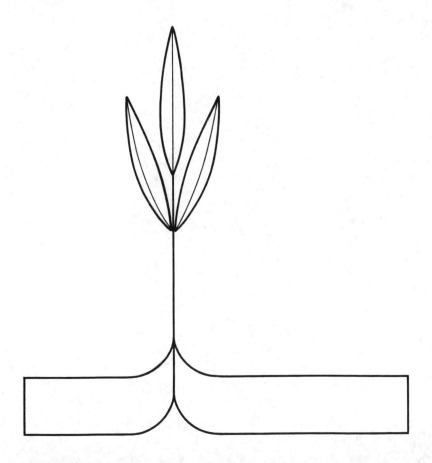

CHAPTER

1

Links of Life

Minerals Are Our Link with the Universe

Without minerals, there would be no universe as we know it, just shapeless swirls of thin gases in the infinite vacuum of black space.

The gold that lured pioneers to California, the iron that was forged into networks of railroads across continents, and the copper that shaped empires in South America are all the result of a colossal burst of fireworks that some scientists believe gave birth to the universe at the beginning of time. From the calcium in our teeth to the chrome on our automobiles, all minerals go back farther in time and space than the mind can comprehend. That applies to the minerals in soil, in our food, and in our bones, blood and skin.

The entire Earth and we, its residents, evolved from just a few dozen basic substances, including minerals. Of the more than 100 elements found in nature, 4 (oxygen, hydrogen, carbon and nitrogen) make up 96 percent of our body. Minerals make up the remaining 4 percent, but a lack of just one of them can make life impossible.

Our bodies and the minerals within them are part of an amazing system that began several billion years ago. Scientists generally believe that the universe was created by a huge, spontaneous blast of energy—the "big bang." That great fireball of intense, brilliant light—light denser than matter—continued to expand, cooling over eons of time, eventually leaving a residue of ordinary matter. The building blocks of matter are tiny units called atoms, which are made of still smaller units called protons, neutrons and electrons. Those units eventually combined in various ways to form the 103 elements, including minerals, that are with us on Earth today. Amazing as it may seem, what gives each element its unique nature—what makes oxygen different from hydrogen, calcium different from magnesium, zinc different from copper—is how many protons each atom contains. The first elements to be formed were probably the gases hydrogen and helium—the two lightest elements.

Gravity pulled the turbulent swirls of gases into stars, which led to the formation of minerals, and later planets, including our Earth. As the earth cooled, water vapor in the atmosphere condensed, and the rain collected in basins to form the ancient oceans.

The rough similarity between seawater and our blood, among other considerations, leads scientists to believe that life originated in those ancient oceans, perhaps about 3½ billion years ago. They can only guess at just how that transition from nonliving to living took place. However it happened, we doubt that it was anything short of a miracle.

Minerals not only preceded life, but made life possible. The first one-celled bacteria and blue-green algae swam in a soup brimming with minerals. As plants and animals evolved and migrated to land many millions of years later, they brought with them that same fundamental need for many minerals. On land, however, minerals are locked into the earth's crust. As land dwellers, our main link with minerals is through a diet of plants (and other animals that eat plants), which are able to extract minerals from the soil as they grow.

Our bodies require large amounts of some minerals, only trace amounts of others, and none at all of several more. The amount we need of each and the amounts present in our bodies are not necessarily in proportion to their importance to health. A few milligrams of zinc, for example, are just as necessary as several hundred milligrams of calcium.

Those minerals that are essential to health in relatively high amounts are often called *macro*minerals. They include calcium, phosphorus, potassium, sulfur, sodium, chlorine and magnesium. Our bodies contain significant amounts of each (see table 1).

TABLE 1   **Minerals in the Body**

	Mineral	Percent of Body Weight
Essential to Human Health		
Major Minerals	Calcium	1.5–2.2
	Phosphorus	0.8–1.2
	Potassium	0.35
	Sulfur	0.25
	Sodium	0.15
	Chlorine	0.15
	Magnesium	0.05
Trace Minerals	Iron	
	Zinc	
	Selenium	
	Manganese	
	Copper	
	Iodine	
	Molybdenum	
	Cobalt	
	Chromium	
	Fluorine	
	Silicon	
	Vanadium	
	Nickel	
	Tin	
Take Part in Biological Reactions, but Essentiality Not Proven	Barium	each less than 0.01
	Arsenic	
	Bromine	
	Strontium	
	Cadmium	
Not Known to be Essential; No Known Biological Function	Gold	
	Silver	
	Aluminum	
	Mercury	
	Bismuth	
	Gallium	
	Lead	
	Antimony	
	Boron	
	Lithium	
	plus 20 others	

SOURCE: Adapted from *Introductory Nutrition,* 4th ed., by Helen Andrews Guthrie (St. Louis: C. V. Mosby, 1979).

Trace minerals, on the other hand, are present in the body in minute amounts; each makes up less than one-hundredth of a percent of body weight. A few trace minerals seem to serve no purpose at all, as far as we know; some can even be harmful if the body gets too much. However, many are just as essential to health as the major minerals, and are required in small but critical amounts, sometimes only a few micrograms. (A microgram is one-thousandth of a milligram). Essential trace minerals include iron, zinc, selenium, manganese, copper, iodine, molybdenum, cobalt, chromium, fluorine, silicon, vanadium, nickel and tin.

What are minerals like calcium, copper and iron from rocks in the earth's crust doing in our living, breathing, moving bodies? A lot. Just a few examples:

• Sodium and potassium regulate water balance. Otherwise, we would swell up with water or dry out and die.

• Iron is part of a substance called hemoglobin, which carries life-sustaining oxygen to our cells.

• Sulfur combines with nitrogen, carbon, hydrogen and oxygen to build protein, the stuff of muscles, skin and organs.

• Calcium, too, is a builder. Calcium gives bones and teeth their strength and rigidity, and also helps nerves to function properly.

• Copper, zinc and cobalt, among other minerals, are necessary for enzyme activities, such as food digestion.

Many minerals do multiple jobs, or overlap in their work. We could give dozens of other examples of the importance of minerals, and such a list is likely to grow. Chromium, for instance, was thought to be nonessential until just a few years ago. Now it's been determined that chromium seems to help regulate fluctuations in blood sugar levels associated with hypoglycemia and diabetes.

Carbon is the most ubiquitous and versatile element in the world, combining with itself as well as with other elements, including minerals, to form a staggering number of substances. In many ways, carbon bridges the gap between minerals and other substances, tying them together into the viable, orderly system called life. Carbon in combination with varying proportions of oxygen, hydrogen, nitrogen and other elements forms the nutrients essential to life: protein, carbohydrates, fats and vitamins. The protein in meat and in our skin, muscles and organs is made of carbon combined with oxygen, hydrogen, nitrogen and sometimes sulfur in more than 20 variations, called amino acids. Potatoes, beans and other plant foods are made primarily of carbohydrates—carbon, oxygen and hydrogen. Fats, too, are made of carbon, hydrogen and oxygen in a slightly different arrangement. Vitamins, likewise, are unique and special combinations of carbon, oxygen, hydrogen and sometimes nitrogen, quite often with a mineral attached.

You'll recall that 96 percent of your body is made of carbon and its sister elements, hydrogen, oxygen and nitrogen. So instrumental to life are combinations of carbon and its compounds that they are collectively christened *organic,* from a very old Greek word meaning tool or instrument. All substances, from potatoes to people, that contain those compounds are also called organic.

Minerals and Vitamins, a Marriage Made in Heaven

Minerals are quite different from vitamins in their structure and the work they do, but the two enjoy an excellent working relationship. Minerals create a healthy environment in which the body, using vitamins, proteins, carbohydrates and fats, can grow, function and heal itself. Some of the B vitamins are active or absorbed only when combined with phosphorus compounds, for example. Zinc facilitates the release of vitamin A from the liver. Some vitamins even contain minerals. Vitamin B_1 (thiamine), crucial to heart and nerve function, contains sulfur. Vitamin B_{12} (cobalamin) contains cobalt.

Conversely, some vitamins are helpmates to minerals. Vitamin C can triple iron absorption. Calcium absorption is impossible without vitamin D. Other vitamin-mineral relationships are explored more extensively in chapter 28, Vitamins and Minerals That Work Together.

A vitamin can be broken down into its basic elements (i.e., carbon, oxygen and hydrogen), but a mineral cannot. It *is* an element. And while many vitamins can be synthesized by animals and plants, minerals cannot. Vitamins A, B_{12} and K, for example, can be manufactured in the body out of substances in the food we eat. Vitamin D is a product of the body's reaction to sunlight. But all minerals must be supplied entirely by our environment. What's more, minerals occur in finite supply. We cannot "make" more calcium. The same goes for nickel, chromium, gold and so on.

Minerals Are Pilfered Away by Today's Food Technology

Drastic changes in our natural environment appeared as civilization arose and technology followed. The tools that revolutionized agriculture were followed by methods of growing and refining food that changed the mineral content of soils and food considerably.

To grow and reproduce, crops take up minerals from water and soil, as plants have done for millions of years. Soil is not made of minerals alone, though. Mixed with minerals is humus, a rich, variegated blend of bacteria, fungi, molds, yeasts, algae, worms, insects and other tiny organisms—not very different from the mixed environment created on land ages ago. Humus-rich soil provides a perfect balance of essential minerals to plants—mosses, grasses, shrubs, wheat and rice, vegetables, fruit trees, redwoods and so on. The health and survival of all plants, domestic or wild, depend on the health of the soil and its ability to provide a constant supply of minerals.

People, like other animals, don't live and grow rooted to one spot like a tree. Our main link with minerals in the rocks and soil is our diet. In the passage of minerals from rocks——▶soil——▶plants——▶people, many things can happen to interrupt the flow of minerals up the food chain. The more technologically advanced the food supply system becomes, the more opportunity there is for minerals to be lost along the way.

The major step toward food technology came when people domesticated plants and animals about 10,000 years ago. Depending on farming and livestock raising instead of hunting and gathering for subsistence meant that families could plan ahead for provisions. The advent of agriculture also meant that households were no longer forced to move on again and again in search of fresh sources of wild food. Shelter became more permanent.

Households were self-sufficient at first, providing for all their own needs, including growing and storing food. No longer dependent on the skill—and luck—required for successful hunting, fewer people starved and populations grew. As communities developed, they grew more efficient: a few people could grow enough food for all, in return for household goods and services provided by the others. Certain individuals milled grain and others baked bread, for instance, in exchange for clothing, tools or other goods. Task specialization gave rise to the market economy, and trade and transportation flourished. Thus, control over the food supply helped make possible the rise of civilization.

But as that control over food increased over thousands of years, nature was increasingly changed and dominated by people to such a degree that much of today's food doesn't even remotely resemble ancient foods. Can you picture a cave family sitting down to bowls of sugarcoated cornflakes at breakfast? Or to those psychedelic cereals hawked by television advertisers? Try to imagine a cave dweller stopping work at midmorning for a Danish and coffee with nondairy creamer. The fact is, our present banquet of fabricated food fare is far removed from what early people plucked and stewed, or sifted and simmered for their tables. It not only looks and tastes very different, it also has far fewer minerals.

Chemical Farming Robs Food of Minerals

Other changes, less obvious but more significant because of their effect on minerals, resulted from people's intensive use of the soil for farming. The mineral content of plants has been drastically altered right in the fields and soil in which they grow. Long ago, farmers discovered that adding compost—decayed plants and animal wastes—kept the soil rich, fertile and productive. Little did they know that they were replenishing the helpful bacteria that are naturally present in humus-rich soil and restoring minerals to be taken up by crops. Because that practice of fertilization was in harmony with nature's own cycles of plant and animal coexistence, it caused no problems. And so it went for thousands of years.

Chemical fertilizers were then developed by making or mining concentrated forms of nitrogen, phosphorus and potassium rather than using compounds as they exist in nature. By adding those artificial fertilizers—nitrate, phosphate and potash—to the soil, crop yields could be greatly increased. But what first appeared to be a blessing has turned out to be a crown of thorns. Man-made fertilizers upset the delicate balance of minerals and organisms in humus-rich soil by killing off the beneficial bacteria and locking in the naturally occurring minerals so they are less available to plants. Chemical fertilizers can also saturate plant roots with too much of one nutrient, making it difficult for crops to pick up other minerals that they need just as much.

Studies have confirmed that chemical farming reduces the mineral content of many foods. In certain soils, according to one researcher, corn raised with heavy use of artificial phosphorus fertilizer is deficient in zinc. Soils in at least 30 states, in fact, have been shown to be seriously depleted of zinc by intensive chemical farming over recent decades. Surveys conducted by West Virginia University show that iron, copper and manganese contents of grain dropped in 11 Midwestern states over a recent five-year period.

In a study using feedlot manure as fertilizer, W. S. Peavy and J. K. Griz found that natural fertilizer produced a spinach crop richer in iron than one grown with chemical fertilizers. "Our results likely came from decomposing organic fertilizer forming organic acids that caused iron to [bind] into forms more readily absorbed by plants," say the researchers (*Journal of the American Society of Horticultural Science,* vol. 97, no. 6, 1972). And in another study, the calcium and phosphorus content of turnip greens increased as the organic matter of the soil increased.

A similar influence on vitamin content of organically versus chemically fertilized crops has not yet been determined. As organic methods of farming receive more attention, both here and in Europe, researchers may find that vitamin levels, too, are higher in organically grown foods. A 12-year study at West Germany's Federal Institute for Quality Research on Plant Products found that vegetables grown by organic methods had significantly higher amounts of vitamin C, along with more potassium, calcium, phosphorus and iron than chemically grown vegetables. "That the consumer would benefit from a higher biological value of such products," concludes Werner Schuphan, director of the Institute, "is beyond question" (*Progressive,* December, 1978).

Disease Is on the Rise
While Minerals Are on the Wane

Those major changes in the way foods are grown and processed have altered the amount and availability of the minerals so essential to life from its very origin. How have we, as consumers of that food, survived those changes?

Not very well, it seems. The results of those severe changes in our food supply, according to mineral researchers, are showing up as widespread health problems. Speaking on the importance of trace minerals, Eric J. Underwood, Ph.D., chairman of an international symposium on nutrition held in 1975, said, "A further feature of recent trace [mineral] research is that mild or marginal deficiencies occur in some human populations, particularly where the dietary patterns include a high proportion of refined and processed foods" (*Proceedings of the Tenth International Congress of Nutrition,* August 3-9, 1975 [Kyoto, Japan: Victory-sha Press, 1976]).

Adding to the quagmire of processed food, artificially fertile fields, and depletion of minerals in our diet is the glut of other man-made combinations, drugs, which are swallowed by Americans. One rarely recognized but far-reaching side effect of many drugs is that they chelate, or bind, with one or more minerals, making those minerals unavailable to the body.

"A great many ordinary drugs are chelating agents," said Henry A. Schroeder, M.D., in a keynote speech at a symposium on trace mineral research in Princeton, New Jersey, in 1973. Penicillin is one of those mineral-binding drugs, pointed out Dr. Schroeder, as are a number of other powerful antibiotics. Other drugs affect minerals in other ways. Diuretics flush potassium out of the body, and deplete magnesium. Sedatives can lower blood levels of calcium and magnesium. Antacids, available without prescription, disturb calcium and phosphorus metabolism. Other examples are discussed more fully in chapter 27, Alcohol, Drugs and Food Ingredients That Meddle with Health-Building Minerals.

That is not to imply that drugs should never be used. What it does say is that doctors need to learn more about long-term effects before prescribing drugs. Drug-induced nutritional deficiencies are preventable. Mineral deficiencies can be corrected by giving doses of the deficient mineral large enough to compensate for the loss. But deficiencies cannot be prevented if doctors aren't aware that they can occur.

Pollution Pumps Harmful Minerals
into Our System

Anything can be harmful in excess. The same goes for minerals.

Paradoxically, even minerals that the body requires for good health can be harmful if we get too much of any of them. That's because taking too much of a mineral, even though it's essential to health, can upset the balance and functions of other minerals and vitamins in the body. If all the potassium the body requires in one day were taken in a single, concentrated dose, for instance, serious illness could result. That rarely happens, though. For essential minerals, too little is more common than too much. Except in the case of a metabolic disorder like iron storage disease (hemochromatosis), the body can excrete much of what it doesn't use of a mineral. But the body cannot possibly make up for what it gets too little of.

Not all minerals are beneficial. A few are quite harmful. Lead, cadmium and mercury are the most common pollutants. Historically, so little of those harmful minerals crept into our food and water that life went on with no alarming effects. Small amounts of insidious poisons like lead, cadmium and mercury are flushed out of the body. Moderate buildups can be countered by an adequate supply of "good" minerals, such as zinc, copper, calcium and manganese. Zinc, for instance, boosts the immune system and lowers body concentrations of both lead and cadmium. It's as if nature provides its own system of checks and balances to help us survive.

That system works fine when the body is infiltrated by manageable levels of toxic minerals. However, large-scale environmental pollution—such as heavy auto exhaust and industrial waste—spewed into our atmosphere, affects every link in the food chain. As harmful minerals continue to be mined out of the earth and find their way into our food, air and water, our bodies may be unable to cope with uncustomarily large amounts of poisons. Chronic exposure to large amounts of lead affects the brain, nerves, blood and digestive system. Cadmium poisoning results in pneumonia and sometimes permanent lung damage. Mercury poisoning can result in bleeding gums, loose teeth, tremors and lack of coordination. The long-term and possibly cancer-causing effects of pollution from those and other toxic minerals, such as certain forms of nickel, are now being investigated (see chapter 25, Canceling Out Lead and Other Harmful Substances).

Minerals in the Fight against Disease

The crux of the matter is that we are getting less of the minerals we do need and more of the minerals we don't need. The science of how all minerals, good or bad, evolved, and how they work in the body is now being applied to the mastery of many diseases.

Scientists have long recognized overt illness due to severe deficiencies of single minerals—iodine in goiter and iron in anemia—and gross deficiencies due to overall malnutrition. Researchers are now pursuing the strong hunch that clear-cut deficiencies are merely one aspect of a more complex relationship between minerals and health. The key to total health may lie in more subtle deficiencies—small deficits of several minerals that are often ignored or overlooked. Infections, for instance, are now fought primarily with antibiotics, and will continue to be treated that way until we understand more about the role of minerals in a strong immune system. Immunity to many diseases may depend on minerals for a great deal of strength, since the body suffers marked changes in the amounts of magnesium, iron, copper, zinc and phosphorus in the blood during infectious attack by viruses and harmful bacteria.

The most vexing problems are the chronic diseases—osteoporosis, osteoarthritis, atherosclerosis and heart disease, diabetes and cancer—which are emerging in epidemic numbers in developed nations. The riddles as to how those diseases develop and how we can prevent or deal with them are complex. Nutrition is receiving more and more attention from medical scientists, whose focus has been predominantly on vitamins. Because minerals and vitamins work so closely together, the solutions to those diseases may very well be found in the way minerals work in our bodies. Our bodies were designed to use both vitamins and minerals to heal themselves. Starve a body of essential minerals or deluge it with toxic minerals, and conditions are no longer right for healing, but for self-destruction.

The Best Is Yet to Come

At first, the only doctors interested in trace mineral nutrition were veterinarians. Livestock raisers quickly found out that cattle and sheep whose diets were deficient in zinc, copper, selenium and other nutrients were less likely to grow strong and healthy. That threatened profits, so livestock diets were soon supplemented with the needed nutrients wherever necessary.

In more recent years, scientists have taken a closer look at those same minerals in humans. And the potential benefits are just as exciting. Dr. M. Kirchgessner of Munich Technical University's Institute of Nutritional Physiology in West Germany explained, "There is a striking increase in the number of outstanding reports on nutritional and medical problems of trace [minerals] in man. . . . Since . . . 1973, about 2,000 scientific reports on trace [minerals] have been published. . . . This means that, per annum, the number of publications on trace [minerals] is about twice as high as 10 years ago and nearly three times as high as 20 years ago."

Dr. Kirchgessner made that remark at the Third International Symposium on Trace Element Metabolism in Man and Animals, in 1977. Two years later an article in a widely read scientific journal stated: "It is probable that trace [minerals] not yet known to be necessary for human health will be added to the 'essential' list in the future, as still newer experimental techniques evolve" (*Chemistry,* March, 1979).

Ironically, it appears that the same high level of technology that brought us chemical farming, artificially fabricated food and industrial pollution will make possible detailed investigation of health problems that technology helped cause.

Not only has there been an explosion of research—and interest—in minerals and health in recent years, but that trend is likely to continue. And so it should be. For never has there been a more clear-cut case of not being able to see the forest for the trees, so to speak, as in the paucity of recognition given to the role of minerals, which not only existed before life was born but actually made life possible. An eminent medical researcher in Birmingham, England, tersely commented on science's sometimes short-sighted approach to the origins and mechanisms of disease by writing, "It is unthinkable that man, who is keenly interested in the nature of the world in which he lives and the contents of the space beyond it, should not have an equal or greater interest in his own body and the diseases which affect it" (*Lancet,* December 15, 1979).

The implications of restoring mineral balance in the fragile ecosystem of our bodies go beyond physical health to total emotional and intellectual health.

The aim of this book is not only to bring to light the effects that changes in mineral distribution in the world have had on us, but to explore what measures can be taken to offset those effects. It's not likely that people will go back to the days of plow horses and horse-drawn carts, or abandon supermarkets for backyard gardens. But there are many ways to put yourself back in control of the minerals in your environment.

This book will help you get a clearer idea of what you are eating and what your personal mineral needs may be. It's likely that you'll want to know if your diet is supplying you with enough minerals. You may wonder whether you should take mineral supplements, and if so, what kinds to look for and how much to take. Many of the nutrition specialists and mineral researchers we spoke to in preparing this book suggest that the best way to be sure that you and your family are getting enough minerals is through a combination of high-mineral foods and mineral supplements. We'll discuss average requirements of individual minerals from chapter to chapter. We'll also talk about foods that are good sources of minerals, and share some recipes for dishes that provide ample supplies of one or more minerals. Other chapters focus on those disorders that either indicate a low intake of one or more minerals or seem to be stalled or relieved by taking extra minerals.

If you are already taking vitamins, but until now have been fuzzy on the importance of minerals, you are now one step closer to rounding out your nutritional education.

PART
II

MINERALS THAT BUILD HEALTH

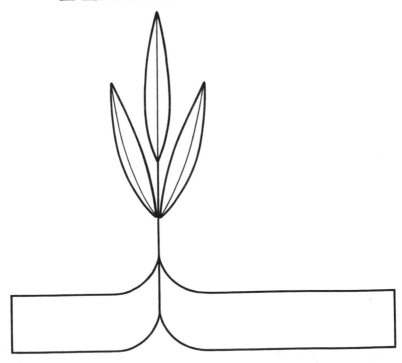

2

Calcium

The Difference between People and Jellyfish

Without calcium, your bones would be so soft they could be tied in knots like ropes of modeling clay. As it is, our bones are about as strong as steel—but far lighter. And flexible enough to absorb the severe sudden impact of a blow without splintering, or of a fall without snapping apart.

Bones owe part of their toughness to superb engineering, too. Our framework of bones follows some of the same principles used by architects to design buildings that will bear up against the forces of wind, weather and earth tremors for hundreds of years. Which makes our internal scaffolding as impressive an engineering feat as the pillars and girders that support the great Gothic cathedrals or modern skyscrapers.

Our remarkable bones are adequate for most practical purposes. Emergencies do arise, however. A bone *will* break under enough strain. And because bones are living tissues, disease can besiege them. Disease of the liver, kidneys, nerves, glands or blood may also affect our bones. So bones must be self-healing. Because bones are made largely of calcium and phosphorus, a diet sparse in those minerals makes growth and good health impossible. Other nutrients—protein and vitamins A, C and D—are important too. But bones can no more do their work without calcium and phosphorus than an open-hearth furnace can produce steel without raw materials of iron and limestone.

People often take their skeleton for granted. Without our custom-designed framework, we would have no means to walk, hold ourselves upright, sit, stand, run or dance. We couldn't do much of anything, as a matter of fact. Without our calcium-rich, remarkably designed skeleton, our bodies would be just as limp and disjointed as a deboned Cornish hen ready to be popped into the oven. Yet some animals do get around quite well without a skeleton for support. Some jellyfish are as big as people, but because they live in the sea, where gravity is neutralized, jellyfish can get around very smoothly without any bones at all. In general, though, most animals, even those who live in the buoyancy of water, need a skeleton of some sort—for support, protection and mobility.

Skeletons aren't always inside the body. Pick up a clamshell the next time you're at the beach. Or a shell left behind by a snail in your garden. Or a conch shell decorating a fireplace mantle. What you hold in your hand is a crude version of your own skeleton. Granted, the clam's shell has 2 sections, and yours has 206 (the approximate number of your bones). But both are skeletons. The simple hinge that opens and closes the clam's skeleton is very much like the joint that enables you to bend your arm at the elbow. And skeletons in all animals, from clams to humans, depend on one special mineral for strength—calcium.

The Grit and Glue of Bone, Calcium and Collagen

Any architect will tell you that the most magnificently designed shelter in the world will collapse if built with inferior materials. And so it is with your skeleton. Like any living tissue, bone contains some water. Other than that, bones owe their hardness to a composition that is one-half mineral (calcium and phosphorus, in a ratio of roughly 2:1) and one-half a gristlelike protein called collagen. Crystals of a calcium compound sandwiched between sheets and fibers of stiff collagen form a bond that's strong, yet flexible enough to absorb the shock waves of jarring impacts, like the repeated stress of running or a fall. Our fast-paced way of life has added new kinds of opportunities for impact unknown to our early ancestors: automobiles, roller skates, skis, skateboards, high-heeled shoes and highly waxed floors, to name a few. Without that tight fusion of grit and glue in bones, we couldn't even type without breaking our fingers, or slap a pal on the back without smashing our hands. The next time someone greets you with a viselike handshake, you can thank calcium and collagen for keeping your fingers intact.

You'll notice it takes a few good whacks with a rock to break a clamshell. That durability may explain why shells have been used as tools, media of exchange and ornaments by primitive people from before recorded history. In a similar way, the human skeleton and teeth, also made primarily of calcium, are all that remain after the rest of the body dies and deteriorates. Detectives rely on bones and teeth to identify bodies of people done in months—or years—before they're found. Archaeologists use the same kind of clues when studying the remains of pyramid residents or our cave-dwelling ancestors. An x-ray of a living person, taken to evaluate a health condition, can help identify the age and sex of that person.

A clam's shell outweighs its body many times over. For that reason, he's restricted to life underwater, where buoyancy helps him get around. Our skeleton, by comparison, is very lightweight—about one-fifth of our total body composition. That's important, because without water to buoy us up, walking on land would be an impossible chore for a heavy frame. Either human life would be limited to lakes, oceans and pools, or we would have to eat far more food in order to produce sufficient energy to carry ourselves around. The earth could support far fewer people if we all had to eat three times as much as we do. It's probable that the demographics of our planet would be quite different if our bones were heavier.

What makes our skeleton so light? And how is such a light skeleton strong enough to withstand the pounding of pavement on a morning jog, falls over coffee tables, or misjudged steps off sidewalk curbs, without twisting and breaking?

The answer lies in two sound engineering principles found in all bones. Architects and builders discovered centuries ago that by setting beams at right angles to each other in latticework fashion, a tall building was able to stand in spite of its great weight. The femur, or thighbone, is the longest bone, and its main job is to support the body. The femur is constructed in a latticework pattern at each end. Toward the center, the femur is hollow. That follows the engineering principle that a column doesn't necessarily have to be solid to be strong. A hollow bone gets the job done without the burden of extra weight. Hollow bones make an effective chassis, for if bones were solid, the skeleton would be much heavier. Making efficient use of the hollow inside is a nursery for red blood cells, which carry vital oxygen to all parts of the body.

Bones, the Ideal Calcium Storehouse

Just as buildings aren't always constructed of steel beams, skeletons aren't always made of bones like ours. We've seen what a far cry from a clamshell our skeleton is. Why did the clam skeleton evolve one way and ours another? Let's take a look.

Obviously, a clam's life is limited by the design of his skeleton. A single, albeit strong, foot makes the clam somewhat mobile—that is, about as quick and nimble as an adult on a toddler's tricycle. A clam gets no farther than a fumbling start if he tries to go after food any faster than the tiny plants siphoned in along with his water supply. And the clam is strictly a defensive player when startled by turbulent tides or enemies: he can either burrow beneath the sand or brace himself within his Tom Thumb tank. As he grows, his shell grows, accruing more and more calcium with age. Truly a sheltered existence.

Fortunately, there's more than one way to build a skeleton. Somewhere along the line, structural design took off in another direction—that of many hinged segments, or jointed shells, in some animals. And—voilà!—the large division of the animal kingdom called Arthropoda (the arthropods) was born. "Arthro" means "joint." You'll recognize the term from the word arthritis, an inflammation of the joints.

Flying and crawling insects like wasps and ants, and sea animals like crabs and lobsters, are just a few familiar arthropods. Arthropods represent sort of a midpoint between animals that have no skeleton and animals that have a bony, internal skeleton like ours. Arthropods live inside their shell, like clams. Their segmented shell consists of a thick, elastic skin called the cuticle. The cuticle consists mostly of an inner layer of a substance called chitin (pronounced "KITE-in"). The inner layer is thick, porous and, in many species, hardened by a buildup of calcium. Very similar to our bones. And the arthropod skeleton is relatively lightweight.

Arthropods get around much better than clams. So much better, in fact, that during the course of evolution many of them were able to migrate to the land and the air. The ants that tote bread crumbs away from your kitchen table and the mosquitoes that dive-bomb your head at a campsite are kin to the lobster you order in a restaurant.

With all of its advantages, however, the exterior skeleton of the arthropod still has real drawbacks. Like the coats of mail worn by medieval knights, the suits are clumsy and awkward. Moreover, arthropods can't simply add on more calcium as they grow, as clams do. The entire skeleton has to be replaced from scratch. That process, called molting, leaves the crab, for instance, very vulnerable during the intervals when his old suit has been discarded and his new suit is being grown.

The need to periodically replace the skeleton limits the size of the arthropods. Science fiction movies thrill audiences with tales of creepy-crawlies dragging their huge horny bodies out of murky swamps to terrorize the countryside with groping antennae and lethal claws. That's all pure fantasy, of course. In comparison to people, most arthropods are quite tiny—shrimps, in a manner of speaking. Perhaps largest are the giant spider crabs, whose bodies weigh only 14 pounds and claws span 12½ feet. That's about as close to monster proportions as arthropods get.

The development of an interior skeleton was a major step in evolution because more sophisticated organs—brain, heart, liver and kidneys—soon followed.

The earliest version of our skeleton first showed up in what was probably one of the first fish. The increased freedom of movement was extraordinary. Fish could dart around after food, explore new areas—broaden their horizons, so to speak. Some of the fish that had little scales of armor plating around their mouths began to eat better than their neighbors. Apparently, the little "dermal teeth" helped them to grab and swallow food. In the cutthroat world of survival by natural selection, that was quite an advantage. Such teeth were passed on, slightly modified, to ensuing generations of fish. The teeth eventually moved inside the body, along with the internal skeleton. Both those traits were passed on to reptiles and mammals.

Teeth are formed from a calcium-laden tissue called dentin, which resembles bone. But it is not true bone, because bone is not strong enough to hold up under the friction of biting and grinding. Teeth solely of bone would wear down in no time. Frequent contact with chemicals in water and food would erode bone, too. For permanence, teeth are modeled out of bonelike dentin but covered with a protective layer of enamel, the hardest substance in the body.

Teeth were not the only updated equipment in early fish. Basic forms of those new organs—brain, heart, liver and kidneys—were passed on, with many, many modifications, from fish to amphibians (frogs and salamanders) to reptiles (snakes and dinosaurs, for instance) to birds, early mammals and, eventually, to people.

Calcium Keeps the Body Running Smoothly

Calcium was—and is—crucial to those new, sophisticated organs. We usually think of calcium in one way and one way only, as the builder of the bones and teeth. While it's true that 99 percent of the calcium in the body is found in the teeth and skeleton, without the other 1 percent, life would be impossible. Every breath you take, every muscle you move, every thought you think depends on the calcium that is redistributed from the skeletal storehouse by your bloodstream to the rest of the body. The nerve cells that power breath, muscle and brain need—and demand—the constant nourishment of calcium to do their jobs.

Looking at the development of the adult human skeleton from a slightly different angle, the growth of bones beginning shortly after conception uncannily parallels the development of the chitin-formed shells of arthropods and the bony framework of fish and mammals. The skeleton of a growing embryo is composed almost entirely of cartilage, a tough fibrous substance partially made of collagen. By birth, much of that cartilage turns to bone. By adulthood, not much cartilage remains. The ears and the tip of the nose are made up of cartilage, vestiges of the embryo skeleton.

Having a skeleton on the inside, as we do, makes things more convenient—and a little more complicated. While the skeleton is continually losing calcium—sort of an internal molting—bones are simultaneously accruing new calcium. That obviates the need to trade them in for new bones as the rest of our body grows during childhood and adolescence. A margin of reserve calcium is held in the bones to provide for short periods of scarcity or extra demands due to injury or disease.

Maintaining that reserve and regulating growth throughout life is controlled by several glands—the thyroid, parathyroid, pituitary, adrenals and sex glands. Among their other functions, the hormones secreted by the thyroid and parathyroid glands regulate the amount of calcium that reaches your bones. Sex hormones, in turn, influence that regulation. Calcium from your diet is absorbed by the upper intestine (just below the stomach), then delivered to the bones and other organs by the blood. At the same time, the blood carries away some calcium, which leaves the body in sweat, urine, feces and tears. As long as new bone growth keeps up with bone loss, as it usually does for the first few decades of life, bones remain hard and strong. If more calcium is lost than is replaced, bones weaken and start to break at the least provocation, such as a slip on the ice. A change in hormone secretion may be one cause. Women past menopause, for example, no longer produce large amounts of estrogen. That makes them prone to degeneration of bone, called osteoporosis (although men are not immune).

Quirks in the workings of some glands and their hormones can result in other, far rarer, conditions. A malfunctioning parathyroid may cause poor uptake of calcium by the bones. Occasionally, disturbance of growth hormone results in a dwarf or a giant.

Exercise Helps Calcium Keep Bones Strong

Perhaps because we walk on two legs instead of all fours, we lack the speed or strength of animals like the cheetah or the elephant. But we can still run, walk and dance with fair agility. And our unique skeleton and muscles which enable us to stand erect also free our arms for finer movements, like playing a violin or tinkering with a model airplane.

But if we allow those finer movements to totally replace more active forms of exercise—walking, running, and maybe a little jumping, kicking, and swinging our arms—our bones begin to dissolve. That's been seen both in bedridden patients and in astronauts who live in weightless space for several days. The stress of exercise, it seems, stimulates the flow of calcium and other nutrients into the bones. With too little use, bones quickly lose calcium and weaken. Few of us expect to do any space traveling in our lifetime, but those same kinds of calcium losses occur in people who give up, say, an active job at manual labor or participation in dance or sports to take up a sedentary job or less strenuous hobbies. Bones lose small amounts of calcium during the hours you lie asleep each night. That's about one-third of your life right there. Add to a night's sleep several hours spent sitting at a desk and lounging in front of a television set, and a lot of calcium can trickle out of your bones due to inactivity. Millions of years of evolution have programmed our bones to build up calcium for the mobility and protection for which they were designed. Our bodies consequently interpret *lack* of mobility as a signal that calcium is no longer needed.

People at any age seem to benefit from exercise, so saying it's "too late" is no excuse. A group of 18 menopausal women was divided in half to see if exercise could modify their bone loss. One group did warm-up, conditioning and circulatory exercises for one hour three times a week. The other 9 women did not exercise. After one year, calcium in the body had *increased* in the exercise group. Body calcium *decreased* in every woman who did not exercise. The researchers learned that aging and frail bones do *not* have to be accepted as a package deal. Even women after menopause could continue to build their bones instead of losing them if they exercised regularly (*Annals of Internal Medicine,* September, 1978).

But men don't lose calcium from their bones because of the effects of menopause. So what happens to weaken their bones?

Catering to Your Body's Calcium Needs

Nutritional factors play a big part. Too little vitamin D (from lack of sunshine) is likely to cause the weak, soft bones of osteomalacia (adult rickets). A lack of vitamin A may result in abnormal growth.

But by far, too little calcium in the diet is the most probable cause. Calcium absorption decreases as we age. That goes for men as well as women. So extra calcium is needed to counteract the decrease in absorption and to prevent bone loss. Researchers at the Mayo Clinic in Rochester, Minnesota, and others who studied the effect of age on calcium absorption—and consequently bone loss—say that because the amount of calcium absorbed into the body does decrease with age, more calcium is needed to make up for poor absorption. Most elderly people do not get enough calcium, which, according to the researchers, might aggravate bone loss due to aging. In osteoporosis patients, needs are even higher (*Journal of Clinical Investigation,* September, 1979).

If you're not elderly—yet—and even if you get lots of exercise, your body needs a good supply of calcium in order to establish good stores. Without enough calcium in the diet, maintaining normal levels in the body in the face of automatic daily losses through sweat, urine, feces and tears means one thing only: the body must steal calcium from its bones to keep the body supplied.

Gum inflammation (periodontal disease) seems to be more prevalent on a low-calcium diet. Along with that goes jawbone deterioration. Without sound supportive gums and jaws, teeth loosen and eventually may fall out. Dentures won't fit right.

Other conditions, such as arthritis, multiple sclerosis and muscle cramps may also be aggravated by too little calcium. That's not surprising, in light of the close working relationship between joints, muscles and nerves, and the fact that all muscles and nerve cells need calcium. Some doctors who happened to be treating osteoporosis reported that some of their patients also had arthritic conditions, and it was their impression that both problems gradually improved over a period of years, with calcium supplementation.

The best source of calcium is diet. Foods richest in calcium are dairy products like milk and cheese. Certain plants, including some dark green leafy vegetables, are also good sources. And the adult dairy cow, which eats no dairy products herself, gets all the calcium she needs from plants. Clams don't dine on milk and cheese, yet they build themselves a shell almost entirely of calcium.

The fact that osteoporosis—which many say is an upshot of calcium deficiency—has risen to epidemic proportions in modern civilization provokes some intriguing questions about our diet.

• Are we eating less calcium than our ancestors, despite the abundance of modern dairy products?

• How does today's official Recommended Dietary Allowance (RDA) for calcium intake of 800 milligrams compare to calcium intake hundreds or even thousands of years ago?

• How did primitive people, without milk and dairy products, get enough calcium from their diets to avoid osteoporosis and to survive generation after generation?

Those questions nagged doctors at the Creighton University School of Medicine in Omaha, Nebraska, in the course of their studies of calcium intake and osteoporosis. Robert P. Heaney, M.D., Robert R. Recker, M.D., and Paul D. Saville, M.D., feel strongly that the current RDA for calcium is, in their own words, "grossly inadequate" for women early middle-aged and older, specifically, and could conceivably be too low for all adults. There is plenty of evidence, they say, to suggest that 1,200 milligrams a day is a more realistic RDA.

Our Ancestors' Diets Yielded More Calcium

That conclusion is based on clinical studies by Drs. Heaney, Recker and Saville, as well as many others. In addition, a few known facts about the calcium requirements of other mammals and man's own historical eating habits add credence to their findings. Data from the National Research Council (the same source that separately sets the human RDAs for calcium) on the calcium requirements of several mammals shows that, based on comparative body sizes, the established RDA for calcium for people is only one-fifth what it would be if human requirements were computed the same way as animal requirements are.

That curious inconsistency between human and animal RDAs wasn't the only thing that bothered the researchers. Facts about the diet of emerging mankind indicate that, historically, people probably ate a lot more calcium ages ago than we do today. Most people would probably assume that without milk and refrigerators, our ancestors didn't get much calcium. Many others might say that since adults very frequently cannot digest milk, their calcium needs are presumably low. Both those assumptions are wrong, according to Dr. Heaney and his fellow researchers at Creighton. "While it is true that dairy products are the principal dietary source of calcium for modern, civilized Western man, this is self-evidently not the case for other cultural situations. . . .[Widely available] fresh milk is a product of high technological civilization (and of refrigeration). For less technologically advanced people, milk is preserved primarily as cheese, in which lactose is predigested" (*American Journal of Clinical Nutrition,* October, 1977).

And even if lactose-intolerant adults *didn't* have a lot of cheese to munch on for calcium, there are plenty of nondairy foods that provided significant amounts of calcium to primitive people, including bones, roots, tubers (potatoes, for instance), seeds and especially the greens of root vegetables like turnips and carrots, plus other vegetables (see table 2 later in this chapter). The researchers go on to say, "Simple calculation, even from our civilized diet tables, reveals that a predominantly vegetarian intake adequate to meet protein requirements would have provided an abundance of calcium—significantly in excess of the current RDA. Furthermore, when such vegetarian sources are supplemented by nuts, seeds and by animal sources such as locusts, termites, grubs and caterpillars . . . all of which are staples even of twentieth century primitive man, the calcium content of the diet may rise to quite respectable levels. Add to this small birds, rodents, and fish, often eaten bones and all, and it becomes clear that calcium intake for most of the human race has not been predominantly determined by dairy products."

Stews of birds, fish and wild game, cooked with the bones, contain significant amounts of calcium even when the bones are removed before they're eaten. The researchers analyzed stews made from chicken and turkey carcasses and found appreciable amounts of calcium—up to 124 milligrams—in each serving. (That's about the amount of calcium in ⅔ cup of cottage cheese.) Dr. Heaney and his colleagues also noted that in India today, some dishes are traditionally served with bones, which are nibbled on after dinner (although the bones are not served when a Western guest is at the table to dine).

Within the perspective of our ancestors' diets, then, an RDA of 1,200 milligrams or more would be much closer to what people used to eat than the current 800 milligrams adhered to by the National Research Council, say the researchers.

Just for the sake of argument, let's say our ancestors *didn't* eat a lot of calcium. Wouldn't osteoporosis have wiped them out? Not necessarily, we're told. It's reasonable to consider that even if osteoporosis as a result of calcium deficiency is nothing new, and that somehow low calcium intake has been a serious and widespread problem in adults for thousands of years, it wouldn't necessarily threaten survival of the species. Dr. Heaney and the others think calcium deficiency could have conceivably come down to us through many generations. While an equally severe deficiency of a critical nutrient such as protein or a B vitamin, for instance, would most likely have meant certain extinction, a low intake of calcium would not. That's because osteoporosis takes a long time—many years—to manifest itself. Because life expectancy of our ancestors was somewhat shorter than ours, people probably died from other causes before osteoporosis became full-blown. Moreover, because osteoporosis doesn't affect women until after their childbearing years, the disease would have no effect on mate selection or reproduction.

What the RDA for Calcium Means to You

By now it's probably rather obvious that short rations of calcium in the diet can have far-reaching effects on health. It's a wise person who takes a few minutes to think about how much calcium he or she is getting. You may be wondering how the government's Recommended Dietary Allowance of 800 milligrams applies to you, and what the best food sources of calcium are. Perhaps you should take supplements to meet your requirements. If so, you'll want to know what to look for.

As comparison of modern and historical diets strongly suggests, the RDA for calcium, established by the Food and Nutrition Board of the National Research Council in the United States, deserves reconsideration. (See chapter 60, The RDAs: What the Recommended Dietary Allowances Mean to You.) First and foremost, any such "standard requirements" are merely estimates. Those estimates for calcium are based on studies in which the calcium content of diets—a big variable—is compared to the amount of calcium excreted in urine and feces. It would seem, then, to be a simple matter of What Goes In Replacing What Comes Out. It's not that simple to calculate, though. For one thing, measuring calcium intake seldom takes into consideration the amount of calcium in drinking water, which may be appreciable in hard water areas. For another, a considerable amount of calcium may be lost in perspiration (and, less so, in tears), which is not analyzed for sheer lack of the technology to do so. You may think that's of little significance, but for people hard at work in high temperatures, it's estimated that calcium lost by perspiration can amount to as much as 1,000 milligrams a day—more than the RDA for intake! So a person who drinks water treated with a softener (which removes calcium from the water and replaces it with salt) and works in a hot, busy kitchen or as an outside laborer in the South is likely to need far more calcium in his or her diet than the person who drinks hard water and works in a cool, air-conditioned office.

Further coloring the matter of calcium needs are individual differences in the way our bodies handle calcium. Without going into all the metabolic factors at length, basically it works like this: we're each endowed at birth with different tendencies to absorb and excrete calcium. Some people adapt to low calcium intake year after year by conserving calcium, either through a higher rate of absorption in the upper intestine, a lower rate of excretion in urine and feces, or changes in digestion. A person accustomed to a daily intake of 500 milligrams could probably also get by with 400 milligrams a day for a while. But the person who is used to 1,000 milligrams a day—from either food, water or the body's own special way of handling the mineral—might not get by on 400 milligrams.

The length of time needed to adapt to lower intake varies. Say you move to a soft water area, decide to cut down on milk and dairy products, or make some other change. Some people may adapt within two months, others much longer—and others, never. Those who adapt slowly or never could be just those people who are vulnerable to weak bones, inflamed gums, muscle cramps and other calcium-related disorders.

Emotional stress can temporarily flush calcium out of your system at a higher rate. If you've been waiting nine weeks for mortgage approval on your new dream house, calcium can go down as your hopes go up.

In spite of their limitations, the estimated RDAs for calcium are the benchmarks for that mineral. Old-fashioned nutritionists argue loudly as to whether or not low intakes matter very much at all. Some say that no clinical condition can truly be classified as a calcium deficiency per se; that any hint of any such deficiency is in reality the result of a vitamin D deficiency. But today, ample evidence shows that not all people do so well on average intakes and, in fact, those people may suffer real harm. Nit-picking aside, then, intake *is* important, according to many studies.

How much calcium is right for you? You'll have to use your own judgment, based on your history of fractures, bone pain, muscle cramps, gum inflammation and perhaps some of the things your doctor may have uncovered during checkups. If you're a woman, chances are that 800 milligrams will not be enough to prevent osteoporosis in your lifetime. Man or woman, if you've been laid up or slowed down by a broken arm or leg, your needs are probably higher. Many people with gum disease or dentures may also need higher amounts of calcium than the average diet provides.

Tally Up the Calcium in Your Diet

How many Americans are getting even the arbitrary RDA for calcium? Not as many as you probably think. According to data from the well-known Ten-State Nutrition Survey completed in 1970, the calcium intake of many Americans falls below minimum standards. If you are concerned about preventing bone, muscle, nerve and gum problems, you may want to check to see how your own calcium intake stacks up against the RDA for your age group and sex given in table 41 in chapter 60.

Ideally, the best way to find out precisely how many milligrams of calcium you get from your daily food would be to add up the calcium values for each mouthful of food you eat. To do that, you'd have to look up those values in books like the U.S. Department of Agriculture's *Nutritive Value of American Foods in Common Units,* available from the U.S. Government Printing Office in Washington, D.C. Handbook No. 456 is a comprehensive collection of nutrient data, with calculations of the amounts of protein, carbohydrate, fat, calories, and some vitamins and minerals of nearly 1,500 of the foods we most commonly eat. To save you time and trouble, though, we've gone through that book and others and listed a few dozen of those foods that are the best sources of calcium (see table 2). Notice that we say the *best,* not the only sources. Refined, processed or "convenience" foods that are high in calcium because of their milk content are also likely to be high in sugar, fat and additives. Baked goods like waffles and chocolate eclairs are two glaring examples of rich but still poor sources of calcium. So is ice cream.

Calcium is present in significant amounts in only certain food groups and practically absent in others. We all know that milk and cheese are the principal sources. Meat is stripped of much of its calcium when it's deboned, which is more often than not. Some vegetables and nuts have appreciable amounts of calcium. Fruit, grains and oils provide very little.

One way to guarantee ample calcium in the diet would be to consume a lot of milk and cheese every day. That can cause problems, however. Many people cannot drink milk because of lactose intolerance, an inability to digest milk sugar. That results in gas, abdominal cramps, bloating or diarrhea. Dairy products also tend to be high in animal fat and calories, and people concerned with weight control and coronary heart disease will want to limit their saturated fat intake. So while cheese is usually a rich source of calcium, it too has its drawbacks. Milk fat in cheese is over 50 percent saturated or animal fat. Most cheeses contain a significant amount of cholesterol and should be used sparingly by people on low-cholesterol diets. Others on modified fat diets should avoid eating whole-milk cheeses and buy only those made with skim or very low-fat milk.

TABLE 2 **Food Sources of Calcium**

Food	Portion	Calcium (milligrams)
Sardines, Atlantic, drained solids	4 ounces	494
Salmon, sockeye, drained solids	4 ounces	365
Milk, skim	1 cup	296
Buttermilk	1 cup	296
Yogurt, skim milk	1 cup	294
Swiss cheese	1 ounce	262
Cheddar cheese	1 ounce	213
Provolone cheese	1 ounce	212
Monterey Jack cheese	1 ounce	209
Brick cheese	1 ounce	207
Muenster cheese	1 ounce	201
American cheese	1 ounce	198
Colby cheese	1 ounce	192
Mozzarella cheese	1 ounce	181
Limburger cheese	1 ounce	167
Dandelion greens, cooked	½ cup	147
Tofu (soybean curd)	4 ounces	145
Pizza, cheese	⅛ of 14-inch pie	144
Blackstrap molasses	1 tablespoon	137
Soy flour	½ cup	132
Collards, cooked	½ cup	110
Kale, cooked	½ cup	103
Mustard greens, cooked	½ cup	97
Watercress, finely chopped	½ cup	95
Cottage cheese, dry-curd, uncreamed	½ cup	90
Almonds	¼ cup	83
Chick-peas, dried	¼ cup	75
Broccoli, cooked	½ cup	68
Soybeans	½ cup	66
Parmesan cheese	1 tablespoon	61
Artichoke	1 medium bud	61
Filberts	¼ cup	60
Eggs	2 large	54

SOURCE: Adapted from *Nutritive Value of American Foods in Common Units,* Agriculture Handbook No. 456, by Catherine F. Adams (Washington, D.C.: Agricultural Research Service, U.S. Department of Agriculture, 1975).

In tracking down our treasures of calcium, we came across some surprises about cheese. Because cheese is such a fundamental source of calcium, we assumed at first that all cheeses were rich in that mineral. Not so. Blue or Roquefort cheese, Camembert and cream cheese do not measure up to brick, Cheddar and Swiss.

Buttermilk and yogurt made from skim milk are reasonably high in calcium but low in cholesterol. Low-moisture, part-skim mozzarella and part-skim mozzarella are also lower in cholesterol than most other cheeses. One tablespoon of grated Parmesan cheese (⅙ ounce) adds some useful calcium to soups, salads and casseroles, but yields only about four milligrams of cholesterol, an extremely small amount.

Other people who are on diets to control high blood pressure must avoid a lot of cheese because of its high sodium content.

Nondairy Sources of Calcium

Don't hastily assume that without a lot of cheese or milk in your diet you're automatically destined for the fracture ward.

Bone, Nature's Own Calcium Bank

Salmon is a great source of calcium as long as the soft little bones are eaten. It's considerably less useful if the bones are discarded. So salmon steak, which has no bones, is not as valuable as canned salmon, with its well-cooked nuggets of bone.

Yet bone is the one source of calcium that is most ignored, although it is probably just as natural for people to eat bone, in one form or another, as it is to eat food fiber. Most primitive peoples around the world make bone a regular part of their diet. The amazingly hardy Eskimos eat small birds, when they can catch them, bones and all. In South America, the Vilcabamba people, who are also fabled for their strength and strong bones, cook beef bones all day with a few vegetables to make a soup that is very high in calcium. (Vinegar or acidic vegetables help get the calcium out of the bones.) Indians also chew up and suck or even swallow small bones in curry dishes.

Bone eating, however, is by no means limited to so-called primitive peoples. Although the habit seems to have fallen off somewhat of late, many people say they can remember, as children, being encouraged to chew soft bones, crack them, and suck out the marrow. Another favorite dish in grandmother's day was soup in which bones had been cooked for hours. In both cases, valuable minerals were being extracted. Our parents or grand-parents probably appreciated the value of bones because they inherited this knowledge from their own parents. So it is likely that people have *always* gotten calcium from bones.

Until recently, that is. Today, much of the meat that we buy has already been cut away from the bone. And then, people today eat about one out of every three meals in a restaurant, where chewing on bones is not exactly considered good etiquette.

To put bones back in your diet, make your own soup from leftover chicken or turkey carcasses instead of buying canned soups. Save the bones from roasts, crack them apart, and make your own soup stock to freeze and keep on hand. Or ask the butcher to save you some bones. As the bones simmer in a big kettle of water, add chopped onions, celery leaves, carrots and a clove of garlic for flavor, plus a tablespoon or two of vinegar, lemon juice, or tamari (a fermented soybean product) to help draw calcium out of the bones. While most vegetables, including beets, beans, celery, squash and carrots are slightly acidic, tomato juice is much more acidic and also enhances calcium uptake from bones. A cup or so of tomato broth or stewed tomatoes added to your soup stock will also add to the calcium content of the soup. Chicken gumbo soup and Russian borscht readily come to mind as hearty—and calcium yielding—soups made with acidic vegetables and animal bones. Recipes for these soups appear in chapter 31, Recipes: Putting It All Together.

Including foods like tofu, yogurt and cheese in soups made with bone stock adds extra calcium to your diet. Use your homemade beef broth for French onion soup, sprinkled with Parmesan cheese and broiled until bubbly and brown. Or stir dollops of yogurt (also acidic) into your borscht. We'll share other versions of mineral-rich soups with you in our recipe section.

Tofu, a New Calcium Source for the West

What is tofu?

Tofu is a high-protein, cholesterol-free food, made from soybeans, which originated in the Orient. Tofu resembles custard, although in the United States it's usually somewhat coarser in texture. And tofu is high in calcium. One-half cup of tofu has 145 milligrams of calcium—about the same as ½ cup of yogurt or buttermilk.

In making tofu, soy milk is extracted from whole soybeans with hot water. Just as rennet is used to curdle animal milk in making dairy cheese, certain salts are used to obtain the same effect in making tofu. When the compounds calcium sulfate or calcium chloride are used in the solidifying process, tofu becomes an exceptionally good source of calcium. Of equal importance, tofu is an alternative to the stock sources of protein in America—meat, poultry and processed cheeses.

Tofu was once found only in Chinatown or in Oriental cooking classes. Now it appears in food co-ops, natural food stores and, increasingly, in supermarkets. Home and family magazines sometimes feature tofu recipes. Because commercial tofu is extracted by various methods, try to choose brands made from the calcium compounds, calcium chloride or calcium sulfate. The solidifiers magnesium chloride and nigari, a salt from evaporated seawater, are okay, too, although the calcium content of the tofu will be slightly lower. Avoid tofu that has had chemical preservatives added to prolong its shelf life. If you are uncertain about what a tofu contains, a note to the manufacturer should elicit the information you want.

When meeting tofu for the first time, it helps to know what to expect. Tofu has a creamy texture, an off-white color, and is stored in small blocks in a tub of water. Some brands of tofu are more crumbly than others, but it shouldn't be difficult to find the firmer, creamier types. Start off by buying a pound or less—that's just under two cups.

When you get tofu home, it requires some special handling, but not much. Simply transfer the tofu from the bag or tub in which it's sold to one of those pint-size freezer containers or a wide-mouthed glass jar for refrigeration. Be sure to add enough water to cover the tofu. (If you buy the prepackaged kind of tofu, you don't need to transfer it to your own container until the seal has been broken.)

Fresh tofu will keep for about a week when refrigerated in a closed container. Replace the water at least every other day to keep the tofu at optimum freshness. With each day that tofu is stored, the flavor grows slightly stronger. That's not a problem, though. Use fresh tofu in recipes where it more or less stands by itself, as in stir-fried tofu and vegetables, and older tofu in dishes where flavors of other foods predominate, such as in casseroles or quiches.

You should never have to throw tofu away, which makes it very economical. If you buy more than you can use right away, freeze it. For best results, first drain the tofu and place it in a plastic bag. Be certain to squeeze all the air from the bag. Tie it securely and freeze it immediately.

Most people's first reaction to tofu can be summed up in two typical comments: "I don't like the way it looks" and "It has no flavor." (A close third is "My family will never eat it.") We're not going to try to kid you by saying that tofu is good enough to eat plain, right out of the bag. That's just not so. Tofu has no real distinct flavor of its own, but readily takes on the rich flavors of other foods cooked with it, which makes it all the more versatile—and valuable—as a source of calcium.

Not only is tofu good for you and relatively inexpensive, but for the many people who cannot tolerate milk products, tofu can be a blessing as an alternate source of calcium. Even those who can eat dairy products are better off with less animal fat in their diets, and can turn to tofu to replace some of the cheese or eggs in quiches, omelets or sauces. Tofu can be cubed and added to soups just like egg noodles. And unlike cheese or sour cream, you can eat a lot of tofu without being swamped with calories. (Tofu dishes can be prepared from recipes given in chapter 31.)

Some Greens Rate Well, Others Fail

Dark green leafy vegetables contain considerable amounts of calcium. They also contain varying amounts of oxalic acid, a substance that combines with calcium during food digestion to form an insoluble compound, calcium oxalate. Calcium bound up with oxalic acid passes out of the body without being absorbed.

Some greens have far more oxalic acid than others, which means some are good sources of calcium and others are not. Beet greens, spinach and Swiss chard have up to eight times as much oxalic acid as calcium. Nearly all of the calcium in those vegetables is carried out of the body without being absorbed, so they are considered poor sources of calcium. According to Philip Washko, Ph.D., of the department of food science and human nutrition at Michigan State University, "Consumption of high-oxalic-acid greens probably does not pose a problem in a typical American diet. While the oxalic acid will decrease the amount of calcium available from the vegetables themselves, it appears that there is little excess oxalic acid available to bind the calcium from other dietary sources. It could be a problem if a person ate a phenomenal amount of chard or spinach every day—without other calcium-containing products, but such a case would be extremely unlikely."

Other greens, notably turnip, mustard and collard, plus kale and the buds and leaves of broccoli, pose no such problem with calcium absorption. In those vegetables, calcium exceeds oxalic acid by a ratio of up to 42:1, making them excellent sources of calcium.

Don't Ignore Beans and Whole Grain Foods

Phytic acid in the outer husks of beans and grains has a similar effect on calcium and other minerals. While the exact effect of phytic acid on minerals in the body is not yet fully understood, chances are that phytic acid will not seriously interfere with mineral absorption if grains and beans are balanced by a variety of other good foods in the diet.

Nutritionists know that people lack phytase, an enzyme capable of digesting the phytic acid in grains and beans. In our digestive tracts, phytic acid binds with calcium, zinc, magnesium and iron to form insoluble compounds called phytates, making a certain amount of those minerals unavailable.

If grains and legumes (beans and peas) make up such a large portion of the diet that those foods are the main sources of minerals, there could be a problem. But in a diet that combines grains and legumes with a variety of other foods—vegetables, dairy products, and fish or meat—no calcium deficiency will result, according to one food scientist we spoke to, whose area of expertise is fiber and mineral metabolism.

"People have been eating whole grains and beans for hundreds of years. Obviously, those foods don't cause mineral deficiencies," says Pericles Markakis, Ph.D., a food scientist from Michigan State University.

Sprouting and leavening neutralize the effects of phytic acid. Adding bean sprouts and alfalfa sprouts to soup, salads and stir-fry vegetables helps to make certain that we're consuming minerals in a form our bodies can use. Tempeh is a fermented soybean food that's produced by the action of molds, which break down phytic acid. Soaking beans and peas in water before cooking also breaks down some phytic acid, although cooking in itself does not.

Calcium and Phosphorus in Good Balance

From time to time, researchers suggest that too much phosphorus in the diet will interfere with calcium absorption. But that may not be true. In a telephone conversation, Herta Spencer, M.D., chief of the Metabolic Section of the Veterans Administration Hospital in Hines, Illinois, told us that phosphorus is of some concern in calcium balance. But Dr. Spencer feels that normal eating patterns spread phosphorus intake over several hours each day and over several days each week. And we feel that regular meals of a variety of wholesome, unprocessed foods are not likely to provide the single, large dose of phosphorus necessary to interfere with calcium absorption. (See chapter 4, Phosphorus, for more on calcium and phosphorus in the diet.)

Supplements Help Guarantee Your Calcium Supply

Tally up your daily totals of calcium intake over the course of a week or so. Choose a fairly normal week—not one in which you eat out more or less than usual or are out of town visiting the home of a relative. Compare your daily totals with the Recommended Dietary Allowance for calcium for your age and sex, given in table 41 in chapter 60, The RDAs: What the Recommended Dietary Allowances Mean to You.

If your calcium intake falls short, you're not alone. When 90 people at Oregon State University were tested, researchers found that 37.7 percent of the men and 84.4 percent of the women consumed less than the RDA (*Nutrition Reports International,* June, 1978). And a U.S. Department of Agriculture survey of 5,500 women over 45 showed that their average intake of calcium was 450 milligrams per day—not even half of what they should have been getting to prevent osteoporosis.

How can you be sure you're not cheating yourself out of calcium?

It could be that you need to pay a bit more attention to what you're eating. Eating enough of those foods closest to the top of table 2 will help. Trying a few recipes that combine two or more of those foods can further boost your calcium intake. Recalculate the amount of calcium you're getting after a week of supplementing your diet with yogurt, buttermilk, tofu dishes and extra servings of greens. (Greens are incredibly low in calories.)

Food sources may not do it in some cases. Remember, you're shooting for a *minimum* of 800 milligrams a day. At least one study says that women would have to consume a quart of whole or skim milk a day (or its equivalent in cheese products) to meet the 800 to 1,000 milligrams necessary to maintain healthy bones after menopause. An alternative, concluded the researchers, is taking a daily supplement of calcium. That study was conducted by Anthony Albanese, Ph.D., Edward Lorenze, Jr., M.D., and Evelyn Wein at the Burke Rehabilitation Center in White Plains, New York.

One of the dentists we spoke to who studied calcium and denture problems feels strongly that periodontal patients and denture wearers both should definitely take calcium supplements.

As a result of other work along those lines, several internationally recognized experts on nutrition and health have warned that the RDA of 800 milligrams for calcium puts many people—and particularly women—in danger of developing problems like osteoporosis, and have urged that a really protective amount would be 50 to 75 percent higher—up to 1,400 milligrams a day. Because getting that much calcium from food alone isn't always easy to do, you may choose to take calcium supplements of some type.

Basically, calcium supplements are simply edible compounds of calcium bound to another substance, as in calcium gluconate, calcium carbonate, calcium lactate or calcium phosphate.

Bone meal is a powder made from the long bones of cattle. It contains calcium, of course. But bone meal goes calcium one better. It also contains small amounts of the important mineral, phosphorus, in the same ratio to calcium that's found in human bones, about 2:1. Because the minerals in bone meal are in a form that's natural to the body, the body makes better use of them.

That's not to say there's anything wrong with plain calcium supplements. Far from it. But calcium may work better—to prevent bone fractures, to relieve muscle cramps, to stave off gum disease—when it's found in bone meal.

Bone meal usually comes in tablet form. But you can also buy it as a powder. One researcher has found that up to 1,800 milligrams of bone meal can be added to one serving of bean soup or beef stew without affecting the taste. You could also try adding it to beef patties. You'd be putting back what nature included in the first place.

Dolomite—one common form of limestone—is a perfectly balanced source of calcium and another important mineral, magnesium, which you will learn all about in the next chapter. As a dietary supplement, dolomite is a perfectly edible and wholesome source of calcium.

Why do some people take both bone meal and dolomite? Simply because one has what the other doesn't. Bone meal gives a natural combination of calcium and phosphorus, while dolomite gives the magnesium in amounts bone meal doesn't provide.

3

Magnesium

Dolomite, a Supplement from Our Prehistoric Past

Dolomite is a very special kind of rock. Not only does it contain calcium and magnesium in just the right ratio in which we need them for good health, but rockbeds of dolomite are a valuable source of information about our past. Deposits of dolomite contain so many fossils of early life, from microscopic algae to sea worms, sponges and shellfish, that layers of dolomite are really a petrified chronicle of the evolution of life and history of the earth. And in an intriguing way, dolomite's role in Earth's history is intertwined with its role in health.

Dolomite is a kind of limestone formed almost entirely by tiny animals and plants. Algae, coral, mollusks and other shellfish contribute their skeletons of calcium carbonate, which sink to the bottom of lakes and oceans when they die. In shallow areas, coral skeletons sometimes form rings and mounds; the results are coral reefs. Certain algae also contribute to layers of dolomitic limestone by secreting the lime for which the rock is named. Limestone, like skeletons and shells, is mostly calcium carbonate. The skeletons, shells and secreted lime pile up on the ocean floor in layers—kind of like geological lasagna.

The skeletons, shells and lime pellets that piled up in tons have little magnesium. Marine skeletons contain about 4 to 8 percent magnesium at most. Yet dolomite contains a much larger proportion of magnesium, about half as much as calcium. How did dolomitic limestone accumulate so much magnesium?

Geologists speculate that nature added it gradually over years and years. Some comes from seawater. Magnesium is the fifth most abundant mineral in the sea, averaging 6,600,000 tons per cubic mile. In cool seawater, at lower depths, animals generally accumulate much less magnesium than those in warm, shallow areas. Apparently, the rate of dolomitization, or accumulation of magnesium by limestone, takes place at a much faster rate in warm water than in cool water.

Not all of the magnesium in dolomite comes from seawater, however. Some is recycled from the land. What seems to have happened is that in the course of several episodes of depositing nice, neat horizontal layers of limestone and other sedimentary rocks on the ocean floor, upheavals in the earth's crust shoved portions of those underwater deposits above sea level to become part of the land.

Water from springs and wells trickling through those layers on land percolates through soil and various kinds of rocks, picking up magnesium along the way and adding it to the limestone sediments. On the surface, meanwhile, wind and rain battering the continents over the years also dissolve limestone and other matter, carrying some of it back to the sea through rivers, lakes and streams.

As magnesium was deposited again and again, the limestone very slowly amassed more magnesium until the ratio of calcium to magnesium reached 1.65:1. Remarkably, that's roughly the ratio of calcium to magnesium that our bodies seem to require for good health. Powdered dolomite is perfectly edible and wholesome—and so almost seems to have been put on Earth as a way for us to reap a correctly balanced supply of both calcium and magnesium.

Apparently very little dolomite is being formed on Earth today. That which is, is found in just a few locations deep in the ocean, where cooler temperatures produce a dolomite with much less magnesium than older dolomite. No one is quite sure why. And where dolomite *is* being formed, the process is so slow as to be imperceptible. Fortunately, turbulent action in our planet's history has left us with almost inexhaustible supplies of dolomite, common throughout the world.

Magnesium's Colorful History as a Health Patron

Over the past several years, scientists have discovered that in populations where the magnesium is delivered by way of dolomite-filtered water, there seems to be a lower incidence of heart disease. Meanwhile, we knew that magnesium was an essential mineral, but we didn't know exactly what it did for healthy hearts, sound muscles, and innumerable other health factors.

At about the beginning of the 1600s, magnesium gained a questionable reputation as a cure-all, although people didn't know it was magnesium they were applauding. They called it Epsom salts. The salts, a compound of magnesium sulfate, are recognized even today as a powerful laxative. For hundreds of years, it was widely believed that daily evacuation of the bowels prevented virtually all disease. So when water high in magnesium sulfate started percolating up through a spring in the small village of Epsom, England, about 17 miles south of London, the locals started drinking the water in quantity, hoping to cure all their internal afflictions—even though they didn't know what it was. But they'd have been better off moving their bowels with a high-fiber diet and exercise routine—the natural, healthful way to keep regular. As a component of Epsom salts, magnesium works strictly in a chemical way, stimulating the wavelike contractions of the intestine that promote evacuation. The magnesium in Epsom salts is not absorbed into the bloodstream, where it could in fact have a remarkable influence on health.

A Mission Doctor Makes an Astounding Discovery

The scene is a hospital in a city nestled among the grasslands and forests of East Africa. Doctors and nurses are treating children who suffer extreme malnutrition, feeding them a diet high in protein and minerals. The results, however, are frustrating. Despite good food and care, many of the starving children—up to 40 percent of them—do not respond at all. Those who do recover soon relapse after returning home to their families in the nearby village. The doctors are completely baffled.

A khaki-clad pediatrician at the hospital first shares the bewilderment of her colleagues. She then begins to suspect that one very crucial mineral has been ignored—magnesium. Working on a hunch, she supplements the diet of some of the sick children with magnesium; other children continue to receive standard treatment alone. In four to ten days, those children taking magnesium are almost miraculously better. Children not receiving magnesium continue to respond poorly.

Our story may sound more like a corny screenplay than a medical journal report, but it's not fiction. What's more, the tale comes to us not from the nutritional Dark Ages of a century ago but from 1965. The pediatrician is an American, Joan L. Caddell, M.D., who at the time was working under the auspices of the Rockefeller Foundation in Uganda. Her discovery that magnesium plays a critical role in the recovery of malnourished children made clear an important point of nutrition previously unrecognized: A diet that is plentiful in nearly every other vital nutrient—protein, carbohydrates, vitamins and minerals—is worthless without magnesium.

The ingenuity that led to Dr. Caddell's discovery makes more than just an intriguing detective story. The clues she used to solve the mystery of a stubborn disease bring to light many of the important health tasks performed by magnesium.

The cause of the children's disease was as obvious as the cure was elusive, and is suggested by its name, kwashiorkor, which means "the disease of the deposed baby when the next one is born." The typical kwashiorkor child is one who is weaned from the breast when the second child is born. The child is put on sugar and water, or a meager diet consisting mostly of cereal and syrup, cornstarch and ground cassava root. Denied the nutritional benefits of mother's milk, the weaned child is starved for protein, vitamins and minerals—barely taking in enough to survive from one day to the next, let alone to thrive. Vegetables, beans and seeds—the most plentiful food sources of magnesium—are usually absent. Up to three-quarters of the children in tropical and subtropical countries like Nigeria and Ghana are likely to suffer this devastating form of malnutrition to some degree. Kwashiorkor tends to be self-perpetuating, for when children become sick with the disease, any magnesium that may get in their food is quickly flushed out of their bodies by vomiting and diarrhea. Dehydration is common, and death may result.

How did Dr. Caddell single out magnesium as the wanting nutrient? Like any good detective and scientist, she began with careful observation. Besides diarrhea, nausea and loss of appetite, most of the children were dull and listless, not even crying or complaining of their discomfort. Their heart rates were weak and unstable. Some suffered tremors or muscle convulsions. Blood pressure was hardly detectable in most. Several children were anemic. Sores didn't heal. Skin became pink and inflamed instead of the usual smooth dark tones of the natives' skin. Faces and ankles swelled. Skin became taut and stretched. Bellies bulged. The children failed to grow normally or gain weight. A condition called fatty liver was common. Almost everything that could go wrong, did.

What impressed Dr. Caddell about this awesome array of symptoms was that many were remarkably similar to symptoms associated with magnesium deficiency.

The first symptom that jogged Dr. Caddell's curiosity was the weak, irregular heartbeat of kwashiorkor children. Dr. Caddell knew that heart tissues are very sensitive to drops in magnesium. She knew, too, that magnesium seems to maintain normal heart rhythm by balancing the stimulating effect of calcium on heart muscle.

In a very similar way, magnesium regulates muscle contraction and relaxation, and lack of magnesium could explain the convulsions. Low magnesium is a known cause of uncontrollable tremors and convulsions.

But convulsions can often result from a vitamin B_6 (pyridoxine) deficiency, as can other nerve problems. And skin sores seen in kwashiorkor are similar to those produced from vitamin B_2 (riboflavin) and B_6 deficiencies. The fact that had been overlooked was that those B vitamins require magnesium to work properly. And magnesium is absolutely necessary for the body to utilize vitamin B_1 (thiamine). Coincidentally, kwashiorkor children are usually low in several B vitamins. Without magnesium, no amount of B vitamin supplements would have done the children any good.

Perhaps the most puzzling part of the problem was that while milk and other foods high in protein, calcium, phosphorus and potassium were the logical regimen for undernourished children, that diet seemed to prolong rather than arrest the disease. Medical intuition told Dr. Caddell that while those nutrients promoted good health in children with healthy magnesium intake, high doses of those same essential nutrients posed special problems for kwashiorkor children. Calcium *competes* with magnesium for absorption sites in the intestine. If only small amounts of magnesium are reaching those sites, as seemed to be the case with the sick children, it's easily elbowed aside by copious amounts of calcium, and never reaches the rest of the body where it's needed.

Phosphorus and protein each increase demand for magnesium. So a high-phosphorus, high-protein diet—like the high-milk diet fed the recuperating children—increases the demand for magnesium still further, in effect creating a deficiency out of marginal intake. Magnesium also helps to regulate the level of potassium, which, along with sodium, controls fluid levels in the body. So low magnesium could also explain the swollen faces and ankles. The net result of a deluge of protein, calcium, phosphorus and potassium in kwashiorkor is a desperate requirement for more magnesium. Which helps to explain the baffling intractability of the disease.

The fatty livers in the children were nearly identical to those seen in chronic alcoholics who subsist on magnesium-free calories, chiefly from alcohol, for months or years. And retarded bone growth is a classic sign of severe magnesium deficiency.

All the pieces fit. Carefully and methodically, Dr. Caddell documented the children's improvement after magnesium supplementation. Their symptoms were dramatically reversed. Skin healed. Heart rates returned to normal. Appetites improved. Diarrhea subsided. Tremors disappeared. The children gained weight. And most important, none died (*Journal of Pediatrics,* February, 1965).

Follow-up studies done by Dr. Caddell and others later confirmed her conclusions. The funny thing is, previous reports had said the opposite— that there was absolutely no relationship between kwashiorkor and magnesium. Quite possibly, that was because magnesium levels in the blood can register normal even when the body as a whole is depleted. And odd as it may seem, at that time doctors weren't exactly sure *why* magnesium was essential. Now, we know that magnesium activates the hundreds of enzyme reactions responsible for a whole spectrum of biological activities that keeps our bodies in working order. Magnesium is also largely responsible for regulating heartbeat and muscle contraction, and for helping to conduct nerve impulses. Magnesium helps to maintain water balance so we don't swell up or dehydrate. Without magnesium, the body systems don't work as smoothly as they should—or they don't work at all. The body suffers in many and varied ways, as seen in kwashiorkor children.

Magnesium, for the Metabolic Manager within Each Cell

While virtually none of us will experience kwashiorkor, a closer look at just what magnesium does will tell us a lot about our needs for the mineral.

Our body is made up of 100,000,000,000,000 cells (more or less), each one bustling with activities that depend on magnesium. In fact, next to potassium, magnesium is the most plentiful mineral inside each cell. In both plants and animals, cells are continually renewing and discarding parts. That simultaneous buildup and breakdown of cells, collectively called metabolism, is controlled by hundreds of protein substances, or enzymes. Acting as metabolic managers, enzymes deftly coordinate each of the many different reactions going on in our bodies by bringing together the right ingredients at the right time and place, much as a good business manager brings together the right people with the right skills to get a job done. Enzymes in both plants and animals depend on energy delivered by magnesium to do their work. Magnesium delivers that energy by activating the production of a special substance called adenosine triphosphate (ATP), which extracts energy from the foods we eat and delivers it to each and every one of those billions of cells in our bodies, whether they be in the heart, lungs, muscles, kidneys, brain, blood or bone.

At the same time, there are hundreds of other jobs to be done. Old tissues must be replaced, damages must be repaired as quickly as possible. Heart, brain and other organs are never at rest, even while we sleep. The muscles that keep lungs pumping oxygen in and carbon dioxide out are working 24 hours a day. Our hearts cannot take a leave of absence for more than five or six minutes if we are to go on living. All in all, magnesium is a catalyst, or activator, to countless physical activities. Without enough magnesium, the energy transport system on which our bodies depend to keep metabolism humming would grind to a halt or be seriously disrupted, resulting in disease or discomfort.

Calcium and Magnesium, Steady Partners for Strong Muscles

Magnesium enjoys a reciprocal relationship with calcium. In our muscles, calcium pushes and magnesium pulls, like two men working a bow saw to fell a tree. Calcium stimulates muscle fibers to tense up and contract. Magnesium, present in the fluids that bathe the nerve cells, responds by encouraging the muscle fibers to loosen up and relax. The regular pattern of *contract, relax, contract, relax* is what enables us to grasp a pencil, reach for the phone, walk, swim, swing a golf club and so on.

When our bodies are low in calcium, they can borrow from ample reserves in the bones. Bones contain magnesium, too—about half the magnesium in our bodies is in our bones. But our bones do not give up as much magnesium as calcium, and instead our bodies are forced to take magnesium from the second best source, muscles, in times of short supply.

Without enough magnesium in muscles to counterbalance the stimulating effect of calcium, they stiffen up or contract at liberty. The result may be cramps, irritability, twitching or even tremors.

That effect of calcium-magnesium imbalance has been seen in dairy cattle for years. Dairy cattle in Australia, New Zealand, England and Holland sometimes suffer from a condition known as grass staggers. Symptoms include an unsteady gait, muscular twitching, and uncontrollable flicking of the tail. All cows with grass staggers have been found to have low magnesium levels in their blood, attributed to disturbed magnesium and calcium metabolism. By giving the animals additional magnesium in their diet, the disorder is both cured and prevented.

Cows are not the only creatures that require calcium and magnesium to avoid painful cramps. People do too. Readers participating in the Calcium Research Project conducted by *Prevention* magazine in 1977 remarked that dolomite, a supplemental combination of about two parts calcium to one part magnesium, often quelled their muscle spasms or cramps. Calcium and magnesium work together to maintain the regular pattern of *contract, relax, contract, relax* in muscles.

Magnesium for a Healthy Heart

Because our hearts are muscles, calcium and magnesium affect the heart in a similar way. Heartbeats, of course, are really a series of contractions and relaxations of that organ. Long before Dr. Joan Caddell's inklings about the effect of low magnesium on heart tissues of kwashiorkor children, South African doctors had begun to successfully treat many forms of heart disease (angina, blood clots and arteriosclerosis) with injected magnesium supplements. That early work in South Africa was prophetic, for in the following years, epidemiologists (scientists who study disease patterns among populations) then began to find fascinating associations between higher levels of magnesium in the soil, water and diet, and lower death rates from heart disease.

Researchers in Finland, for instance, have compiled some intriguing data in regard to magnesium deficiency within their country. Eastern Finland has a higher rate of coronary heart disease than western Finland. The average content of magnesium in Finland's soil is low, *especially* in the eastern areas. Magnesium in the diet and drinking water there is also lower than other areas. Researchers examining Finland's drinking water observed a definite relationship between the hardness (amount of magnesium and other minerals) of drinking water and heart disease death rates. In hard water areas there were fewer deaths related to heart disease than in soft water areas. Soft water lacks the minerals of hard water, which picks up calcium and magnesium as it passes through soil and dolomitic limestone in the earth's crust (*Advanced Cardiology,* vol. 25, 1978).

Other studies in England, Wales, Sweden, Ireland, Canada and the United States have further established that death rates from heart disease are lower in areas with hard water. Many feel that magnesium is a decisive factor, but that has been overshadowed by the controversy over the role of dietary cholesterol in heart disease.

A Mineral of the Future

Like cholesterol and heart disease, sodium and potassium have received a lot of publicity for their role in a related condition, high blood pressure, which can lead to heart attack, stroke or kidney problems. While sodium and potassium are important, magnesium's ability to help control blood pressure has long been acknowledged but, until recently, shrugged off.

Magnesium's hypotensive, or blood pressure-lowering effect, is the result of one of two possible actions. Either magnesium neutralizes the stimulating effect of calcium in the arteries and blood vessels, slowing down contractions, or magnesium acts on nerves to relax those muscles. Either way, the net result is that with more magnesium, the heart becomes a more efficient unit, pumping more blood with less effort.

Similarly, when magnesium is low in blood vessels of the heart, a spasm in the vessel may trigger a heart attack. (For more on magnesium and heart health, see chapter 26, Hard and Soft Water: The Inside Story, and chapter 33, Heart Disease.)

Magnesium protects more than the heart. Evidence over the past few years supports earlier findings that magnesium helps prevent formation of kidney stones. Ongoing research is gathering evidence that magnesium may play a role in other medical mysteries, such as cancer.

Why Plants Are Green and Blood Is Red

Plants, like animals, have adopted magnesium as their patron mineral. Plants owe their customary green color to chlorophyll, a substance similar to a substance called heme in our blood. Both pigments, in fact, are made the same way, out of the same basic substances. Our blood isn't green, though, so obviously there's a difference at some point along the way. In plants, those basic substances (glycine and succinic acid) bind with magnesium from rocks, soil and water to form chlorophyll, which carries out the plant's main energy process, photosynthesis. Chlorophyll harnesses energy from sunlight, which is needed to convert carbon dioxide in the air, and water in the soil to carbohydrates, which the plant stores or uses later for food and growth.

In people and animals, the same basic substances that form chlorophyll in plants bind instead with iron to form heme, a substance that gives blood its characteristic red color. When we eat plants, the magnesium from their chlorophyll helps ATP to liberate energy from our food.

The Strange Case of Magnesium Drain

Chemical farming creates a magnesium debt. Plant roots draw magnesium out of the soil and carry it to the rest of the plant. When plants grow and die in the wild, decaying plant matter replaces magnesium "borrowed" from the soil while the plants were growing. In traditional agriculture, addition of organic compost—decayed plant matter and animal wastes—recreates that natural cycle. Chemical farming, however, returns only nitrogen, potassium and phosphorus, but neglects to replace magnesium. Unfortunately, chemical fertilization has become the most common farming method. Foods grown on chemically fertilized soils, as most today are, have 10 to 12 percent less magnesium than food grown by traditional organic methods of fertilization. Consequently, food composition tables put out by the U.S. Department of Agriculture (the major source of dietary information in our country) quite probably overestimate the magnesium content of foods by a corresponding 10 to 12 percent (*Water Hardness, Human Health, and the Importance of Magnesium,* National Research Council of Canada, 1979).

Food Processing Adds to the Magnesium Debt

Magnesium is one of those minerals lost in food processing that is not replaced by enrichment at the factory. Unprocessed fruits, vegetables and grain products have a lot more magnesium than pared-down, refined versions of the same foods. For example:

• Whole wheat bread has 3 times as much magnesium as white bread, including French, Vienna and raisin breads.

• Whole wheat flour has about 4½ times as much magnesium as white flour. Rye flour has about 3 times as much magnesium as white flour.

• Brown rice has 3½ times as much magnesium as white rice.

• Blackstrap molasses has over 5½ times as much magnesium as light molasses.

• Whole grain barley has over 3 times the magnesium of pearled barley.

• Potatoes in their skins have about 1½ times as much magnesium as peeled potatoes.

Whether you choose white bread or whole grain bread, then, or white rice or brown, will certainly make a difference in your magnesium intake.

Even simple home cooking steals some magnesium from food. Up to 40 percent of the magnesium in food leaches out during cooking. Fresh‧ green peas, for example, lose about 33 percent of their magnesium when frozen and 42 percent when canned. And frozen turnip greens have less than half the magnesium of fresh greens.

Many of Us Get Less Magnesium Than We Should

To meet heavy demands for magnesium's talents, our bodies need at least 300 milligrams a day for women and at least 350 milligrams a day for men, according to the official Recommended Dietary Allowances set for us by the Food and Nutrition Board of the National Research Council. A few mineral researchers, however, insist that 400 to 450 milligrams is more realistic. Mildred S. Seelig, M.D., of the Goldwater Memorial Hospital at the New York University Medical Center in New York City argues that people are deficient in magnesium when intake drops below 420 milligrams a day, and that deficiencies of magnesium are more common than most nutritionists believe. Below 420 milligrams, says Dr. Seelig, we excrete more magnesium than we take in, losing small amounts of the mineral every day. Dr. Seelig has amassed a great deal of data to support her theory. Supporters of Dr. Seelig's position say that magnesium balance is not only required for optimum health, but that extra magnesium may have definite advantages. They cite magnesium's many and varied roles in the body, especially its link with lower incidence of heart disease, control of blood pressure and prevention of kidney stones.

One would think that with magnesium available from a veritable smorgasbord of dolomite, water and plants that a deficiency, even by the government's standards, would be practically nonexistent. Until recently, most nutritionists believed just that.

Well, they were wrong. While magnesium is supplied generously in green leafy vegetables, nuts, beans, whole grains, brown rice, soybeans and molasses, the typical Western diet doesn't usually include enough of those foods to provide even the established, albeit low, RDA for magnesium. Our story of undernourished children in underdeveloped countries may lead you to assume that below-par magnesium intake in our own country occurs only among the poor and disadvantaged, but that's not true. While one study found magnesium levels to be as low as 200 milligrams a day in low-income families, the same study found that people considered well off had "higher" levels of only 245 and 288 milligrams—still inadequate (*The Food and Health of Western Man,* John Wiley, 1975).

According to one nutrition text, "It is estimated that a typical American diet provides 120 milligrams per 1,000 [calories]—a level that will barely provide the recommended intake" (*Introductory Nutrition,* C. V. Mosby, 1979). Various other studies also indicate that Western table fare in general—high in meat and refined grains like white flour, and low in nuts, beans and fresh vegetables—yields about 200 to 260 milligrams a day of magnesium—roughly half of what we really need.

Why Momma Always Said, "Eat Your Vegetables!"

Aware of such evidence, nutritionists at the University of Montreal, in Canada, grew curious about the magnesium content of meals served in their own university cafeteria. The team of Srivastava, Nadeau and Gueneau from the university's department of nutrition went into the dining room and analyzed food selections made by students at the three main meals of the day. Breakfasts freely chosen by the students from the foods offered included combinations of juice, toast, eggs, ham, bacon, oatmeal, cornflakes, milk, sugar and coffee. Lunches and dinners were chosen from a variety of dishes: meat, lasagna, juice, soup, dessert, tea and coffee. Menu selections, in each case, were fairly typical of most North American tables.

Nutritional analysis showed that men students took in an average of about 247 milligrams of magnesium a day, and women took in about 224—not only lower than the RDA, but way below the 400 to 450 milligrams deemed adequate by some nutritionists. Their recommendation: ". . . it will be advisable to increase the magnesium content of the three main meals by including the foods rich in magnesium; i.e., cereals, spinach, maize [corn], sugar beets, fruits and vegetables" (*Nutrition Reports International,* August, 1978).

Take a lesson from your pet cat. If Mittens starts munching your houseplants, she may not necessarily be up to pure mischief. Cats need chlorophyll-containing foliage for its magnesium just like people, and may resort to nibbling on your indoor greenery if they don't get their fill outdoors.

Besides green leafies, other good sources of magnesium are nuts, legumes, grains, potatoes and some fruits. See table 3 for a more comprehensive list of magnesium sources.

TABLE 3 **Food Sources of Magnesium**

Food	Portion	Magnesium (milligrams)
Soy flour	½ cup	155
Soybeans, dried	¼ cup	138
Tofu (soybean curd)	4 ounces	126
Buckwheat flour, light	½ cup	112
Black-eyed peas, dried	¼ cup	98
Wheat germ, raw	¼ cup	97
Almonds	¼ cup	96
Cashews	¼ cup	94
Lima beans, large, dried, raw	¼ cup	81
Brazil nuts	¼ cup	79
Pecans, halved	¼ cup	77
Kidney beans, dried	¼ cup	75
Whole wheat flour	½ cup	68
Shredded wheat	1 cup	67
Peanuts, roasted, chopped	¼ cup	63
Walnuts, black, chopped	¼ cup	60
Beet greens, raw, chopped	1 cup	58
Banana	1 medium	58
Avocado	½	56
Peanut flour	¼ cup	54
Blackstrap molasses	1 tablespoon	52
Potato	1 medium	51
Oatmeal	1 cup	50
Spinach, raw, chopped	1 cup	48
Salmon, sockeye, drained solids	4 ounces	43
Rye flour	½ cup	37
Swiss chard, raw, chopped	1 cup	36
Milk, skim	1 cup	34
Chestnuts	½ cup	33
Collards, raw	1 cup	31
Brown rice	½ cup	28
Ground beef, lean	4 ounces	28
Peanut butter	1 tablespoon	28

SOURCE: Adapted from *Composition of Foods,* Agriculture Handbook No. 8, rev. ed., by Bernice K. Watt and Annabel L. Merrill (Washington, D.C.: Agricultural Research Service, U.S. Department of Agriculture, 1975).

That sounds like a lot of food. Won't I gain weight? you ask.

No, probably not. Plant foods, the richest sources of magnesium, are low in calories. Food and nutrition researchers Greger, Marhefka and Geissler, who conducted a study of 150 common supermarket foods at Purdue University in 1978, calculated the ratios of magnesium to total calories in basic food groups. "Generally, the ratios were higher in vegetables than in meat, milk and [refined] cereal products," they report. Put another way, that means you can get more magnesium and fewer calories from vegetables than from meat. A quarter-pound burger will give you 28 milligrams of magnesium at a caloric cost of 324, while you can get almost double that amount of magnesium from a medium-size baked potato at only 111 calories.

A closer look at that study's data shows that a diet heavy in cereals and vegetables could yield about 40 percent more magnesium than one emphasizing meat, eggs and dairy products (*Journal of Food Science,* September/October, 1978). A vegetarian who dines primarily on grains, beans and fresh vegetables is likely to get more magnesium than his steak-loving dinner partner, especially if the partner passes up brown rice and vegetables for white dinner rolls and ice cream. It's interesting to recall that the undernourished children with kwashiorkor, who ate lots of starch and few or no vegetables, did not improve on high-protein food until magnesium was introduced into their diet.

Supplements Help Take the Guesswork Out of Magnesium Resources

You can obtain magnesium supplements in which the mineral is usually bound together with another substance. Magnesium oxide and magnesium gluconate are two common examples. But remember, magnesium works best when accompanied by about two parts calcium. You can get that proportion by taking a calcium supplement or bone meal along with your magnesium, aiming for about twice as much calcium as magnesium.

Dolomite is a simpler alternative. It happens to provide both magnesium and calcium in good balance, so you don't need to wrestle with calculations.

The other magnesium "supplement" may be in your water tap, if you're fortunate enough to live in a hard water area and can avoid using a "softener" on your drinking water supply. In addition to robbing the water of magnesium and calcium, water softeners add sodium (salt) to the water, which contributes to high blood pressure. Although there's not much you can do about living in a soft water geographical area, choosing foods high in magnesium and keeping supplements of dolomite in the kitchen will best assure you of an adequate supply of magnesium.

CHAPTER

4

Phosphorus

Phosphorus and the Marathon of Daily Life

Most, but not all, of the two pounds of phosphorus in our bodies is tied up with calcium to give strength and rigidity to bones and teeth. Much of the rest is distributed in each cell and all body fluids as part of that special substance, adenosine triphosphate (ATP), which controls energy release. In our bodies, the phosphorus in ATP takes up where magnesium leaves off: magnesium sparks energy release and phosphorus controls it. After proteins, carbohydrates and fats in food are oxidized, phosphorus compounds release the bound-up energy slowly and evenly, like a control valve.

That's important, because with too little phosphorus we'd have to eat nonstop just to maintain basic metabolism. To eat while playing the cello is gauche, if not downright awkward. To eat while giving a speech is impolite, not to mention dangerous. And to eat while sleeping—just plain impossible. Yet if it weren't for phosphorus, we'd have no choice. For while we speak, eat and sleep, our bodies are continuously running a silent, internal marathon. And for that we need energy. Just as long-distance runners know the importance of pacing themselves, so do our bodies. Starting the contest with a gush of unbridled energy means the marathon runner will stall out long before he reaches the finish line. The marathon runner has only so much energy to expend in the race. Energy must be meted out judiciously, conserved for the home stretch—and the hills between start and finish. Similarly, if our bodies used up all energy from protein, fats and carbohydrates immediately after a meal, there'd soon be none left to feed our brains, hearts, lungs and other organs for the rest of the afternoon or overnight as we slept. It's easy to see the sense in having an internal governor to store energy for later use, gradually dispensing it at just the right rate, so that we only have to refuel every few hours. Phosphorus is that governor.

Our bodies can't use protein, fats and carbohydrates just as they are, straight from our dinner plates. Our blood isn't equipped to transport them in raw form. Proteins are directly broken down by enzymes. Fats and carbohydrates, however, are first "phosphorylated" during digestion. In other words, as part of the energy release process, some phosphorus latches onto molecules of each, changing them into forms the body can use. Fats become phospholipids, oily droplets which can easily slip into the blood-stream and be carried to the rest of the body, where they're needed.

Some phospholipids give off choline, a vitaminlike substance. Many of the B vitamins have adopted phosphorus and are only active in phosphate form. Phosphorus bound to thiamine (vitamin B_1), called thiamine pyrophosphate, is vital to healthy nerves. Phosphorus bound to nicotinic acid (vitamin B_3) is, aside from being a real tongue-twister—nicotinic adenine dinucleotide, or NAD—important to good digestion and emotional health. Bound to pyridoxine (vitamin B_6), phosphorus becomes pyridoxal phosphate, helpful to immunity, steady nerves and water balance. Riboflavin (vitamin B_2) functions chiefly in combination with another phosphorus compound, phosphoric acid, and is essential for growth.

A Realistic Look at Calcium:Phosphorus Balance

The critical factor in phosphorus intake is balance—specifically, balance with calcium. Some nutrition researchers suggest a 1:1 ratio between dietary calcium and phosphorus. Their recommendations are based on animal studies that indicate any excess phosphorus prompts calcium to be pilfered from the bones, contributing to the bone loss occurring with osteoporosis in later years. Consequently, the Recommended Dietary Allowance (RDA) for phosphorus has been matched to that of calcium—800 milligrams a day.

Looking at the calcium:phosphorus ratio in our food, however, shows that more often than not, phosphorus is higher than calcium.

The baking industry uses calcium phosphate and sodium phosphate as leavening agents (baking powder) in commercial baked goods like refrigerator rolls, doughnuts and cake mixes. Those compounds of phosphorus make dough rise by reacting with baking soda to generate hundreds of tiny bubbles of carbon dioxide. (In yeast breads, enzymes produce the same kind of gas bubbles.)

Calcium phosphate is no significant threat to calcium balance. Calcium phosphate, however, is faster acting than sodium phosphate, so manufacturers usually use sodium phosphate alone or in addition to calcium phosphate because it doesn't fizzle out so readily and still reacts after batter is held for considerable periods of time, as in restaurant batters and frozen bread doughs. Using both kinds of phosphate leavening together, of course, takes advantage of the slow release of the sodium type and the faster action of the calcium type. But the sodium type does add phosphorus with no calcium.

Bubbles, too, are what give carbonated soft drinks their fizz. Bottlers add small amounts of another compound of phosphorus, phosphoric acid, to some soft drinks because it keeps carbon dioxide bubbles intact longer and prevents the soda from going flat. Some researchers blame bone loss of osteoporosis in many women past menopause on too much phosphorus and too little calcium, brought on by drinking soft drinks instead of high-calcium milk. That theory is based on several studies of adult rats fed twice as much phosphorus as calcium. But other studies contradict the theory (*Journal of the Canadian Dietetic Association,* April, 1977).

We took a closer look at the phosphorus levels in soft drinks and found that even the highest didn't exceed the amount in most unprocessed foods (see table 4 for examples). A whole bottle of Dr. Pepper contains about as much phosphorus as a cup of orange juice. You'd have to drink four Cokes to get the amount of phosphorus in a cup of milk. The problem, say researchers, is that soft drinks have no calcium at all to balance out the phosphorus. And those beverages tend to be gulped down many times a day, every day, replacing high-calcium milk and other foods. Long-term studies of the effects on people haven't been done yet.

Still, blaming osteoporosis on soda seems a little too simple. After all, an estimated six million Americans have osteoporosis. Are they *all* quaffing down lots of soda? Probably not. And besides, it would take six Cokes to equal the phosphorus in four ounces of cod, four Dr. Peppers to equal half a cup of chopped chicken, and five Pepsis to equal the phospho-

TABLE 4 **Phosphorus in Some Foods**

Food	Portion	Phosphorus (milligrams)
Cod	4 ounces	312
Beef	4 ounces	290
Milk	1 cup	227
Yogurt	1 cup	213
Chicken, chopped	2½ ounces	158
Brewer's yeast	1 tablespoon	140
Cottage cheese	½ cup	127
Brown rice	½ cup	71
Pepsi-Cola	12 ounces	61
Whole wheat bread	1 slice	57
Coca Cola	12 ounces	53
Orange juice	1 cup	42
Dr. Pepper	12 ounces	41

SOURCES: Adapted from
   Nutritive Value of American Foods in Common Units, Agriculture Handbook No. 456, by Catherine F. Adams (Washington, D.C.: Agricultural Research Service, U.S. Department of Agriculture, 1975).
   Research News, U.S. Department of Agriculture, Science and Education Administration, June 10, 1980.

rus in four ounces of beef—all foods with very little calcium. Nobody's discouraging us from eating them. True, soda has other serious faults—sugar, sodium and sometimes caffeine—but as for causing bone loss, what really matters is total diet.

Phosphate additives are as popular with meat processors as they are with bakers. Phosphates are added to many meats to retard spoilage and to give them an appealing but artificial pink color. Such compounds add phosphorus to cured beef and pork products like ham, Canadian bacon, corned beef, cold cuts, sausages and frankfurters.

In addition, many salad dressings, most processed cheeses, and snacks like potato chips contain added phosphates as preservatives.

Eating Unprocessed Foods
Helps Keep Phosphorus in Check

A few foods—some citrus fruits and dark green leafy vegetables—have more calcium than phosphorus. Milk, dairy products and other fruits and vegetables have approximately equal amounts of each. Most other foods have a surplus of phosphorus (see table 5). Grains, nuts, beans, white potatoes and some fish range from about 1:2 to 1:10. Poultry and other fish are lower, about 1:10 to 1:12. Beef liver has one of the lowest ratios of calcium to phosphorus, about 1:45. In most diets, in fact, phosphorus

TABLE 5   Calcium:Phosphorus Ratio of Some Foods

Food	Ratio (calcium to phosphorus)
Turnip greens	5:1
Collards	4:1
Mustard greens	4:1
Watercress	3:1
Cheddar cheese	2:1
Yogurt	1:1
Milk	1:1
Tofu (soybean curd)	1:1
Apples	1:1
Broccoli	1:1
Soybeans	1:2
Cottage cheese, dry-curd	1:2
Orange juice	1:2
Tomatoes	1:2
Almonds	1:2
Filberts	1:2
Whole wheat bread	1:2
Bananas	1:3
Peanuts	1:6
Oatmeal	1:6
Haddock	1:6
Brewer's yeast	1:8
Lamb	1:18
Beef	1:20
Pork	1:23

SOURCE: Adapted from *Nutritive Value of American Foods in Common Units*, Agriculture Handbook No. 456, by Catherine F. Adams (Washington, D.C.: Agricultural Research Service, U.S. Department of Agriculture, 1975).

exceeds calcium to some extent. And it seems that eating only those foods that contain a low ratio of phosphorus to calcium would mean completely eliminating some very nutritious foods from our diet. Liver, for instance, may be high in phosphorus, but it's also an exceptionally good source of protein, zinc, copper and iron.

A calcium:phosphorus ratio of up to 1:2, then, is more practical, and can be maintained by avoiding cured meats, soft drinks and commercial baked goods. While there is some dickering about effects of smaller imbalances of phosphorus and calcium, most nutritionists would agree that a diet high in foods which yield an oversupply of phosphorus is undesirable.

Researchers in the departments of food science and animal nutrition at the University of Illinois, in the course of studying the physiological effect of phosphorus, found out just how much unwanted phosphorus could be avoided by eating foods free of phosphate additives. R. Raines Bell, Ph.D., H. H. Draper, Ph.D., and three associates compared two diets in eight people over two four-week periods. During the first period, the group ate foods free of added phosphates. During the second period, processed cheese was substituted for natural cheese; soft drinks for fruit juice; quick breads for yeast breads; and cured meats for phosphate-free meats. The first diet contained about 1,000 milligrams of phosphorus a day, the trial diet about 2,100—more than twice as much. Calcium intake, on the other hand, rose only slightly. The calcium:phosphorus ratio, as a result, was pushed from 1:1.4 in the first diet to 1:3 in the second diet. Levels of phosphorus in blood and urine increased; calcium levels decreased (*Journal of Nutrition,* January, 1977).

Drs. Bell and Draper feel that, combined with the fact that calcium absorption is known to decrease in older people, a high-phosphorus diet like that eaten during the second period of their experiment may contribute to bone loss as people age. Some, but not all, of the phosphorus surplus may be countered by calcium supplements. Evidently, steering clear of cured meats and processed foods is a simpler way to keep phosphorus in reasonable equilibrium. Read food package labels to find out what contains phosphate and what doesn't. Fruit juices almost never contain phosphates and are worthier thirst quenchers than soda.

Aside from concerns with calcium:phosphorus balance, pure comfort is an added consideration in keeping clear of phosphate additives. In the University of Illinois study, everyone reported soft stools or mild diarrhea and abdominal discomfort when they started eating phosphate additives. For some, the symptoms abated; for some, they did not.

Bone Meal, the Food Supplement That Matches Our Bones

A food supplement made from the long bones of cattle, bone meal is primarily taken to insure calcium intake. Bone meal also contains some phosphorus, however, in a ratio that matches the ratio of those minerals in our own bodies. For that reason, calcium may work better when it comes from bone meal. In any case, bone meal is a perfectly balanced—and very useful—combination of both minerals.

CHAPTER

5

Sodium

Salt is the oldest food preservative in the world, adopted because the sodium in salt draws water out of food, removing moisture on which harmful bacteria depend to live, grow and reproduce. Before refrigeration, salt was the only practical way to keep meat and fish from going bad. The modern habit of seasoning food with salt at the stove or table probably followed the discovery that salt not only preserved meat, but also disguised bad flavors had it already begun to spoil.

There's much debate over whether our craving for salt is an acquired or an inborn taste, but it seems likely that the practice of adding salt to food was adopted only after its preservative qualities were stumbled upon. Although sodium is essential to health, primarily for water balance, added salt is rarely needed. Sodium is so widely distributed in food and drinking water that short of outright starvation or severe illness, minimum needs—about 200 milligrams a day—are easily met. Most Americans today consume about 10 to 35 times our actual need for sodium, most of it from salt added at the factory, stove or table. (One gram of salt contains about 400 milligrams of sodium.)

Salt was unknown in several central American countries up until the Spanish conquest, and in many parts of Africa before European exploration there. The ancient Egyptians actually forbade the use of salt. In ancient China, only the rich could afford salt. And it's relatively recent that Greeks began to use salt. Evidently, people managed to survive for thousands of years without salting their food. They derived all the sodium they needed from what was found naturally in food. When salt's preservative qualities were discovered in Europe and China, whole economies sprang up around salt mining and trade. Roman soldiers were paid in salt, and our word "salary" stems from *sal,* the Latin word for salt. By the 1700s and 1800s, the salt industry had become a rich source of revenue for England and Bavaria.

Today we're still paying a high price for salt—not in dollars, but in health. For reasons still unknown, certain people seem to react to high salt intake by developing high blood pressure, or hypertension. That is, the arteries carrying blood around the body are in a state of tension which makes it difficult for the heart to pump blood through the system. Hypertension speeds up atherosclerosis, or hardening of the arteries, often leading to heart attack or stroke. Hypertension also tends to damage walls of the arteries pumping blood to the kidneys, causing kidney failure. That can be fatal, as toxins normally filtered out of the body by the kidneys back up and poison the system. In any case, life expectancy is shorter for people with chronic, or essential, hypertension. And the younger a person is when hypertension develops, the shorter life may be.

Salt doesn't cause hypertension. No one is sure what does. But those people who eat the most salt, like the Japanese, also happen to develop high blood pressure more often. Those who eat little salt, like Australian aborigines, Greenland Eskimos and Panamanian Indians, seldom have high blood pressure. The pattern is the same, all over the world, with no exceptions.

Our early ancestors ate about 240 milligrams of sodium a day from vegetarian fare—somewhat more when the hunt was successful since meat contains more sodium than vegetables and fruit. For hundreds of thousands of years, our kidneys functioned efficiently on about 1,200 to 1,600 milligrams of sodium a day at most.

Today we consume much more—from 10 to 30 times as much. About one-fourth of that total still comes from sodium naturally present in foods. A large share of the remainder comes from salt added in the kitchen or at the table. One teaspoon of table salt alone contains over 2,000 milligrams of sodium. A still larger amount is added to food at the factory, added primarily for flavor, not as a preservative. Americans, on the average, lug 11 pounds of sodium home from the supermarket each year, in the form of table salt or food additives. On a daily basis, that boils down to 4,000 to 5,000 milligrams or more a day per person.

Hypertension, Stormy Weather in the Sea within Us

Since sodium plays a major role in regulation of body fluids, it's reasonable to assume that salt is capable of influencing blood pressure. Some argue that salt can't be the noxious villain in high blood pressure, for supposedly nature wouldn't have us crave something that is so harmful. But that may not be true. Hypertension may result from the fact that we've started eating too much salt, too quickly, without giving nature enough time to adapt. Our kidneys were programmed for thousands of years to process three or four grams of salt a day. When that amount is suddenly and greatly exceeded, the kidneys may work less efficiently. The apparent result is hypertension, especially in people who come from ancestors who used no added salt. Blacks, for instance, are more susceptible to hypertension than nonblacks, perhaps reflecting the fact that salt was not used in many parts of Africa until introduced by Europeans. Likewise, people who leave a home country where little salt is used are likely to develop the disease after moving to the United States and adopting our high salt intake.

Although sodium and salt are often used synonymously, the two are not quite the same. When people speak of salt, they are usually referring to sodium chloride, or common table salt—the most common compound of sodium, found abundantly all over the world. Plants and animals as well as our bones, blood and body fluid all contain sodium chloride. Chlorine is important in its own way, but sodium is the most active ingredient in salt.

Rock salt as it's mined from underground deposits is used in coarse form to clear highways and sidewalks of ice. Sodium reacts quickly with water, giving off heat and melting ice. Table salt is a refined form of rock salt.

The sea is the ultimate source of all salt. When we swim in the ocean and return to our beach chairs to dry off in the sun, we notice a salty residue left on our skin. Salt deposits on Earth were formed by a similar process of evaporation in ocean lagoons and shallow inland seas.

30 Million Years of Experimental Kidneys

Our blood, sweat and tears are salty like seawater, a legacy from the sea where all life originated. When marine animals migrated first to freshwater ponds and later to dry land, they retained that salty internal sea. Like all animals, we need a certain amount of water and salt to survive. With too little of either, we'd shrivel up and die. With too much, we'd swell up, drowning in our own fluids. To keep our internal sea in constant balance, we have a pair of highly sophisticated kidneys.

Kidneys also prevent us from poisoning ourselves with harmful wastes produced during digestion and metabolism. Every plant and animal, from the smallest microbe to the largest mammal, must rid itself of waste products, and most use water as a flushing agent.

In the sea, where life began, getting plenty of water was no problem. The first fish that swam upstream to freshwater rivers and ponds probably swelled up and died, due to a spontaneous action, called osmosis, between salty water in blood and cells and fresh water rushing into the body. Simply put, "water goes where salt is." Water tends to be drawn through a membrane to an inner area containing a higher concentration of salt, in order to equalize the amount on each side of the membrane. That happens to the organism as a whole because it happens within each cell.

Through trial and error, fish developed specialized organs to excrete some salt along with water and waste products, retaining just enough to maintain life. Those organs were forerunners of our own kidneys.

With more trial and error, nature found ways to help animals survive the comparative drought on land by modifying kidney-like organs to better economize water for waste flushing. Most reptiles, birds and mammals—including people—rely almost entirely on kidneys to maintain water and salt balance.

Our kidneys are the shape and color of their namesake, the kidney bean, and are about the size of a fist. Without such efficient kidneys to purify and recycle body water, we'd have to drink over 40 quarts of water a day to assure our bodies of an adequate water supply unpolluted by our own wastes, leftover drugs and other unwanted toxins that find their way into our bloodstream. Our bodies contain 42 quarts of salt water, distributed in blood, water inside cells (intracellular fluid) and water bathing the cells (extracellular fluid). We normally experience slight fluctuations in both water and salt, excreting more after meals and less during the night. If we drink a lot of fluid, we excrete more of each. If we perspire freely due to intense heat or fever, we excrete more salt through sweat. If we drink a lot on a hot day, after exercise, or when we run a fever, water and salt usually balance out under regulation by our kidneys.

Kidneys filter up to a quart of blood per minute, 15 gallons per hour, or 360 gallons per day, relying on the heart to pump blood to tiny filtering beds, called nephrons, by way of larger renal arteries and smaller capillaries. Around the clock each day, blood delivers used body water, digestive wastes and harmful contaminants to the kidneys for disposal and at the same time picks up purified water, minerals, and the right amount of sodium for redelivery to the cells. Excess salt, along with waste water, is stored in the bladder for later discharge as urine. Some water—about a quart—along with wastes and salt is also lost through sweat, feces and exhaled air, but most leaves the body in the one or two quarts of urine passed daily.

Sodium, Necessary in Moderation, Dangerous in Excess

There's no such thing as an actual sodium deficiency, although extreme circumstances may call for replacement.

Sodium losses run high when prolonged vomiting, diarrhea or sweating due to fever, intense heat or exercise flush so much water out of the body that the kidneys cannot keep up the job of holding back on sodium. It must then be replaced. During pregnancy, on the other hand, water retention—or edema—is common. At one time, pregnant women were advised to restrict salt intake, but obstetricians now recognize that needs actually go up, for the body is holding back on fluid losses in an effort to conserve sodium. But those are about the only circumstances that call for added sodium in the diet.

Like phosphorus, too much sodium in the diet is more of a problem than too little. One out of every five Americans has or will get hypertension. Although it would seem prudent for everyone to avoid high sodium intake, diet is not always given serious consideration, for a variety of reasons.

Not all physicians prescribe low-sodium diets for people who are clearly diagnosed as hypertensive. Instead, they treat high blood pressure with drugs, including diuretics, which force the kidneys to pump more water and sodium out in urine, lowering blood pressure the same way low-sodium intake would. Commenting on that approach, George R. Meneely, M.D., and Harold D. Battarbee, Ph.D., write, "Although low-salt diets are obviously effective in most hypertensives, it appears that physicians prefer to prescribe pills rather than diets" (*Present Knowledge in Nutrition,* Nutrition Foundation, 1976).

Potassium is nearly as critical to water balance as sodium (something we'll take up in the next chapter) and work by Dr. Meneely and others supports the theory that low potassium along with high salt intake may contribute to high blood pressure. (For a more complete discussion of the role of minerals in hypertension, see chapter 34, High Blood Pressure, in Part 5.)

Salt, the Insidious Seasoning

Pretzels have so much salt clinging to them that it falls off and collects in our laps. Few other foods, however, give such a clear indication of their salt content. Consequently, most people don't know which foods are high in sodium and which aren't. We took a long, hard look at just about every food likely to be carted home from the store, and found some revealing data. Sample comparisons of what we found are presented in tables 6 through 16.

Unprocessed foods generally have less sodium than processed foods. Most vegetables and nearly all fruits and grains are quite low; milk and meat tend to be higher (see table 6). We take in about three grams of salt a day from basic, unprocessed foods—meat, fish, poultry, fruit, vegetables, rice, beans, potatoes and so on. That's about how much our early ancestors ate.

To those three grams of salt naturally present in food, four to six more are added by food processors. Salt is the most widely used food additive. Much is added to foods for flavor; some, however, is used as a preservative—often when freezing or canning (minus the salt) would serve the same purpose.

TABLE 6 Sodium in Some Foods

Food	Portion	Sodium (milligrams)
Buttermilk	1 cup	319
Haddock	4 ounces	200
Milk	1 cup	122
Yogurt, whole-milk	1 cup	115
Swiss cheese	1 ounce	74
Chicken	4 ounces	72
Roast beef	4 ounces	65
Egg	1 medium	54
Celery, raw	1 stalk	50
Cantaloupe	¼ melon	16
Green pepper, raw, diced	½ cup	12
Endive, chopped	1 cup	7
Potato, baked	1 long	6
Lettuce, shredded	1 cup	5
Brown rice	½ cup	4
Radishes	5 medium	4
Tomato	1 medium	4
Onions, raw, minced	¼ cup	4
Applesauce	½ cup	2
Apple	1 medium	2
Plums	5	1
Apricots, fresh	3	1
Grapefruit	½	1
Orange	1 medium	1
Strawberries	½ cup	trace
Wheat germ, toasted	¼ cup	trace

SOURCE: Adapted from *Nutritive Value of American Foods in Common Units*, Agriculture Handbook No. 456, by Catherine F. Adams (Washington, D.C.: Agricultural Research Service, U.S. Department of Agriculture, 1975).

Cured meats

Sausage, salami, ham, bacon, frankfurters, corned beef and other cured meat products are reservoirs of added sodium. Most of the 200 or so cured meat products on the market spend a good part of their life at the factory soaking in a salt brine similar to the sea brines that formed the earth's salt deposits. Salt brine breaks down muscle protein and binds it into the characteristic gel of meat, moisture and fat that makes a salami a salami. Incidentally, both the words "salami" and "sausage," like "salary," are derived from *sal*, the Latin word for salt.

Salt and other sodium compounds provide that "cured" taste and pink color of processed meat. Salted meat products retain water, which reduces shrinkage. The added salt also helps retard rancidity and inhibits growth of botulism, a deadly organism, while the meat sits in the super-market. Table 7 shows how much sodium can be avoided by choosing untreated beef and poultry over cured, processed meat products. Sodium in unprocessed roasts, stew meat or fryers can be reduced by braising and discarding the cooking liquid, which draws sodium out of the meat.

TABLE 7   **Sodium Content of Processed vs. Unprocessed Meats**

Meat	Portion	Sodium (milligrams)
Processed		
Bologna	3 slices	1,107
Corned beef	4 ounces	1,069
Ham	4 ounces	848
Hot dog	1	627
Bacon, Canadian	1 slice	537
Sausage	4 links	500
Bacon	3 medium slices	229
Unprocessed		
Beef liver	4 ounces	208
Chicken, light meat	4 ounces	72
Lamb	4 ounces	70
Roast beef	4 ounces	65
Pork	4 ounces	64

SOURCE: Adapted from *Nutritive Value of American Foods in Common Units,* Agriculture Handbook No. 456, by Catherine F. Adams (Washington, D.C.: Agricultural Research Service, U.S. Department of Agriculture, 1975).

Salted fish

Some fish products contain proportionately more salt than the seawater from which they're harvested. Kippered herring, smoked salmon (lox), caviar, anchovies and dried codfish are too salty to be considered healthful foods—despite their low fat and high healthful mineral content. Stick to less exotic but tasty varieties like broiled haddock, codfish, flounder, halibut, perch or salmon, which are high in all the good things but lower in sodium (see table 8).

TABLE 8   Sodium in Fish

Fish	Sodium (milligrams per 4 ounces unless specified)
Cod, dried, salted	5,806
Lox (smoked salmon)	2,132
Salmon roe, salted	1,633
Anchovy paste	1,540 per 1 tablespoon
Whitefish, smoked	1,474
Herring, pickled	1,168
Anchovies	1,140 per 5
Crab, king, canned, drained solids	1,137
Sardines, canned, drained solids	932
Caviar	624 per 1 ounce
Salmon, canned, drained solids	439
Tuna, canned, drained solids	384
Scallops	301
Flounder	268
Lobster	238
Oysters	232
Shrimp	212
Haddock	200
Perch	172
Halibut	152
Salmon	132
Sturgeon	124
Cod	124
Bluefish	116
Mackerel	113
Shad	88
Trout	78

SOURCE: Adapted from *Nutritive Value of American Foods in Common Units*, Agriculture Handbook No. 456, by Catherine F. Adams (Washington, D.C.: Agricultural Research Service, U.S. Department of Agriculture, 1975).

Canned fish, like canned vegetables, contains added salt. Canned salmon contains a hefty 439 milligrams of sodium per serving from added salt, while salmon from the fish market contains only 132 milligrams of sodium per four ounces, making it a wiser choice for salads and antipasto. Similarly, canned tuna fish, regular pack, contains 384 milligrams of sodium per four-ounce serving, while low-sodium pack yields only 41 milligrams.

Cheese

Like meat, cheese often contains added salt, chiefly to inhibit undesirable bacteria, but also for various other reasons. Added to basic

TABLE 9 **Sodium in Cheese**

Cheese	Sodium (milligrams per 1 ounce)
Parmesan, grated (1 tablespoon = .18 ounces)	528
Roquefort	513
Swiss, cheese food, pasteurized process	440
American, pasteurized process	406
Blue	396
Swiss, pasteurized process	388
American cheese spread, pasteurized process	381
Romano	340
Feta	316
American cheese food, cold pack	274
Edam	274
Provolone	248
Camembert	239
Gouda	232
Limburger	227
Cheshire	198
Brie	178
Muenster	178
Cheddar	176
Colby	171
Brick	159
Monterey	152
Mozzarella, part skim	132
Cottage, low-fat (2%)	115
Cottage, low-fat (1%)	115
Cottage, creamed	114
Mozzarella	106
Gruyere	95
Cream	84
Swiss, unprocessed	74
Cottage, dry-curd, unsalted	4

SOURCE: Adapted from *Composition of Foods: Dairy and Egg Products,* Agriculture Handbook No. 8-1, rev. ed., by Consumer and Food Economics Institute (Washington, D.C.: Agricultural Research Service, U.S. Department of Agriculture, 1976).

milk curd in just the right amount, sodium is one factor that helps give each type of cheese its distinctive texture and flavor. Too much salt produces a dry, brittle texture; too little, a bland, pasty cheese. Obviously, then, some cheeses have more sodium than others, depending on how sharp or mild, moist or dry they are, and what specific flavors they impart. In the production of Roquefort or blue cheese, milk curd is highly salted to inhibit the growth of undesirable organisms but to allow a desirable, salt-tolerant penicillin mold *(Penicillium roqueforti)* to grow. Special bacteria are added to lightly salted cheese, like Swiss, for instance, to yield the characteristic holes and sweet flavor. As a result, Swiss cheese contains only 74 milligrams of salt per ounce, while Roquefort contains 513 and blue contains 396. Most other cheeses fall somewhere in between (see table 9).

If a person is restricted by a physician to 500 milligrams or less of sodium daily, cheese should be eliminated entirely from the menu. However, most people can avoid a lot of cheese-based sodium by choosing certain varieties over others. One cup of low-fat cottage cheese contains 918 milligrams of sodium, and a cup of creamed cottage cheese contains 850 milligrams. Buy unsalted, dry-curd cottage cheese, however, and the sodium content is reduced to just 19 milligrams per cup. Parmesan is relatively high in sodium, but since its concentrated flavor allows a little bit to go a long way, it adds lots of flavor at only 93 milligrams a tablespoon.

Canned vegetables

Even though heat destroys harmful bacteria when vegetables are canned, salt is usually added, ostensibly for flavoring. Vegetables and other foods intended for specific use on low-sodium diets list the amount of sodium; the rest rarely do. Frozen vegetables, with the exception of peas and beans, are more likely to be salt-free. Lima beans, butter beans and peas, however, are usually salted before freezing, sometimes to preserve their color. See table 10 for comparison of some fresh vegetables with frozen and canned versions.

Fruits

Fruits generally escape the salt line at the factory. Both fruits and vegetables are good sources of potassium, which is important in offsetting the effect of high sodium in the diet.

Fermented foods

Fermented foods, like pickles and sauerkraut, are either fermented by action of salt or contain salt for flavor—or both. Salt helps make sauerkraut out of shredded raw cabbage by drawing out the water and providing the proper environment for specific bacteria conducive to fermentation, while certain unwanted bacteria are thwarted. One-half cup of plain cabbage has a scant 7 milligrams of sodium, while its fermented form, sauerkraut, is chock-full at 877 milligrams. In a similar way, the sodium content of cucumbers jumps from 18 as they linger on the vine to 928 as they're stuffed into the pickle jar.

TABLE 10 **Sodium Content of Fresh vs. Processed Vegetables**

	Sodium (milligrams per ½ cup)		
Vegetable	Fresh	Frozen	Canned
Asparagus	1	1	288
Beets	36.5	(NA)	200
Broccoli	8	14	(NA)
Brussels sprouts	8	11	(NA)
Carrots	25.5	(NA)	183
Cauliflower	5.5	9	(NA)
Collards	18	13.5	(NA)
Corn	trace	1	248
Kale	23.5	3.5	(NA)
Lima beans	1	86	292
Mustard greens	12.5	7.5	(NA)
Peas	0.5	50	115
Snap beans	2.5	0.5	282
Spinach	45	53.5	274
Squash, winter	1	1	(NA)
Sweet potatoes	13	(NA)	61
Tomatoes	5	(NA)	156

SOURCES: Adapted from
   Nutritive Value of American Foods in Common Units, Agriculture Handbook No. 456, by Catherine F. Adams (Washington, D.C.: Agricultural Research Service, U.S. Department of Agriculture, 1975).
   "Sodium and Potassium," by George R. Meneely and Harold D. Battarbee, *Nutrition Reviews,* August, 1976.
NOTE: (NA) Information not available.

Soup or salt brine?

Sitting down to a hot, steaming mug of salt brine is a sure way to add to your chances of high blood pressure. Sound unlikely? Soups are one of the richest sources of unwanted salt in the diet. One instant bouillon cube contains nearly a full gram—1,000 milligrams—of sodium. Canned and powdered soup concentrates aren't any better. One package of instant chicken rice soup powder we looked at contained more salt than chicken! People who are accustomed to the homemade variety and happen to fall back on a canned or powdered soup concentrate in an emergency are

TABLE 11   Sodium in Commercial Soups

Soup (prepared according to package directions)	Sodium (milligrams per 1 cup)
Canned	
Onion	1,051
Vegetable beef	1,046
Chicken vegetable	1,034
Minestrone	995
Chicken noodle	979
Tomato	970
Cream of celery	955
Cream of mushroom	955
Clam chowder	938
Chicken with rice	917
Vegetarian vegetable	838
Chicken consomme	722
Dehydrated	
Tomato vegetable with noodles	1,025
Bouillon, from cube	960
Pea, green	796
Onion	689
Chicken rice	622
Chicken noodle	578
Bouillon, from powder	480
Beef noodle	420

SOURCE: Adapted from *Nutritive Value of American Foods in Common Units,* Agriculture Handbook No. 456, by Catherine F. Adams (Washington, D.C.: Agricultural Research Service, U.S. Department of Agriculture, 1975).

often amazed at how salty commercial soups taste in comparison. Table 11 shows the sodium content of some popular varieties. Make your own and cut down salt intake considerably.

Bread and baked goods

Few breads have a distinctly salty taste, yet up to 400 milligrams of sodium in our daily diet come from bread. Most people eat about three slices a day, or the equivalent in muffins and rolls. Although the level of sodium in wheat flour is quite low (a fraction of a percent), most bakery products contain substantially larger amounts from added salt, baking soda and baking powder.

Quick breads (biscuits, muffins, pancakes, waffles and others) contain not only added salt but sodium bicarbonate (baking soda) and either calcium phosphate or sodium phosphate or both (baking powders). Baking powder reacts with baking soda to release bubbles or carbon dioxide gas, which gives bread or batter lightness of grain, texture and volume.

Yeast breads rise due to an enzyme action that produces similar bubbles, but these breads still contain added salt for flavor.

Bread is probably the most relied-upon convenience food. Even those people who love to bake bread don't always have time to supply all their bread needs by home baking. Most major commercial bakers produce some salt-free breads. Finding time to bake some of your own bread, too, can help control the amount of salt that goes into your diet. (See chapter 31, Recipes: Putting It All Together, in Part 4, for some good-tasting salt-free breads.)

Snacks

Snacks, like salted nuts, pretzels, potato chips and such are the most obvious caches for lots of added salt. If you must nibble, unsalted popcorn, sunflower and pumpkin seeds are the best all-around munchies. And if you can't resist nuts, unsalted are the best (see table 12).

TABLE 12 **Sodium in Snack Foods**

Snack	Portion	Sodium (milligrams)
Pretzels, thin twisted	10	1,008
Rye wafers	10	573
Crackers, cheese	10	325
Saltines	10	312
Potato chips, salted	10	up to 200
Peanuts, roasted, salted	¼ cup	150
Ice cream, soft	½ cup	54
Ice cream	½ cup	42
Pumpkin seeds	¼ cup	17
Sunflower seeds	¼ cup	11
Cashews	¼ cup	5
Peanuts, roasted, unsalted	½ cup	3
Popcorn, unsalted	1 cup	trace
Walnuts, English, halved	¼ cup	trace

SOURCE: Adapted from *Nutritive Value of American Foods in Common Units,* Agriculture Handbook No. 456, by Catherine F. Adams (Washington, D.C.: Agricultural Research Service, U.S. Department of Agriculture, 1975).

Condiments

Condiments are where people can easily run into unexpected salt. Mustard, ketchup, mayonnaise, salad dressings, Worcestershire sauce and steak sauce add significant amounts of unwanted salt to food (see table 13). The best way to enjoy them is to make your own. Salt-free recipes for many household condiments also appear in our recipe section.

TABLE 13 Sodium in Condiments

Condiment	Portion	Sodium (milligrams)
Salt	1 teaspoon	2,132
Baking soda	1 teaspoon	1,123
Soy sauce	1 teaspoon	440
Baking powder	1 teaspoon	349
Steak sauce	1 tablespoon	273
Salad dressing, French, commercial	1 tablespoon	219
Worcestershire sauce	1 tablespoon	206
Mustard	1 tablespoon	189
Ketchup	1 tablespoon	156
Pickle relish, sweet	1 tablespoon	107
Kelp powder	1 teaspoon	100
Mayonnaise	1 tablespoon	84

SOURCE: Adapted from *Nutritive Value of American Foods in Common Units,* Agriculture Handbook No. 456, by Catherine F. Adams (Washington, D.C.: Agricultural Research Service, U.S. Department of Agriculture, 1975).

How to Read Food Labels for Hidden Salt

You don't have to be a mathematician to see at a glance that packaged and processed foods can easily add the equivalent of a full teaspoon or more of salt (1,600 to 2,400 milligrams of sodium) to your diet each day. Yet people aren't always aware of factory-added salt.

C. Jane Wyatt, Ph.D., of the department of food science and technology at Oregon State University, interviewed 40 people who had been put on sodium-restricted diets by their doctors. Most knew that snack foods like potato chips and crackers, as well as onion salt, ham and sauerkraut, are high in salt. Many, however, were not aware that several other foods—instant chicken noodle soup mix, ketchup, mustard, fried chicken TV dinner, salad dressings, meat tenderizer, nondairy creamer and gelatin dessert—are also high in sodium. Yet most of them claimed they read labels.

Part of the problem could be the many forms that sodium takes as a food additive, says Dr. Wyatt. Aside from salt itself, some of the most common sodium-containing additives are: sodium citrate, sodium nitrate, sodium benzoate, monosodium glutamate (MSG), sodium ascorbate, sodium caseinate, disodium metabisulfate, and sodium EDTA. Additives collectively referred to as stabilizers, emulsifiers and preservatives are also likely to contain sodium (*Journal of Food Science,* March/April, 1980).

One would think that with sodium so heavily implicated in high blood pressure, a disease more common than cancer and just as deadly, foods would be clearly labeled for sodium content—or contain very little sodium. Not so, however. Only foods intended for use in doctor-ordered diets are low in sodium and tell you so. The rest is guesswork. Low-sodium foods are not only harder to find, they usually cost more as well, which contributes to the erroneous belief that the low-sodium diet is a bland, therapeutic diet for the weak and sickly.

Reading labels helps to a great degree. Avoiding packaged foods whenever possible is better. Table 14 shows the sodium content of several convenience foods, and table 15 shows just how much unwanted sodium can be avoided by choosing wholesome, unprocessed foods.

Salt, the Taste Buster

Adding salt doesn't stop at the factory. Up to a third of our total sodium intake comes from salt added by the cook or the dinner guests.

The cry of many salt-tooths faced with a cutback in table salt—voluntary or doctor-prescribed—is, "But food tastes so bland without salt!" Not so. The food isn't bland, we are. After 30 or 40 years or more of sprinkling salt on everything from soup to nuts—literally—sure, we notice something different. What's happened is that we probably haven't learned to identify food's true flavors over the years because salt has always been there like gangbusters to muscle aside more subtle flavors. Take away the copious amounts of added salt, and the flavors that were there all the time slowly begin to emerge for our gastronomical appreciation.

But not everyone can go off salt cold turkey. Simply begin by holding back on salt at the stove, then tasting food before adding salt at the table. When you do reach for the shaker, go easy. Remember, that's a dinner plate, not an icy sidewalk. Over a few short weeks, most people notice that they need less and less salt to enjoy their food. After three months or so, you probably won't miss salt at all, according to one researcher who observed the comparatively low-salt diets of Eskimos some years ago.

You might want to add a third shaker with an herb combination to the salt and pepper shakers on your table. A sample blend is given in our recipe section (chapter 31).

TABLE 14   **Sodium in Convenience Foods**

Convenience Food	Portion	Sodium (milligrams)
Canned		
Beans and frankfurters	1 cup	1,374
Chili con carne, with beans	1 cup	1,354·
Spaghetti	1 cup	1,220
Shrimp chow mein	1 cup	951
Chicken chow mein	1 cup	924
Macaroni and cheese	1 cup	730
Frozen Dinners		
Fried chicken	11 ounces	1,865
Cheese enchilada	12 ounces	1,856
Fillet of fish	12 ounces	1,822
Salisbury steak	15 ounces	1,810
Veal parmigiana	11 ounces	1,450
Meatloaf	11 ounces	1,380
Beans and frankfurters	11¼ ounces	1,370
Beef stroganoff	9¾ ounces	1,300
Pizza	7 ounces (½ pie)	1,285
Sliced beef	14 ounces	1,220
Lasagna	10½ ounces	1,200
Beef enchilada	12 ounces	1,200
Spaghetti and meatballs	12½ ounces	1,150
Ham	10¼ ounces	1,105
Turkey	11½ ounces	1,060
Linguine	10½ ounces	1,010
Frozen Pot Pies		
Tuna	8 ounces	1,120
Turkey	8 ounces	1,115
Chicken	8 ounces	1,070
Beef	8 ounces	1,040

SOURCE: Information supplied by companies.
Values also adapted from *Nutritive Value of American Foods in Common Units,* Agriculture Handbook No. 456, by Catherine F. Adams (Washington, D.C.: Agricultural Research Service, U.S. Department of Agriculture, 1975).

Fast Foods Add to the Salt Deluge

Stroll into any fast-food restaurant (presumably to use the telephone) and look around. What appears to be a sleet storm behind the counter is an employee salting the french fries. Back in the kitchen, neither hamburgers nor apple turnovers escape the salt wizard's wand. Even the milk shakes have more than their share of salt. Table 16 shows the sodium

TABLE 15 **Comparison of Sodium in Two Meals of Processed vs. Unprocessed Foods**

		Portion	Sodium (milligrams)
Meal I	Corned beef	4 ounces	1,069
	Potatoes, hash brown, frozen	6 ounces	463
	String beans, canned	½ cup	159
	White bread, soft-crumb	1 slice	142
	Butter	1 tablespoon	140
	Peach pie	⅛ pie	316
	Milk, whole	1 cup	122
	TOTAL		2,411
Meal II	Roast beef	4 ounces	65
	Potato, baked	1 medium	3
	String beans, fresh	½ cup	2
	Whole wheat bread, firm-crumb	1 slice	132
	Butter, unsalted	1 tablespoon	1
	Peaches, fresh sliced	½ cup	1
	Milk, whole	1 cup	122
	TOTAL		326

SOURCE: Adapted from *Nutritive Value of American Foods in Common Units*, Agriculture Handbook No. 456, by Catherine F. Adams (Washington, D.C.: Agricultural Research Service, U.S. Department of Agriculture, 1975).

levels of several fast-food items. You may want to review that information the next time you vacation and plan on grabbing a bite to eat "on the road." And if short lunch hours land you there for meals, you may be facing needless dietary salt. Brown bagging it in either case can save you from getting zapped by the salt.

Fast-food restaurants aren't the only places that use salt heavyhandedly. Restaurant cooks in general tend to use anywhere from a pinch to a fistful of salt—and measure with little exactness. As a result, salting tends to be overdone.

As we eat more meals outside the home, we inadvertently take in more sodium. But we may have a bit more control over salt intake in a regular restaurant than in a fast-food place. When ordering your meal, specify "no salt, please." Or call ahead. Some restaurants can arrange it, some cannot. And a special order may mean a slight delay, since portions are often made up ahead of time and simply reheated as the food is ordered.

TABLE 16   Sodium in Fast Foods

	Sodium (milligrams per 1 serving)
Arthur Treacher's Fish & Chips	
Fish Sandwich	836
Chowder	835
Chips	393
Cole Slaw	266
Gino's	
Cheese Hero	739
Cheese Sirloiner	618
Vanilla Milkshake	283
Hot Chocolate	158
Gino's Kentucky Fried Chicken	
Chicken Legs (2)	792
Potato Salad	599
French Fries	134
Dinner Roll	72
Jack In The Box	
Bonus Jack Hamburger	1,171
French Toast Breakfast	1,130
Ranchero Style Omelette	1,098
Super Taco	968
Lemon Turnover	404
Onion Rings	318
Strawberry Shake	268
McDonald's Restaurants	
Quarter Pounder with Cheese	1,209
Hot Cakes with Butter and Syrup	1,071
Egg McMuffin	914
Pork Sausage	464
Cherry Pie	456
Chocolate Shake	329

SOURCE: Information supplied by companies.

Sodium in Our Drinking Water

For every ton of salt added to food, two tons are used to soften water and ten tons are used to de-ice highways. As a result, says the Environmental Protection Agency, "Sodium in drinking water may constitute a significant percentage of the total sodium intake of many Americans" (*Journal of the American Medical Association,* December 7, 1979).

Highway salt sometimes leaches into water supplies and may indirectly add sodium to drinking water. Softeners, however, are added intentionally, to sequester "hard" minerals, calcium and magnesium, making water a more effective cleaning agent and reducing mineral buildup in pipes. There's no question that softeners add a significant amount of sodium to the diet of many Americans. On the average, one cup of softened water contains about 100 milligrams of sodium. One cup of hard water, its natural mineral content untampered with, contains about 5 milligrams of sodium. The amount of sodium in your own water supply, of course, depends on how hard it was to begin with and how much sodium, if any, is added as softener.

If you find that a water softener is absolutely necessary to reduce pipe scale and help soap lather easily, the best bet is to treat only the water used for washing, not for drinking and cooking.

If you have a well or want information on testing your drinking water for sodium, see chapter 26, Hard and Soft Water: The Inside Story.

Should Salt Be Put on Probation?

In 1977, the Senate Select Committee on Nutrition and Human Needs stated that in light of the evidence against sodium as a hypertensive agent, salt consumption should be reduced to a prudent 3 grams a day (about a teaspoon) from the higher average of 10 or 12 grams usually eaten. The Committee's recommendation was one of the long-awaited Dietary Goals of the United States.

In rebuttal, a task force of 14 scientists from the Council for Agricultural Science and Technology (CAST), which represents food corporations and trade associations, said that three grams was far too low and would leave people with only a few tasteless foods to eat.

The Senate Select Committee appeased them by raising its recommendation to 5 grams a day. Senator George McGovern, chairman of the Committee, subsequently stated in a letter to the president of the Salt Institute, a trade association, that the limit, whether 3 grams or 5, was meant to pertain only to salt added at the factory, kitchen stove or dining table, over and above what nature put there in the first place. When the new 5-gram limit is applied to added salt, it still brings the total sodium intake to 8 grams a day, not all that much below the 10 to 12 grams most people usually get anyway. What the new limit did, in effect, was undo the work of the McGovern Committee.

In spite of all that number crunching, the fact remains that high sodium intake can lead to high blood pressure in vulnerable people. Whether we do anything about it is up to us. Read labels, and think twice before reaching for the saltshaker.

CHAPTER

6

Potassium

Too much salt isn't the only factor in hypertension. What also seems to do us in is getting too little potassium.

Our kidneys are geared to flush potassium out of our bodies, because, at least in nature, most foods contain plenty. On the other hand, our bodies are in the habit of hoarding sodium, because natural foods contain so little. Unfortunately, though, modern diets run contrary to the way our kidneys were designed to handle potassium and sodium. A diet high in processed foods and low in fresh fruits and vegetables—the best sources of potassium—feeds us extra, unwanted salt and starves us of potassium—the reverse of what we need. The result, apparently, is showing up as higher rates of hypertension, or high blood pressure, among people in industrialized countries like our own.

Potassium, the Natural High Blood Pressure Preventive

Sodium and potassium are called electrolytes because they carry tiny electrical charges in water. And electrically charged water is the key to cell function.

Cells contain and are surrounded by water—the two water bodies being separated by a thin membrane, which, like a screen with thousands of infinitely small holes, allows water, minerals and wastes to pass through. Potassium is the chief electrolyte inside the cells, while sodium occurs mainly in the outer fluid. The tiny electrical charges carried by potassium on the inside and sodium on the outside form an electrical pump across the cell membrane, providing energy to zap cells into action.

In nerve cells, for example, that electrical charge between potassium and sodium sparks a chain reaction of impulses that carry messages from cells to our brain and back. In muscles, that action stimulates contractions, which enable us to walk, talk, and—most critically—sustain a heartbeat. In glands, tiny charges set off the release of hormones, such as estrogen from ovaries, adrenalin from the adrenal medulla, and so forth. And the electrical pump created by potassium and sodium is the power generator for activities within each cell and organ.

The potassium-sodium pump works in arteries as well as muscles, nerves and glands. There's a certain amount of necessary resistance or "blood pressure" between blood and arteries, presumably influenced by the amount of potassium and sodium present in blood, arteries and the muscles that squeeze and dilate arteries as the heart pumps blood through them. Too much sodium in the diet seems to increase that pressure in many people, making the heart work harder to push blood through. The result is high blood pressure.

Enough potassium, however, may act as a natural high blood pressure preventive, exerting a relaxing influence on the arterial stress caused by extra sodium. In some instances, sodium (salt) restriction alone may lower blood pressure, but extra potassium may lower it further. In a few cases, extra potassium has lowered pressure from high to normal without any restriction of salt intake. The connection between blood pressure and sodium and potassium, apparently, is even stronger than the link between high sodium intake and high blood pressure alone.

Exactly how potassium protects against high blood pressure is not clear. One of the leading scholars of hypertension, Lewis Dahl, M.D., wrote in one of his many studies, "Of all the possibilities, the most appealing to us is that added potassium modifies smooth muscle activity in [the small arteries], the major resistance arteries" (*Journal of Experimental Medicine,* vol. 136, 1972).

Another theory says that potassium increases salt excretion, acting as a natural diuretic to assist the kidneys in flushing excess salt from the body. Herbert Langford, M.D., of the University of Mississippi Medical School at Jackson, feels the amount of potassium we take in may determine to some extent just how much salt we can rinse out of ourselves.

Plenty of Potassium in Plant Foods

Because potassium is a major plant nutrient, many vegetables are good sources of the mineral. And fruits are excellent. Potassium is drawn from the soil by the roots of plants and accumulates in stems, leaves, buds, seeds and fruit. As a nutrient, potassium helps form strong stems and is vital to plant growth. Most importantly, potassium balances nitrogen and phosphorus, two other crucial plant nutrients. Balanced nutrition enables the plant to resist cold, disease and insect attack.

Compost (decayed plant and animal wastes) and rocks (granite and greensand) contain potassium in two forms of potassium chloride, both called potash, and are used as fertilizers to return potassium to the soil. Wood ashes—the major plant source of potash—quickly release potassium into the soil. Hay, straw, shredded bark and tree leaves release potash less quickly, and granite or greensand, pulverized into a fine powder, releases potash very slowly. All are easily absorbed by plants. Mixing plant and rock potash combines long-lasting effects with immediate availability.

A plant that gets plenty of potassium is not only healthy, but tastes better. Fruit trees, particularly apples, need lots of it. There's a good chance that any fruit that tastes watery or lacks sweetness, lacks potassium. And, incidentally, the potassium absorbed by plants can be reintroduced into the soil as the plant decays. Banana peels, orange rinds, cantaloupe skins and pea pods make great fertilizer, although they aren't likely to be on hand in large quantities as are wood ashes or granite dust.

One nutrition professor credits the high-fruit, high-potassium diet for the good health of hunters and gathering people. In a review of the nutritional value of the wide variety of fruits eaten by primitive people, John R. K. Robson, M.D., D.P.H. (doctor of public health), at the Medical University of South Carolina, says that when people left hunting and gathering for farming, the wide variety of foods eaten decreased considerably. Intake of fruits and berries, in particular, was often halved. Dr. Robson concludes, "It may be surmised that the abandonment of wild fruits as a dietary component may be responsible for some of the present-day problems of modern man" (*Journal of Human Nutrition,* February, 1978).

Knowing that fruits and vegetables are the best sources of potassium, heavy reliance on those foods could be part of the reason that vegetarians tend to have low blood pressure. Surveys of vegetarian Seventh-day Adventists and nonvegetarians consistently show that vegetarians have lower blood pressure than average meat-eaters. Bruce Armstrong, Ph.D., and other researchers from the departments of medicine and clinical biochemistry at the University of Western Australia, conclude one such study by saying, "Dietary potassium could be the explanatory variable" (*American Journal of Clinical Nutrition,* December, 1979).

Others are far less tentative when it comes to primitive diets and hypertension. A prominent physician in Britain noted in a letter to the medical journal *Lancet* that hypertension is almost nonexistent among hunting and food gathering people, who eat a high-potassium, low-sodium diet. Hugh Trowell, M.D., scolded the journal for an editorial on salt and hypertension that failed to mention the protective action of potassium.

Food processing is especially hard on potassium, points out Dr. Trowell. "Food preparation today involves not only the addition of salt but also the reduction of potassium by leaching into water during the cooking of vegetables and by the milling and preparation of cereal foods. . . . Whole cereals, all fruits and most vegetables contain 10 to 100 times [more potassium than sodium] and meat and fish contain 2 to 10 times more potassium than sodium. On the other hand, modern diets contain more sodium than potassium" (*Lancet,* July 22, 1978).

Punctuating Dr. Trowell's remarks is a minichart listing seven food items and their sodium and potassium content before and after processing (see table 17). As a result of overprocessing, the ratio of sodium to potassium is too high—about 3:1 or 4:1.

TABLE 17 **Sodium and Potassium in Unprocessed vs. Processed Foods**

Unprocessed Food (100 grams)	Sodium (milligrams)	Potassium (milligrams)	Processed Food (100 grams)	Sodium (milligrams)	Potassium (milligrams)
Flour, whole meal	3	360	White bread	540	100
Pork, uncooked	65	270	Bacon, uncooked	1,400	250
Beef, uncooked	55	280	Beef, corned	950	140
Haddock, uncooked	120	300	Haddock, smoked	790	190
Cabbage, uncooked	7	390	Cabbage, boiled	4	160
Peas, uncooked	1	340	Peas, canned	230	130
Pears, uncooked	2	130	Pears, canned	1	90

SOURCE: Adapted from *McCance and Widdowson's The Composition of Foods,* 4th ed., by A. A. Paul and D. A. T. Southgate (New York: Elsevier/North-Holland Biomedical, 1978).

Unprocessed food provides a ratio of potassium and sodium that's just right for us. "In nature, there is a relatively small amount of sodium in any diet and . . . there is much more potassium than sodium in all natural diets," wrote George R. Meneely, M.D., in one of his pioneer studies of the protective effect of potassium on blood pressure (*American Journal of Cardiology*, October, 1961). Dr. Meneely, a professor of medicine and of physiology and biophysics at the Louisiana State University School of Medicine in Shreveport, has been working on the topic, off and on, since 1950.

"Primitive man ate a high-potassium diet . . . with no more than a gram or so of salt a day," says Dr. Meneely. We eat the reverse.

There's no evidence that our bodies are even beginning to adapt to that reversal. Our kidneys hoard sodium because, historically, we ate much less. Potassium is wasted because our bodies are designed to get more. Nature changes slowly. It would take hundreds of thousands of years of small, subtle evolutionary changes to develop kidneys that treated sodium and potassium in the reverse. With high blood pressure showing up earlier than ever (in children and young adults) and in increasing numbers, we cannot afford to wait. It's impossible to change our kidneys, but quite easy to change our diet.

Dr. Meneely is very outspoken on that point. "Are we then permanently committed to the high sodium–low potassium environment? Can we not devise a strategy to get out of it? It does not seem sensible to continue indefinitely to consume . . . a dietary mix of sodium and potassium that is toxic for many" (*Nutrition Reviews*, August, 1976).

Put Potassium Back in Your Diet

Modern diets hardly come close to the wide variety of fresh fruits and vegetables that were staples for our early ancestors. Supermarket baskets are cornucopias of soda, TV dinners, canned soups and vegetables, doughnuts, refrigerator biscuits, luncheon meats, and other processed foods. Fruits, when purchased, are often disguised as pie fillings, jams, sauces and artificial juice-type drinks.

We seem to have lost altogether the fine skills of hunting and gathering. Years ago, market day was a major event, with whole families riding into town, going from store to store, choosing the best for the household—the freshest greens, the ripest fruit, the greenest peas. Today, the average shopping excursion lasts 30 minutes. Again and again, we're advised to "make a list and stick to it"—an approach directly opposed to our innate urge to hunt and gather, to see, smell and touch a variety of fresh foods, picking what seems best. Often, fresh fruits like apples, oranges and lemons are prechosen for us, packaged in cellophane wrappers. Pictures of vegetables and fruits on canned goods are our only clue as to what they may look like inside.

The first move toward boosting potassium while cutting back on unwanted sodium in our diets is simply to bypass those factory products and seek out the fresh versions. A simple comparison of peas shows what happens when peas leave the pods and head for our table by way of the food processor: sodium goes up while potassium goes down.

TABLE 18 ## Sodium and Potassium in Peas

Peas (one cup)	Sodium (milligrams)	Potassium (milligrams)
Fresh	0.9	380
Frozen	100	160
Canned, drained	230	180

SOURCE: Adapted from "Sodium and Potassium," by George R. Meneely and Harold D. Battarbee, *Nutrition Reviews,* August, 1976.

Many fruit-flavored drinks and carbonated beverages contain little or no natural fruit juice—and little or no potassium. Natural fruit juices, in contrast, contain only traces of sodium and lots of potassium. Real fruit juice is the wiser choice. Don't be fooled by labels that boast a small percentage of real juice. If juice contains, say, 10 percent natural juice, you'd have to drink ten glasses to get the amount of potassium in one glass of the real stuff.

Bring out the bananas . . . and the oranges, tomatoes, cabbage, celery, carrots, grapefruit, apples and beans. Those foods are all brimming with potassium. Blackstrap molasses is practically a potassium supplement, at 585 milligrams per tablespoon. Potatoes, squash, fish, lean meat and brewer's yeast are also good sources. See table 19 for a more complete list of food sources of potassium.

There's no official Recommended Dietary Allowance (RDA) for potassium, but the National Research Council (which recommends the RDAs for many other minerals) suggests that most adults need at least 1,875 milligrams a day. Needs, however, go up as sodium intake goes up, so many people need much more than that, especially if they're prone to hypertension. Athletes or laborers who sweat profusely may need up to 6 grams of potassium a day. People who take diuretic drugs, which flush both sodium and potassium out of the body, should ask their doctor whether or not their prescription is for a potassium-sparing diuretic and, if not, should be sure to include potassium-rich fruit in their diet. Bananas and orange juice are the classic chasers for diuretics, because both are exceptionally high in potassium, but several servings of other potassium-rich foods will also fill the gap.

TABLE 19   Food Sources of Potassium

Food Group	500 milligrams and more	
Dairy products (1 cup unless otherwise stated)		
Meat, Fish, Poultry (4 ounces)	Sardines, drained solids Flounder Salmon, fillet, fresh, cooked	668 664 504
Vegetables, legumes and nuts (½ cup unless otherwise stated)	Potato, 1	782
Fruits	Avocado, ½ Raisins, ½ cup	680 553
Grain products		
Other foods	Blackstrap molasses, 1 tablespoon	585

SOURCE: Adapted from *Nutritive Value of American Foods in Common Units,* Agriculture Handbook No. 456, by Catherine F. Adams (Washington, D.C.: Agricultural Research Service, U.S. Department of Agriculture, 1975).

300-499 milligrams		100-299 milligrams	
Skim milk	355	Cottage cheese, low-fat	
Whole milk	351	(2% fat), ½ cup	109
Buttermilk	343		
Chicken	466		
Cod	460		
Beef liver	431		
Turkey	416		
Round steak, trimmed of fat	398		
Haddock	396		
Pork, trimmed of fat	377		
Leg of lamb, trimmed of fat	365		
Perch	324		
Tuna, drained solids	300		
Squash, winter	473	Spinach, cooked	292
Tomato, raw, 1	444	Carrot, raw, 1	246
Beans	374	Almonds, slivered, ¼ cup	222
Sweet potato, 1	342	Brussels sprouts	212
		Broccoli, cooked	207
		Beets	177
		Asparagus	165
		Cashews, ¼ cup	163
		Peas, fresh, cooked	157
		Mustard greens, cooked	154
		Mushrooms, raw	145
		Celery, 1 stalk	136
		Walnuts, chopped, ¼ cup	135
		Radishes, 5 large	131
		Cauliflower, cooked	129
		Peanut butter, 1 tablespoon	100
Orange juice, 1 cup	496	Orange, 1 medium	263
Banana, 1 medium	440	Pear, 1	219
Apricots, dried, ¼ cup	318	Apple, 1 medium	167
Peach, 1 medium	308	Grapefruit, ½	132
Apricots, fresh, 3	301	Cherries, sweet, 10	129
		Strawberries, ½ cup	122
		Pineapple, ½ cup	113
		Plum	112
		Tangerine, 1 medium	108
		Brown rice, 1 cup	137
		Brewer's yeast, 1 tablespoon	152

Some vegetables rival bananas and orange juice as potassium stars. A baked potato will add a hefty 782 milligrams of potassium to a meal. Just ½ cup of baked butternut squash yields 624 milligrams, and acorn squash does almost as well at 492. Beans, too, have a lot of potassium to offer. Cooked soybeans contain 486 milligrams, and navy beans, just under 400 milligrams.

We don't need to get our total supply of potassium at one meal. It's a good idea to include high-potassium foods throughout the day. Table 19 is arranged in major food groups to help in meal planning. So many foods have good amounts of potassium that looking for them isn't like stalking the wild asparagus. It's easy. Remember, fruits and berries were the convenience foods of hunters and gatherers.

Eat Better, Not More

People may worry that adding foods like potatoes, beans, bananas and raisins to their diet will make them gain weight. That won't happen, however, because we don't have to add *more* food to our diet, but simply be sure that the foods we eat are worthwhile; that is, that they pay for themselves in terms of nutrition. Think plants:

• A handful of raisins instead of honey or sugar on your oatmeal adds over 350 milligrams of potassium at breakfast.

• Pour yourself a cup of tomato juice instead of coffee at break time, for 413 more milligrams.

• Try a banana instead of a doughnut, for 440 milligrams, or a fresh peach instead of a Danish pastry, for over 300 milligrams.

• Half a cantaloupe dressed with a dollop of cottage cheese at lunch will add a hefty 734 milligrams to your daily total of potassium.

• Treat yourself to a tall, refreshing glass of chilled grapefruit juice instead of iced tea or a soft drink in the summertime, for almost 400 milligrams of potassium.

• Reach for a crunchy raw apple instead of gooey apple pie at dinner, for 152 more milligrams at dessert.

Choices like that not only add up to two or three grams of potassium to your daily diet, they reduce sodium by cutting out some processed foods. Planning meals that combine wholesome, unsalted meats, vegetables, salads and potatoes also helps to bring the sodium:potassium ratio back to what nature intended it to be. Plan on chicken instead of frankfurters for the family barbecue (and be careful of those bottled barbecue sauces!). Choose lean meat or broiled fish instead of ham or corned beef, and serve it with squash, baked potato, cauliflower or broccoli. Homemade soups are a good way to combine several potassium-rich vegetables and avoid the unwanted sodium of canned soups. See our recipe section (chapter 31) for tasty *Tomato-Pumpkin Soup, Blender Breakfast* and other potassium-laced dishes.

CHAPTER

7

Zinc

Every August, thousands of youngsters come home from summer camp, their arms and legs painted with blotches of pink, foamy calamine lotion, the badge of a mean brush with poison ivy. Zinc is the healing ingredient in calamine lotion, first used as a balm for skin irritations—like the itchy, weepy rash of poison ivy—by the ancient Egyptians. For centuries since, ointments made with zinc have been used to treat all kinds of skin problems. Now we are seeing that inner health problems, too, can be prevented or helped by zinc.

The Small but Mighty Healing Mineral

We each carry within us just about 2½ grams—about ½ teaspoon—of zinc. Yet you could fill a bookcase with reports on the amazing and versatile powers of zinc that have been discovered over the past few years. Zinc is not only critical to the prevention of rare diseases like acrodermatitis enteropathica and Crohn's disease, but essential for normal growth, wound healing, resistance to infections, healthy prostate function, keen night vision, and sharp senses of taste and smell. Zinc also seems to reduce inflammation, reduce body odor and clear up acne. And the list is likely to grow. More research is being published on zinc than on any other trace mineral. Just two decades ago, however, few people—including doctors and nutritionists—were even aware of zinc and its role in health.

Every part of our bodies contains some zinc, most of which is distributed among muscles and bone. The rest is concentrated in the eyes, male sex organs, blood, skin, liver, kidneys and pancreas. And of the hundreds of enzymes that regulate metabolism in our bodies, 90 require zinc to function.

Deficiencies of zinc are most commonly signaled by weight loss, loss of appetite, listlessness, and rough and scaly skin. Poor night vision, dull sense of taste, or white spots on fingernails may also indicate that zinc is low. Too little zinc retards wound healing. Borderline intakes aren't good enough, either; accidental injury, a burn, surgery or unexpected illness, superimposed on an intake of zinc that's just so-so, sets us up for prolonged recovery.

While it's not entirely clear why zinc deficiency causes what it does, zinc's special role in protein manufacture seems to be one reason for its diversity of power. Such dissimilar processes as night vision, wound healing, growth, immunity, taste perception and prostate function all depend on zinc. Because of zinc's versatility, researchers expect to find other, still unsuspected functions for it.

Zinc Spurs Growth and Sexual Maturity

Zinc is found not only throughout our bodies, but everywhere else in life—in all other animals and plants, down to the tiniest microorganism. It was the discovery of zinc's presence in molds back in 1869, in fact, that gave science the first clue that zinc is essential to growth. Over the years, studies of pigs, chicks, lambs, turkeys and dogs showed that animals deprived of zinc lost their appetite and didn't grow very well. When zinc was restored, they resumed normal growth.

Zinc is critical not only to the growth of pigs and hens, but to people as well. One of the many enzymes dependent on zinc takes part in the activity of DNA, a substance necessary for manufacture of new cells. Without zinc, growth is stunted. By far, the best-known studies of the effect of low zinc on growth in people were done in the early 1960s in Iran and Egypt by Ananda S. Prasad, M.D., Ph.D., and colleagues. Certain young men in those countries had grown up on a diet that consisted almost entirely of unleavened bread and consequently was low in zinc, protein and other nutrients. They also ate clay—an odd habit called geophagia—which added to their nutritional problems. The young men grew just so much on that diet, then stopped. Not only were they exceptionally short for their ages, their sexual organs had never fully developed either. A normal diet and zinc supplements prompted normal growth and sexual maturity in the men within a few months (*Trace Elements in Human Health and Disease,* vol. 1, Academic Press, 1976).

Growth-related problems in this country began to crop up shortly after the two Middle Eastern studies. Not that they didn't exist beforehand, but zinc deficiency low enough to affect growth has long been considered impossible in the United States—until investigators started looking around. Much to their surprise, they discovered that a number of children from middle-income families in Denver who seemed to lag behind their classmates in height also lagged behind them in zinc (*Trace Elements and Iron in Human Metabolism,* Plenum, 1978).

As bones grow, so must skin and muscles. Otherwise, we'd split out of our covering like a butterfly emerging from its cocoon. Zinc is critical to enzymes that synthesize new protein from which skin and muscle, as well as liver, kidney, pancreas and other organs, are made. Stretch marks in the skin of growing adolescents and pregnant women, according to one doctor, are engraved legends of skin expansion with too little zinc. Stretch marks are common not only after growth spurts during adolescence and abdominal expansion of pregnancy, but after intensive body-building by weight lifters or considerable weight gain and subsequent loss of extra pounds in dieters. Carl C. Pfeiffer, M.D., Ph.D., says, "We think . . . that this is a sign of zinc deficiency [in these people]. In other words, they have increased their muscles, and increased their hip size, at a time when zinc was low. This is of interest because all women do not get stretch marks on their abdomen at the time of pregnancy, only some" (*Clinical Applications of Zinc Metabolism,* Charles C Thomas, 1974).

Other doctors say they haven't noticed any zinc-related stretch marks. But then, they haven't been looking for them, either. Zinc's known powers of protein manufacture, compounded by the fact that pregnant women, teenagers and dieters all have higher zinc needs than usual, lend much credence to Dr. Pfeiffer's association between low zinc and stretch marks.

Zinc Rushes in to Heal Wounds and Fight Disease

Wounds are more serious business. Zinc is as critical to growth of new protein around a wound—from an injury, ulcer, burn or surgical incision—as it is to a growing child. Spongy connective tissue in skin and underlying tissues throughout the body are made of a tough, fibrous protein called collagen. When those tissues are damaged, collagen must be repaired quickly. Within hours, zinc rushes to the wound site to rebuild collagen. Zinc is also needed for the release of vitamin A, another nutrient crucial to healing.

Zinc accumulating at a wound site saps it from the rest of our body, however, putting stress on every system. Not much zinc is stored in the body at any one time, and the relatively little that is present in blood, bones, muscles and other organs is not all available for mobilization. The stress of wound healing quickly depletes zinc levels in the body unless supplies are continually restored by diet. Surgical incisions close up cleaner and faster when zinc is plentiful. Bed sores, canker or cold sores and chronic leg ulcers respond well to zinc. The whole body benefits, because other organs aren't forced to sacrifice precious zinc to mend the damaged tissues. If the body runs low on zinc, on the other hand, healing is slowed down and recovery is prolonged.

Zinc serves double duty at the wound site by also fighting infections. While wounds are healing, damaged tissues are especially vulnerable to attack by harmful bacteria, viruses and other disease-producing organisms unless zinc is there to help foil them. By keeping key immunity cells in the blood functioning in top form, zinc boosts our resistance to infection whether we're wounded or not.

A tangle with poison ivy or an overdose of sunbathing elicits a different kind of immune response—inflammation. The familiar warmth, redness, swelling and pain of inflammation are produced when blood vessels dilate to deliver extra protein and fluid to heal irritated tissues. Sunburn and poison ivy are only two of many offending agents that can cause inflammation. Others are disease, bacteria, injury, chemicals or allergens.

Inflammation is a healing process, but it's no picnic. Zinc can speed healing of irritated tissues, thereby reducing the need for inflammation. Applied externally, calamine lotion helps to soothe the discomfort of poison ivy inflammation partly because it contains zinc to heal irritated skin. Many sunburn salves also contain zinc to help restore blistered skin the same way it heals wounds.

Zinc also seems to relieve some cases of inflammatory acne and crippling arthritis, possibly by producing anti-inflammatory effects on the irritated membranes around the affected tissues.

Zinc's knack for tempering those flareups may, in a similar way, prevent some of the gum inflammation of periodontal disease. In an unprecedented report, researchers in Stockholm, Sweden, determined that low zinc could be a big factor not only in gum inflammation, but in the accompanying jawbone deterioration that later leads to wobbly—or lost—teeth. Sticky food plaque that builds up between teeth apparently irritates gums, sparking inflammation. Inflammation breaks down collagen (that tough protein material we mentioned earlier) in gums. And because zinc promotes collagen-reliant healing and soothes inflammation elsewhere in the body, the researchers have good reasons to believe that low zinc contributes to gum disease. Their observations are based on a survey of 51 patients at the School of Dentistry, Karolinska Institute in Stockholm (*Acta Medica Scandinavica,* vol. 207, no. 1, 1980).

Zinc boosts immunity in other, less visible ways. By preventing the body from absorbing lead, a harmful element in automobile exhaust, zinc shields us against pollution. And evidence is accumulating that, in a similar way, zinc can help fight some forms of cancer. By interacting with other nutrients to make animals less susceptible to chemical carcinogens that produce cancer of the throat and lungs, zinc may prevent cancer from taking hold.

Zinc Sharpens Our Senses of Taste, Smell and Sight

Food is such an integral part of life that losing our sense of taste is a real handicap. Days are divided into regular intervals marked by mealtimes. Over the course of our lives, each of us will probably eat more than 80,000 meals and snacks. To meet that task, we're bountifully endowed with about 10,000 taste buds. But without adequate zinc, we might as well have none. Food would slip right past our lips and into our stomachs without giving us so much as a hint of its flavor.

Taste buds are slender cells of a very specialized kind of protein, generously distributed over our tongue, throat and the roof of our mouth. They enable us to distinguish sweet from sour, salty from bitter, and the thousands of subtle combinations of those flavors. As people age, many tend to lose their sense of taste somewhat. Often, they don't realize that their taste is gone. Perhaps they feel they're just getting old and can't enjoy their food as much as when they were younger.

That's pretty hard to swallow, for although some of our taste buds do die off as we age, a supply of 10,000 should serve out a lifetime. The real problem seems to be a deficiency of zinc. While the taste mechanism is complex, zinc seems to be as critical to the protein in taste buds as it is to the protein that heals wounds. As older people eat fewer foods high in zinc—meat, nuts, beans and whole grains—and more refined foods, which are low in zinc, their sense of taste becomes dulled.

Many people, young or old, can trace their loss of appetite—and sometimes loss of smell—to a bout with the flu, a bad cold, pregnancy, or a stint in the hospital. Fighting flu or cold germs quickly drains zinc reserves. Hormonal changes during pregnancy drive zinc needs up. Certain drugs bind with and inactivate zinc, often wiping out our sense of taste—sometimes for months after the drugs have been discontinued. Changes in zinc levels brought on by those situations have been known to either erase sense of taste for months or distort it to the point where meals are no longer enjoyable. Food may taste hopelessly bland, or flavors may simply be "off."

Low zinc may affect odor receptors the same way it withers taste buds, and smell, too, may be affected. Fresh tomatoes, for instance, may smell rotten.

Stripped of discriminating taste by any of those conditions, you could just wait it out. Sooner or later, taste and smell will return to normal. The better alternative would be to restore zinc levels by eating a diet rich in zinc or by taking supplements.

Besides taste and smell, our sense of sight depends on zinc. There may be a kernel of truth to the ancient Egyptian belief that eating ox liver cured night blindness. Liver, like carrots, is an excellent source of vitamin A, which helps us to see better at night. But liver is also an excellent source of zinc, which is needed to release vitamin A from our livers. Some cases of vitamin A-deficient night blindness have been cured by giving zinc.

Then there's zinc's power to sweeten our scent. What gives zinc its deodorant powers remains a mystery, but many people suffering from socially incapacitating perspiration odor are grateful for the success achieved in beating the problem with extra zinc.

When Planning Meals, Think Zinc

Only recently has the attention paid to zinc in nutritional circles caught up to its importance in health. When the Food and Nutrition Board of the National Research Council hammered together its revised version of the U.S. Recommended Dietary Allowances (RDAs) for key vitamins and minerals in 1974, zinc was included for the first time. The recommended amount is 15 milligrams. Double that amount is needed for optimum healing of wounds, fighting infection and inflammation, correcting poor night vision, or restoring lost sense of taste.

Long supposed to be in adequate supply in the American diet, zinc now appears to run low. Thanks largely to overuse of chemical fertilizers, farms in at least 30 states have zinc-deficient soils and plants, the U.S. Department of Agriculture reports. Farmers pour on the nitrogen and phosphates. Plants suck up those major nutrients in large quantities and miss out on needed zinc. Worldwide, zinc deficiency in soil is more widespread than any other mineral deficiency.

Refining robs bread and other grain foods of zinc. "Whiter, softer, smoother and sweeter" make great food ads, but woeful diets. Breads, rolls, cereals, noodles and pastries of refined white flour are outrageously low in zinc, yet serve as a staple in many diets.

Hearty slabs of whole wheat bread were the Parker House rolls and croissants of the masses in earlier days. Until the 1840s, stone mills pulverized whole wheat grain into flour. The entire seed of the wheat kernel, including the outer husk, or bran, the starchy endosperm and the oily germ in the center, went into the flour—along with zinc and other valuable minerals and vitamins. Stone mills were then replaced with iron rollers, which squeezed the grain in such a way that the endosperm popped out of its coating. The zinc-rich germ and fibrous bran layer were discarded. Without the wheat germ and oil, the flour, no longer a soft brown but a barren white, could be stored for longer periods of time without turning rancid. And the new roller-milled flour took less time to grind. White flour greatly pleased millers, bakers and shopkeepers, but swindled the poor, who depended on bread for the mainstay of their diet, out of zinc and other nutrients.

Each year in this country, 5 million tons of wheat are milled into flour. Of that, 1.4 million tons of bran and wheat germ—the most nutritious part—goes to make food for pigs. We get what's left, in airy, springy, lily-white sliced bread and powder puff-like dinner rolls sold in stores—unless we seek out whole wheat.

Rice has undergone similar refinement, also affecting its zinc status. Rice, like wheat in the West, is a staple in the Orient, eaten with breakfast, lunch and dinner. Beginning in Asia toward the end of the 1800s, its drab outer sheath, similar to the germ of wheat, was torn away and discarded during processing, taking much zinc along with it. As this "polished" rice became more popular, serious nutritional deficiencies cropped up among people who depended on rice as a daily staple.

The Japanese had a chance to change that during the Second World War, when rationing led to the distribution of brown or partially milled rice. But many preferred the eye appeal and extra fluffiness of the white variety so much that they rigged up crude home mills to beat out the last vestiges of brown goodness from their wartime rice. Table 20 shows what that kind of treatment, at home or in the factory, does to the zinc content of rice.

TABLE 20 **Zinc in Rice**

Rice (½ cup, cooked)	Zinc (milligrams)
Brown	0.6
White	0.4
Parboiled white	0.3
Precooked white	0.2

SOURCE: Adapted from "Provisional Tables on the Zinc Content of Foods," by Elizabeth W. Murphy, Barbara Wells Willis and Bernice K. Watt, *Journal of the American Dietetic Association*, April, 1975.

Zinc is not among the handful of vitamins and minerals put back into either bread or rice by enrichment at the factory, so assurances from food processors that refined grains are nutritionally as valuable as whole grains ring hollow. People who prefer white bread over whole grain, white rice over brown, and other refined grain products over whole versions are cheating themselves out of zinc.

That worries nutritionists. Leslie M. Klevay, M.D., and fellow researchers at the University of North Dakota, looked at 20 hospital diets as well as diets consumed by the public at large and found that zinc levels averaged 35 percent lower than the minimum RDA of 15 milligrams of zinc. The researchers are convinced that the average diet consumed by most people both in and out of hospitals is quite probably low not only in zinc, but also in copper, another important mineral (*Journal of the American Medical Association,* May 4, 1979). Zinc is lost from the diet as people in industrialized countries adopt white bread, refined cereals and sugared pastries, often at the sacrifice of whole grains, nuts, seeds and other whole foods.

Low intake of zinc can also block absorption of folate, an important B vitamin. Researchers at the University of California at Berkeley have found that among a group of six otherwise healthy men, experimentally decreased zinc levels reduced folate absorption by an average of 53 percent (*Federation Proceedings,* March 1, 1978).

Modern notions that white food connotes nutritional wholesomeness are not only wrong, they lead to serious trouble. Two tribes of Australian aborigines who abandoned their traditional diet of meat, vegetables, fruit, dairy products and whole grains for a diet heavy in white bread, processed cereals and refined sugar soon developed serious health problems, most likely due to low zinc intake, say medical researchers from the Royal Children's Hospital Research Foundation in Australia who studied the effects of that change. Zinc status was further undermined by temperatures that often ran over 100°F for several days in a row, for in hot climates, much zinc can be lost through sweat in addition to that routinely lost through urine and feces. And the soil in those particular areas of Australia is depleted of zinc, contributing to low zinc content of food grown there. In short, conditions were right for widespread zinc deficiency.

As a result of low zinc intake, nearly a third of the infants born died before their second birthday. Children who survived didn't grow as they should have. Immunity among all the tribespeople dropped right off the chart: children and adults alike were prone to infections, viruses and intestinal parasites (*American Journal of Clinical Nutrition,* January, 1980).

Eat Better, Think Zinc

The Royal Children's Hospital researchers are silent on just what should be done to solve those problems among the aborigines. We know, however, that although zinc deficiency may cause endless problems, it can easily be corrected through diet, supplements, or both. Because the main cause of zinc deficiency is not eating enough zinc-containing foods, it is wise to include liver, lean meat and poultry, beans, nuts, seeds and whole grain bread and cereals in the diet (see table 21 for a list of foods rich in zinc).

TABLE 21 Food Sources of Zinc

Food	Portion	Zinc (milligrams)
Beef, lean	4 ounces	7.0
Calf liver	4 ounces	6.9
Beef liver	4 ounces	5.8
Lamb, lean	4 ounces	5.7
Chicken heart	4 ounces	5.4
Turkey, dark meat	4 ounces	5.0
Ground beef, lean	4 ounces	5.0
Chicken liver	4 ounces	3.6
Soybeans	½ cup	3.2
Pumpkin seeds	¼ cup	2.6
Turkey, light meat	4 ounces	2.4
Chicken, dark meat	4 ounces	2.2
Sunflower seeds	¼ cup	2.0
Brazil nuts	¼ cup	1.8
Wheat berries	¼ cup	1.7
Cashews	¼ cup	1.5
Black-eyed peas	½ cup	1.5
Oats, rolled	½ cup	1.4
Tuna fish, drained solids	4 ounces	1.2
Peanuts, roasted	¼ cup	1.2
Fish, white varieties	4 ounces	1.1
Swiss cheese	1 ounce	1.1
Cheddar cheese	1 ounce	1.1
Peas, dried, cooked	½ cup	1.1
Chicken, light meat	4 ounces	1.0
Chick-peas	½ cup	1.0
Lentils	½ cup	1.0
Filberts	¼ cup	1.0
Lima beans, dried, cooked	½ cup	0.9
Wheat germ, toasted	1 tablespoon	0.9
Mozzarella, part skim	1 ounce	0.8
Walnuts	¼ cup	0.8
Muenster cheese	1 ounce	0.8

SOURCES: Adapted from
  "Zinc Content of Selected Foods," by Jeanne H. Freeland and Robert Cousins, *Journal of the American Dietetic Association,* June, 1976.
  "Provisional Tables on the Zinc Content of Foods," by Elizabeth W. Murphy, Barbara Wells Willis and Bernice K. Watt, *Journal of the American Dietetic Association,* April, 1975.
  "Zinc and Copper Content of Seeds and Nuts," by Kenneth G. D. Allen, Leslie M. Klevay and Hugh L. Springer, *Nutrition Reports International,* September, 1977.

Although meat is a rich source of zinc, it also tends to be high in cholesterol and saturated fat, blamed for a high incidence of heart disease. And fatty meats are definitely not for calorie counters. Choose meat wisely. Meat needn't always be a thick chop or sizzling steak. Well-trimmed pot roast or lean ground beef gives just as much zinc for less fat. Bacon, sausages and frankfurters are also too fatty to be considered good food sources of either zinc or protein. Even among our meat-eating ancestors, fatty meats were not a standard diet. Wild game like deer and antelope is leaner than beef or pork. When those were hard to get, hunters were happy to bring home smaller game of rabbits, pigeons or wild turkeys. Chicken and turkey, modern counterparts of those leaner-fleshed animals, are good sources of zinc.

Liver is perhaps the one red meat that should definitely be included in our diet. Liver is an excellent source of not only zinc, but also iron, copper and potassium, making liver truly an antistress, healing and strengthening food. Liver doesn't have to be the tough stringy piece of dinner meat we battled with as children. See our recipe section (chapter 31) for easy, tasty ways to prepare liver.

Other sources of protein also help bolster zinc intake. Oysters are exceptionally high in zinc, but since they're harvested near polluted water and have been blamed for some cases of hepatitis and shellfish poisoning, we don't recommend them. Fish and cheese are good sources of zinc, although they provide less zinc than meat and poultry. Plant foods, too, supply some zinc. Wheat germ added to your cereal in the morning, to yogurt or fruit at lunch, or to meatloaf, rice, casserole or salad can add a few milligrams. Or make wheat germ a main attraction: half a cup of toasted wheat germ mixed with fruit, oats, seeds and milk or yogurt in the morning gets the day off to a fresh, tasty start with ten milligrams of zinc. It makes a great midnight snack, too.

Who Needs Zinc?

Almost everybody. "There's a large number of people in the USA who would benefit from an increased zinc intake," wrote a leading trace mineral researcher, Walter Mertz, M.D. (*Clinical Application of Zinc Metabolism,* Charles C Thomas, 1974). Certain people in particular need to pay special attention to zinc intake. In these cases, food sources alone may not meet requirements, and supplements can take over.

• The aged, the poor and hospital patients are most likely to be low in zinc, according to studies done throughout the country. Absorption and utilization of zinc decreased significantly after age 50. Poor diet, especially one low in protein and high in refined foods, aggravates zinc deficiency.

• Mothers-to-be share a good part of their zinc intake with their unborn babies and need at least 20 milligrams of zinc a day during pregnancy. Nursing mothers need 5 milligrams more than that.

• Growing children and teenagers need zinc for proper growth. A tendency to snack on junk food and soft drinks or to crash diet puts teenagers, especially young women, at special risk.

• Women taking oral contraceptives (birth control pills) may require extra zinc as the result of hormonal changes, similar to those that take place during pregnancy, which increase zinc needs.

• Surgical candidates would do well to boost zinc intake before their operations. People recovering from surgery need zinc even more, to promote fast wound healing and stave off infection. The same goes for any other kind of wound, burn or accidental injury.

• Dieters may fall short on zinc because they often avoid meats, bread, nuts and seeds to cut down on calories. Vegetarians, too, may find that a nonmeat diet does not always give them the zinc they need.

• Runners who load up on carbohydrates at the expense of meat in the diet could be at special risk because of excessive losses of zinc through sweat.

• Blue collar laborers or persons who live in a hot, steamy climate likewise need to replenish the zinc lost through sweat.

• Heavy drinkers suffer zinc losses. Alcohol flushes zinc right out of the system. Cutting back on alcohol and adding extra zinc reverses those losses.

• People beefing up their calcium intake to avoid osteoporosis or other problems also need adequate zinc. Increased calcium increases the need for zinc.

Zinc Supplements Take the Guesswork Out of Diet

Because zinc and protein often go hand in hand in food, eating a fair share of protein may help assure you of zinc intake—but it won't guarantee it. So discovered U.S. Department of Agriculture nutritionists in a study of freely selected diets of 22 people over two-week periods. Although protein intake—from meats, cheeses, and milk—was generally more than adequate, both zinc and copper were low. Sixty-eight percent of the people studied took in less than two-thirds of the RDA of 15 milligrams for zinc. (Deficiencies of zinc and copper often show up together, as we saw in Dr. Klevay's study earlier. The implications of low copper are addressed in the next chapter.) Joanne M. Holden, Wayne R. Wolf, Ph.D., and Walter Mertz, M.D., conclude, "Data from this study suggest that diets which provide adequate levels of . . . protein do not guarantee levels of zinc and copper. Careful attention must be paid to the nutritional density [including the zinc content] of food items selected" (*Journal of the American Dietetic Association,* July, 1979).

Even with a sensible diet, then, it may be difficult to meet zinc requirements, especially under demanding circumstances. Correcting a deficiency doesn't take long, since zinc is absorbed very rapidly after a period of low intake.

Many multivitamin-mineral tablets and antistress formulas contain zinc. As a supplement in itself, zinc in the form of zinc sulfate or zinc acetate is sometimes prescribed by doctors, but zinc gluconate is preferred by most people because it doesn't cause stomach distress as other forms sometimes do.

CHAPTER

8

Copper

Without copper, nerves would fray like worn toaster cords. Copper helps forge the protective myelin sheath around each of the millions of nerve fibers in our bodies. Calm nerves and clear thinking depend on it. Copper also builds proteins that give blood vessel walls the strength and flexibility to accommodate the forceful rivers coursing through our veins and arteries. Copper activates a number of enzymes important to energy metabolism. And copper seems to share some of zinc's anti-inflammatory powers, augmenting that mineral's role in healing. Taste perception, too, may be partially influenced by copper.

Next to iron and zinc, in fact, copper is the most intensely studied of the trace minerals (minerals of which we only require only a tiny amount). And while there is still a lot of unknown about copper, what *is* known is exciting.

Copper Keeps Coronary Arteries Strong and Supple

The heart and its arteries are primary targets of copper action. Copper is the key mineral in a special enzyme, lysyl oxidase, which weaves together the tough, elastic fibers of collagen and elastin, two main connective tissue proteins in the body. A blend of collagen and elastin is particularly useful in tissues like tendons and blood vessels, which must be strong, yet flexible. In the aorta and other main coronary arteries, collagen supports the vessel walls, while elastin—as the name implies—gives them elasticity.

Lysyl oxidase obligingly knits together the fibers of collagen and elastin in cross-link fashion for reinforced strength and resilience. As blood gushes through the vessels, the walls widen and then contract, yielding to changes in blood volume. Without copper, the enzyme gets lazy, and no longer builds up the strong cross-links of elastin and collagen, which soon dissolve and wash away. Weak spots develop in walls. If the blood vessels deteriorate too much, the weaker areas thin out and rupture, spurting blood like water from a split garden hose.

A diet totally devoid of copper would cause hemorrhage severe enough to end life. That's not likely, though. The practical question is, can major blood vessels—particularly the heart's aorta—survive short periods of low copper without serious harm? Or do the patches heal over? Edward D. Harris, Ph.D., a Texas A & M University biochemistry professor, speculates that copper deficiency during the early stages of growth could leave a person more susceptible to damaged blood vessels later on in life. Speaking at the 30th Annual Texas Nutrition Conference in 1975, Dr. Harris said, "It is reasonable to suspect that lysyl oxidase must function continuously in the early development of the aorta. A [short lull] in activity during development could give rise to an adult protein structure with intrinsic weaknesses throughout, much the same as a bricklayer who, in constructing a wall, omits certain bricks, leaving gaps in the wall." Such weak spots, says Dr. Harris, are quite vulnerable to rupture. Later on, such a rupture in the aorta could mean trouble for the heart.

Low copper may add insult to injury by raising blood levels of cholesterol, a waxy fatlike substance which raises the risk of coronary heart disease. Leslie M. Klevay, M.D., working for the Human Nutrition Laboratory set up by the U.S. Department of Agriculture in Grand Forks, North Dakota, purposely to study the effects of trace minerals on health, says, "Consumption by children and adults of diets containing too little copper may further contribute to [high blood cholesterol] and atherosclerosis."

The problem, Dr. Klevay proposes, is a high ratio of zinc to copper—caused by too little copper, he says—and he blames poor food choices for that imbalance. "Many diets in the U.S. and perhaps other industrialized countries contain considerably less than the two milligrams [of copper] thought to be the daily requirement for adults," writes Dr. Klevay (*Lancet,* June 4, 1977). High consumption of processed foods, especially white bread and flour, and low consumption of liver, nuts and legumes, and green vegetables (good food sources of copper) are the norm in industrialized countries, where heart disease is the number one cause of death. Dr. Klevay's theory fits in very well with the other primary risk factors for heart disease: high fat and sugar intake, low dietary fiber and water softness (lack of beneficial minerals), as well as smoking, hypertension and lack of exercise (*Nutrition Reports International,* March, 1975, and *American Journal of Clinical Nutrition,* July, 1975). Dr. Klevay's theory is acknowledged as an impressive observation in nearly every full-scale report on copper, but it remains just a very strong theory until more work is done.

Understanding Copper's Special Quirks

Part of the reason for that kind of gap in research is that scientists cannot intentionally deprive people of copper in order to see what happens to their coronary arteries over the years. So chicks, pigs and other animals whose systems seem to most closely resemble our own have been studied. In those cases, copper deficiency causes not only arterial abnormalities, but bone abnormalities, anemia, and degeneration of the brain, spinal cord and heart muscles as well. Our only direct clues about copper deficiency in humans come from people who suffer low copper as a result of some other medical problem—children with severe malnutrition, hospital patients on long-term intravenous feeding, or those with Menke's syndrome, a fatal, inherited inability to absorb copper.

Deficiency of copper, as is the case with other minerals, almost never occurs alone. Above all, what has become obvious is that copper interacts with other nutrients, often in complex ways. Understanding the most important of those interactions helps nutritionists—and us—know what makes a diet good (or not so good).

Best known is the effect of copper deficiency on iron absorption. Low copper, due either to poor diet or to defects in absorption, interferes with the body's uptake of iron, which is needed for the manufacture of hemoglobin, the oxygen-carrying part of our red blood cells. Without both iron and copper, iron deficiency anemia results. And it won't let up until copper is restored, no matter how much iron is pumped back into the system.

Large, single doses of vitamin C enhance iron absorption and provide other health benefits, but at the same time can interfere with copper absorption. To maximize its benefits while minimizing its effect on copper, the day's vitamin C allowance should be divided into smaller doses taken at several intervals. Of course, it's equally important that the diet doesn't fall short of copper. People taking vitamin C supplements for whatever reason need to pay close attention to the copper sources in their diet, according to Dr. Harris.

Getting Your Fair Share of Copper

Zinc requires an underpinning of adequate copper, like a nutritional alloy for our bodies. While considerable amounts of zinc are lost in sweat, only small amounts of copper leave the body. That is one reason why we need more zinc than copper—15 milligrams compared to just 2 or 3 for copper. But both compete for the same absorption sites in the intestine. If one is exceptionally high, it elbows the other aside. That antagonism between the two has been seen most clearly in people given zinc while on I.V. feeding for several weeks. When zinc levels rise, copper seems to bow out. Restoring copper to normal levels of 2 to 3 milligrams a day is all it takes to compensate for very large doses of zinc—up to 100 milligrams a day in those people. Evidently, intake of copper doesn't have to go up in the same proportion as zinc, says Philip A. Walravens, M.D., of the University of Colorado Health Sciences Center, since the body does have some means of regulating the balance. For people taking extra zinc to speed healing of an injury or surgical incision (or for other reasons), eating a diet that provides at least 2 milligrams of copper will do the trick, Dr. Walravens told us. That is easy to accomplish, as many foods rich in zinc—liver, for instance—are also rich in copper. Others are raisins, nuts, beans and peas (see table 22 for a more complete list).

Drinking water may add a significant amount of copper to our diet, depending on whether it's hard or soft. Soft water may add as much as 1.4 milligrams of copper a day to our intake, assuming we drink about two quarts a day, from copper naturally present in soft water or copper eroded from pipes by more-corrosive soft water, or both. Hard water, on the other hand, adds other good minerals but only as little as 0.05 milligrams or less of copper. To determine just how much copper your water tap is giving you, you may wish to have your water tested for minerals (see section on "Cleaning Up Your Drinking Water" in chapter 25 for suggestions on how to go about it).

It's not impossible, through poor choice of foods, for someone to take in too little copper, especially if he or she lives in a hard water area. While the standard thinking for years has been to assume that everyone is getting plenty of copper, that's changing. The authoritative National Research Council says in *Recommended Dietary Allowances,* "Copper is widely distributed in foods, but the older analytical data reporting a daily intake of two and three milligrams from most diets are being reexamined and questioned. Recent surveys of a variety of diets have indicated much lower intake, often substantially below one milligram a day" (*National Academy of Sciences,* 1980).

One of those surveys was conducted by Dr. Leslie M. Klevay and colleagues as part of their work with the Agricultural Research Service. The researchers studied 20 diets typical of both hospital patients and the public in general, and estimated most to be considerably low in copper. The average daily intake was just 0.76 milligrams—far short of the 2 milligrams required by most adults. Not surprisingly, zinc too was low, though less severely than copper. Drinking water was not taken into consideration (*Journal of the American Medical Association,* May 4, 1979).

"The possibility that diets in the U.S. contain too little copper seems to have escaped general notice," said Dr. Klevay at the Third International Symposium of Trace Element Metabolism in Man and Animals, Germany, 1977.

What's happened here? Our great-great-grandmothers didn't stand before their cast-iron stoves fretting over zinc-copper imbalances while stirring pots of lamb stew or baking loaves of whole grain bread. They didn't have to. After all, they didn't prepare supper by popping TV dinners into the oven, defrosting refrigerator rolls and whipping up gelatin dessert from a box.

Unprocessed foods are rich in copper; refined foods are poor. And that's what makes the so-called rich nations poor. "Dietary intake of copper from prepared foods . . . in industrialized countries is much lower than the RDA values," says Dr. M. Abdulla of the University Hospital in Lund, Sweden (*Lancet,* March 17, 1979).

White flour is one reason. Breads, noodles, muffins and cereals— staples of the diet in developed countries—are, as a rule, made with refined white flour, which has only two-fifths the copper of whole wheat.

Liver is to copper what orange juice is to vitamin C. Yet liver is rarely eaten. Several kinds of fish are rich in copper. So are nuts, beans and peas, mushrooms, avocados and green vegetables. In the diets surveyed by Dr. Klevay, however, those foods were almost nowhere to be found. What people *did* eat were: Swiss steak, sausage, veal and poultry; milk and eggs; white bread, crackers, noodles and cereal; potatoes, other vegetables and fruit; salad dressing, canned soup and turkey gravy; jelly, margarine and butter; pies and pudding; coffee and sugar.

In short, a menu typical of foods eaten by many people every day in this country. And certainly not the "grossly distorted diet" that more conservative nutritional texts say is the only way a copper deficiency can possibly occur. Yet the selections yield very little copper. Because copper deficiencies pave the way for serious health problems, surveys like Dr. Klevay's represent a troll under the bridge for advocates of the Four Food Groups approach to nutrition. Noel W. Solomons, M.D., assistant professor of clinical nutrition at the Massachusetts Institute of Technology, put it in more scholarly terms: "Zinc and copper deficiency states probably represent an under-recognized segment of human nutritional problems both in clinical practice and at the population level" (*American Journal of Clinical Nutrition,* April, 1979).

If you think copper deficiency can only happen to the next person, compare your diet to the above list. Then take a look at foods rich in copper, given in table 22. If you find you tend to eat more of the first diet (especially white flour products, dairy products and desserts) and little of the second, you could be playing a losing game of tag with copper.

Breakfast is a good time to introduce yourself to copper-rich foods. Say goodbye to sticky buns, fried eggs and coffee. Try oatmeal with walnuts and raisins instead.

For lunch, turn to an old favorite, peanut butter on whole wheat bread. (Look for the natural nut spread, without hydrogenated oil, salt, and sugar or corn syrup.)

TABLE 22　Food Sources of Copper

Food	Portion	Copper (micrograms)
Beef liver	4 ounces	3,267
Cashews	¼ cup	760
Sunflower seeds	¼ cup	708
Mushrooms, raw	½ cup	627
Beans, dried	¼ cup	480
Whole wheat flour	½ cup	470
Chicken, dark meat	4 ounces	467
Almonds	¼ cup	436
Barley, raw	¼ cup	410
Pecans	¼ cup	367
Banana	1 medium	350
Walnuts	¼ cup	300
Chicken, light meat	4 ounces	307
Halibut	4 ounces	257
Peanuts	¼ cup	223
Wheat germ, toasted	1 tablespoon	143
Prunes	¼ cup	130
Sesame seeds, unhulled	1 tablespoon	127
Apricots, dried	¼ cup	114
Raisins	¼ cup	80

SOURCES: Adapted from
"Zinc and Copper Content of Seeds and Nuts," by Kenneth G. D. Allen, Leslie M. Klevay and Hugh L. Springer, *Nutrition Reports International,* September, 1977.
"Copper Content of Foods," by Jean T. Pennington and Doris Calloway, *Research,* August, 1973.

Served raw and unsalted, nuts are a superb copper food. But nuts supply large amounts of calories, so they should be eaten in moderation. Add them to a main dish as a stuffing. Garnish a salad or dessert. Use them in meatloaf, soup or granola.

Beans and peas are also good, with fewer calories. Feast on split pea or lentil soup instead of noodle-with-a-hint-of-chicken from the supermarket shelf. And don't pass by lima beans when making baked bean casserole for the Sunday cookout.

If plain liver sounds stark and unattractive, try our delicious *Polynesian Liver,* or *Paté Meatloaf* in the recipe section (chapter 31).

Diet is by far the best way to get our quota of copper. Desiccated liver, a supplemental food rich in iron and zinc, is also a fairly good source of copper. Copper supplements are available, but shouldn't be used as freely as iron and zinc. When intake of copper exceeds 15 milligrams a day, there can be problems: nausea, vomiting, diarrhea and intestinal cramps. And above 5 milligrams a day, there are no particular benefits to extra copper. While the *Recommended Dietary Allowances* says an occasional intake of up to 10 milligrams is safe for adults, both a biochemist and a medical doctor we spoke to agreed that copper-rich foods, like liver, are highly preferable to copper supplements, even if you take zinc in supplement form.

"Remember, the RDA for copper—two or three milligrams a day—is meant to be spread out over a 24-hour period, not dumped into the system all at once," says Dr. Harris, of Texas A & M University. "So diet is the more natural approach."

There is some concern that copper leaching into drinking water from copper plumbing may push copper intake to the other extreme—too much copper taken in over and above what we get from food. Having your water tested is the best way to find out how much you're getting, although actual copper poisoning occurs only under farfetched circumstances. Acidic liquids (vinegar, carbonated soft drinks and citrus juices) stored in copper containers for a long time, although an improbability, can conceivably load the body with unwanted copper—far more than that found in water supplies. Pots should have copper only on the outside—copper cladding, it's called.

CHAPTER

9

Iron

Remember what happened to Superman every time he got near a chunk of kryptonite? He turned pale. Started to go weak in the knees. And most of all, he felt tired. *Really* tired—easily exhausted by the slightest effort. Not at all the way a Man of Steel should feel.

We all know what caused Superman's problems—the kryptonite. But sometimes many of us feel the same way and don't know why. Besides paleness and fatigue, we may also suffer:

> Irritability
> Heartburn
> Dizziness
> Headaches
> Loss of appetite
> Heart palpitations
> Sore tongue

Overall itching
Hair loss
Constipation or flatulence
Diarrhea
Nausea after meals

Not exactly eager to leap tall buildings, in other words.

If any of those problems are your problems, then you might be a victim, not of kryptonite, but of iron deficiency. To feel like the Man of Steel, you need iron. And the Woman of Steel needs even more.

Iron Perks Up Worn-Out Blood

How can lack of just one mineral smother so much zest and leave a legacy of so much discomfort? The answer to that is in the workings of our red blood cells. Hemoglobin, the most essential component of our red blood cells, is a pigmented substance—a protein ("globin") embellished with a special form of iron ("heme"). Hemoglobin is what makes red blood cells red. But most importantly, it's what gets life-sustaining oxygen from point A in our lungs to points B through Z in every cell and tissue in our bodies. Every time we take a breath, oxygen molecules are sucked through the membrane of the lung walls into the microscopic pouches of hemoglobin and whisked off by the bloodstream to nourish all the body cells.

Without iron, however, there would be no hemoglobin, no way to distribute oxygen, and cells would die. A small but still inadequate supply leaves every system of the body gasping for oxygen. Our bodies feel cheated and react in the ways listed above. Symptoms read like an excerpt from a hypochondriac's diary, but the condition is real—iron deficiency anemia.

Milder deficiencies may not be quite so debilitating. Yet a feeling that something's "not quite right," little nagging discomforts, or a shortened attention span can result from even a small lack of iron in our bodies.

What's more, putting more iron into your diet can increase your level of energy even if you have no symptoms whatsoever of iron deficiency. And even if a blood test shows your iron is normal. Because besides its function of delivering oxygen to tissues, iron may also be working in an enzyme inside muscle. Studies have shown that iron improves muscle function independent of anemia (*British Journal of Hematology*, vol. 40, no. 179, 1978).

In one little-known but important study carried out a few years ago in Sweden, scientists studied the effect of iron supplementation on the work capacity of healthy, nonanemic men and women between the ages of 58 and 71. Half were given iron supplements twice daily for a period of three months, and half were given a placebo (a pill containing nothing of value). Their capacity for work was measured throughout the three months using an exercise bicycle, and the performance of the two groups was compared. While the average work performance improved in both groups as a result of regular exercise, the improvement was about *four times greater* in the group taking iron. That in itself is extremely important, because all these people appeared to be perfectly healthy before taking iron. But there's more. Researcher Per Ericsson reported that, "In spite of the fact that there was a significant increase in physical work capacity in the iron-supplemented group, no correlations were found between the increases in physical work capacity and the initial values or changes of other measures of the state of iron nutrition" (*Acta Medica Scandinavica,* vol. 188, 1970).

In other words, despite the astonishing improvement in endurance experienced by the group, blood tests failed to show that hemoglobin levels were going up. It's possible that the extra iron consumed by those older folks in Sweden didn't show up on blood tests because it was hard at work helping to produce energy in muscles.

Why Eve Needs More Iron than Adam

How much iron do we need to keep hemoglobin humming? Or energy levels up to par?

To build up healthy reserves and replace daily losses, men need about 10 milligrams and women about 18 milligrams, according to the Recommended Dietary Allowances (RDA). In both men and women, old iron-carrying red blood cells pass out of the body. Skin, which contains some iron, is shed. Losses through skin, urine and gastrointestinal tract are tiny—about 1 milligram a day.

For most men, diet can easily replace that small loss. But if you're a woman, you could be balancing on a precarious tightrope. First of all, women lose additional iron in blood flow of menstruation. And women eat less; consequently, they take in less iron. That spells double trouble right from the start. And it doesn't take into account special circumstances, like the excessive blood loss of menorrhagia (heavy or prolonged menstrual bleeding), caused by physiological problems or the use of certain intrauterine devices for contraception.

Pregnancy, too, drains maternal iron stores. Most women don't carry enough stored iron or eat enough to see them safely through pregnancy and childbirth.

During the second half of pregnancy, the growing fetus begins to draw larger and larger amounts of iron from the expectant mother every day. During the last few months of pregnancy, a total of about 500 to 700 milligrams of iron is transferred across the placenta to the baby. Most women, however, have only 400 milligrams of iron stored in bone marrow and other body tissues. So, more likely than not, the mother-to-be becomes iron deficient during pregnancy.

During labor and delivery, iron demands are intensified. Not only is a lot of blood lost during childbirth, but the physical exertion of labor demands more oxygen—and more iron. Commenting on that, a general practitioner from Holt, Norfolk, England, Dr. M. Jolliffe, says, "No athlete would expect to sustain optimum performance over 12 minutes, let alone 12 hours, without optimum hemoglobin levels. Are we justified in denying a woman in labor the same benefits of an efficient oxygen transport system?" Dr. Jolliffe adds that he tests pregnant women for adequate iron levels at eight weeks, usually followed by giving supplemental iron in preparation for the feat of endurance ahead (*British Medical Journal,* December 2, 1978).

A footnote to the *Recommended Dietary Allowances* urges pregnant women to supplement their diet with 30 to 60 milligrams of iron a day. Don't stop when the baby arrives, though. It takes at least two or three months of continued supplementation to replenish reserves.

Yet, pregnant or not, women in general are not getting enough iron. Preliminary data from a nationwide survey by the Department of Health, Education and Welfare in 1974 revealed that 95 percent of American women aged 18 to 44—the childbearing years—are getting only a little more than one-half of the RDA for iron (*Ob. Gyn. News,* April 15, 1974).

Part of the reason may be sporadic attempts to lose extra pounds. At one time or another, each of us has probably decided to go on a diet. There comes a point when we decide we want to be slimmer and trimmer—if not for life, then for a special occasion: a fiancé's homecoming, a daughter's wedding, a forthcoming vacation at the beach. And invariably we start out the same way: by eating less. That usually means less meat, especially, and more yogurt, cottage cheese and skim milk. Meat, however, is one of the richest sources of iron; dairy products are not. So without it, dieters lose valuable iron while they lose pounds.

Other conditions also require more iron. Blood lost during surgery—even a messy tooth extraction—can deplete iron in anyone, man or woman. The regular use of aspirin, which tends to cause irritation and bleeding of the stomach lining, can also push needs higher than the RDA. So can a number of common conditions, including hiatal hernia, peptic ulcers, diverticular disease, colitis or hemorrhoids. Antacids, often taken for ulcer distress, indigestion or other stomach upsets, block iron absorption.

Children need iron for growth. At the other end of the life span, absorption of iron may decrease with age, putting the elderly, too, at special risk. Scientists in Britain have found that the surface area of the small intestine available for the absorption of food is greatly reduced with age—a factor, they say, that "could be nutritionally important where the intake of any nutrient is marginal" (*Lancet,* October 14, 1978).

The "tea and toast" syndrome, common among elderly people who live alone, has the same effect on iron intake that dieting does in younger members of the family, only for different reasons. Iron-rich foods, such as meat and green vegetables, are relatively expensive—a factor that may prevent older people on limited incomes from getting enough. Even if income is no problem, eating alone or lack of mobility may prevent some older people from cooking the kind of meals they should. Tea and toast is the easy way out, but leaves older people low in iron—and stamina—further discouraging them from planning and cooking more elaborate meals. It's a vicious circle.

Tea in itself is a culprit. One way to increase iron intake is to cut down on tea. A study done by nutritionist Lena Rossander and two professors of medicine at the University of Göteborg in Sweden clearly illustrates the inhibiting effect of tannic acid in tea on iron absorption. Blood tests showed that, in 129 people eating typical Western-type breakfasts, tea reduced iron absorption by half, while orange juice instead of tea increased iron absorption 2½ times. Yet the actual iron content of the breakfasts varied little (*American Journal of Clinical Nutrition,* December, 1979). More about vitamin C's own special effect on iron follows shortly.

Cutting down on processed foods may revive your iron stores. Phosphate food additives used in soft drinks, ice cream, baked goods, candy, beer and many other products actually cut down on the amount of iron we absorb. So does the preservative EDTA, which is on practically every food label on the grocery shelves.

Processed foods, especially breads and cereals, have much iron removed by refining. Alarmed over the iron famine, the government asked the food industry to please put some back. And food manufacturers obeyed. But they put in the wrong kind of iron. Ferrous iron, the type found in mineral supplements like ferrous sulfate, is most like the iron found in food and is similarly absorbed. But the food industry doesn't use ferrous iron. Instead, it prefers another kind, ferric iron, which is much like the iron in rust—and poorly absorbed by our bodies.

Even if manufacturers could add enough ferric iron to turn muffins into magnets, it wouldn't do us much good. They can't fool our bodies. So when doctors or dietitians tell us that white bread or refined cereal is just as good as whole grain because it's "fortified" or "enriched," we have good reason to be skeptical.

It's not that food manufacturers don't know any better. They purposely shy away from absorbable forms like ferrous iron because, they claim, those types of iron shorten a product's shelf life, discolor white bread with a gray tinge, and ruin the "baking performance" of enriched flour.

Meat and Vitamin C Make the Most of Iron in Food

Fortunately, plenty of other foods supply us with iron, as shown in table 23. Remember Mom telling you to "eat your spinach" when you were a child? Well, if you think spinach has a lot of iron, take a look at liver. Or beef, chicken and fish. Or apricots. And prunes. Raisins. Cooked lima beans and kidney beans. Broccoli. Nuts. And most of all, that super iron supplier, blackstrap molasses. Just one tablespoon of this black gold offers us 3.2 milligrams of iron.

With all that iron around, it may seem odd that it's the most common nutritional deficiency, vitamin or mineral. Much of the iron

TABLE 23 Food Sources of Iron

Food	Portion	Iron (milligrams)
Beef liver	4 ounces	10.0
Roast beef	4 ounces	4.1
Ground beef, lean	4 ounces	4.0
Blackstrap molasses	1 tablespoon	3.2
Lima beans, dried, cooked	½ cup	2.9
Sunflower seeds	¼ cup	2.6
Turkey, dark meat	4 ounces	2.6
Soybeans	½ cup	2.5
Kidney beans, dried	½ cup	2.2
Apricots, dried	¼ cup	1.8
Broccoli, raw	1 stalk	1.7
Spinach, raw, chopped	1 cup	1.7
Almonds, slivered	¼ cup	1.6
Chicken, white meat	4 ounces	1.5
Peas, fresh, cooked	½ cup	1.5
Brewer's yeast	1 tablespoon	1.4
Beet greens, cooked	½ cup	1.4
Turkey, light meat	4 ounces	1.3
Raisins	¼ cup	1.3
Haddock	4 ounces	1.2
Cod	4 ounces	1.2
Prunes	¼ cup	1.1
Endive or escarole, shredded	1 cup	1.0

SOURCE: Adapted from *Nutritive Value of American Foods in Common Units*, Agriculture Handbook No. 456, by Catherine F. Adams (Washington, D.C.: Agricultural Research Service, U.S. Department of Agriculture, 1975).

problem has to do with whether or not it's absorbed. There are two kinds of iron in food: heme iron, which is in the ferrous form (like the heme iron in red blood cells), and is easily absorbed; and nonheme iron, which is not. About a third of the iron in meat is the readily-available heme type; the rest is nonheme. And all of the iron in green vegetables, nuts, dry beans, prunes and raisins is nonheme.

Unlike the heme iron in meat, nonheme iron in those foods needs a little shove to enter our bloodstream. There are two things that coax iron into our blood: a "meat factor" found in beef, poultry and fish (but not in eggs or dairy products), and vitamin C. To do their best work, one or the other should be included with *every* meal. In other words, the vitamin C-rich orange juice drunk by people in the Swedish study mentioned earlier enhanced absorption of iron in their breakfast rolls, but did nothing to enhance the absorption of iron from spinach at dinner.

Popeye would have done well to take a swig of orange juice along with his spinach before coming to loggerheads with his constant foe, Bluto. Scientific studies illustrate that. In one study, the addition of 60 milligrams of vitamin C—the amount in half a cup of orange juice—to a meal of rice more than tripled iron absorption. In another, adding papaya, which is also high in vitamin C, to a meal of corn boosted iron absorption by more than 500 percent!

You don't need a computerized formula to get the same results. To make the most of the nonheme iron in your meal, simply include one of the following *with each meal:*

> 3 ounces of meat, poultry or fish
> or
> 75 milligrams of vitamin C
> or
> 1 to 3 ounces of meat, poultry or fish *plus* 25 to 75 milligrams of vitamin C.

Table 24 lists a few vitamin C-rich foods which, if eaten with meals, improve iron absorption. Including a savory summer tomato salad with your steak, or a hefty serving of broccoli with your roast chicken, could quadruple the amount of iron you absorb from those meats.

In a more subtle, ongoing way, adequate copper in the body makes iron absorption possible. Some cases of iron deficiency don't respond to added iron until low copper levels are also raised to normal. Because liver is a good source of both iron and copper, including liver and other copper-rich foods in the diet also helps iron absorption (see chapter 8, Copper). Outright copper deficiency by itself, however, is rare, due both to its wide occurrence in food and to its presence in water from copper plumbing.

TABLE 24   Food Sources of Vitamin C

Foods providing 75 milligrams or more per serving	Cantaloupe, *½ melon* Orange juice, *1 cup* Peppers, *diced, ½ cup* Strawberries, *1 cup* Grapefruit juice, *1 cup*
Foods providing 25-75 milligrams per serving	Cabbage, cooked, *½ cup* Tomato, *1 large* Tomato juice, *1 cup* Sweet potato, *1 baked* Potato, *1 baked* Broccoli, *chopped, cooked, ½ cup* Brussels sprouts, *½ cup* Cauliflower, *cooked, ½ cup* Collards, *cooked, ½ cup* Mustard greens, *cooked, ½ cup* Spinach, *cooked, ½ cup*

SOURCE: Adapted from *Nutritive Value of American Foods in Common Units,* Agriculture Handbook No. 456, by Catherine F. Adams (Washington, D.C.: Agricultural Research Service, U.S. Department of Agriculture, 1975).

Don't worry that by increasing your absorption of dietary iron, you'll overdose on the mineral. The percentage of iron we absorb from food is regulated by the amount of iron we have stored in our bodies. If reserves are low, we'll absorb more. If we've already got a good supply, then we'll absorb less. Our bodies know how much they need to function best. But it's up to us to provide an ample available supply—and that, as we've mentioned, depends not only on the amount of iron in our diet, but also on the type of iron we eat and the other foods with which it is eaten. See accompanying box, Factors That Influence Iron Absorption.

When iron absorption goes up, hemoglobin levels usually go up, too. Whether our energy level and sense of well-being also go up, or whether we get sick less often, is not as easy to measure. But with survey upon survey showing that iron deficiency is the most common nutritional deficiency, especially among children, women and older people, it's quite likely that more iron means more pep and energy for many, as long as underlying disease has been ruled out.

Eating liver once a week goes a long way toward meeting iron requirements for most people. If you want to be absolutely sure of sailing around the doldrums of an iron deficiency, the best bet is iron supplements. Look for the word "ferrous" on the label. Ferrous compounds contain considerably more absorbable iron than ferric compounds. Two tablets of ferrous gluconate, for example, contain 70 milligrams of iron, of which about 25 milligrams will be utilized by the body. That amounts to more iron than you could get from eating 14 steaks.

Factors That Affect Iron Absorption

Paying special attention to iron enhancers while avoiding the iron inhibitors is the best way to step up iron absorption from the food we eat.

Iron Enhancers	Iron Inhibitors
Vitamin C, eaten with meals	Tea
Heme iron in meat, poultry and fish eaten at meals	Phosphate additives in food
	EDTA, a common food preservative
Adequate dietary copper	Antacids, especially when taken in large quantities
	Advancing age
	Copper deficiency

CHAPTER

10

Selenium

"A catalyst, par excellence."

That's how one scientist describes this trace mineral. Because a whole variety of enzymes depend on selenium to:

- Keep muscles sound and healthy
- Protect cells against harmful oxidation—in much the same way that rust-proofing protects our cars
- Stimulate the manufacture of antibodies, our own natural defense against infection
- Guarantee heart function
- Synthesize protein in both liver and red blood cells
- Activate DNA and RNA—the "code of life" substances in cells
- Link oxygen to hydrogen—key elements in many body compounds

Debunking the Cancer Myth

With all that ability going for it, it's hard to believe that selenium once had the unjustified reputation of not promoting health, but of actually causing harm. Erroneously deemed to be cancer-causing 20 years ago—on the basis of just a handful of flimsy, inaccurate studies—it's taken a landslide of research to bury that myth. What's more, selenium is not only a required nutrient, but it looks like it may even help *prevent* cancer.

Perhaps more than any other mineral, selenium owes its new-found status as a healthful mineral to animal science. Veterinarians in the United States and abroad have known for 20 years or more that cattle and sheep grazing on low-selenium pastures develop lameness and muscular weakness, skin problems and infertility. Young ones fail to grow properly. So selenium supplements are routine items in the country vet's little back bag.

Why People Need Selenium

The idea that selenium-poor diets can cause problems for people is just taking hold, long delayed by the stigma attached to the mineral by those early incorrect reports. But nutritionists who keep up on the latest vitamin and mineral research have tried very hard to clear up the historical confusion about selenium. The job has been an uphill battle at times, because of one main problem: potential toxicity in animals at very high doses. Certain plants are selenium-accumulators—which means they suck inordinately high amounts of selenium from the soil. Normally, accumulators are interspersed with non-accumulators on grazing land, so there's no big problem. Occasionally, though, animals will be let out to graze on pastures covered almost exclusively with selenium-accumulator plants, and they simply get too much selenium. Furthermore, those same accumulator plants are also high in alkaloids, which are also poisonous.

In any case, the problem is rare, and the levels of selenium that do cause problems in livestock range from about two to ten parts per million, or ppm (the common units of measure for substances that occur in very tiny amounts). Some researchers estimate that those levels equal about 2,400 to 3,000 micrograms a day for people, according to the National Academy of Sciences. Everyday nutritional levels for people are estimated to be 50 to 200 micrograms a day, with somewhat larger doses used in some experiments to control cancer, with no apparent ill effects. In any event, neither recommended nutritional nor therapeutic amounts in animals or people approach the toxic level. According to the National Academy of Sciences, there have been no confirmed reports of selenium toxicity from food or food supplements in people.

We can't do without selenium—there's absolutely no question about it. Selenium's essential role in human nutrition became most obvious in New Zealand. Residents there have the second lowest blood selenium levels in the world (next to Finland), reflecting the fact that they live on some of the world's lowest-selenium soil.

Average selenium intake in New Zealand is very low—about 28 micrograms a day. And for years, New Zealanders have been coming down with muscular aches and pains similar to those that plague their selenium-deficient livestock. Plain old horse sense told them that what works for Elsie the Cow may work for Farmer Jones. The New Zealanders' pains disappeared after selenium supplementation.

Much of that was dismissed as merely anecdotal by the scientific community—until doctors started to notice that the same aches and pains showed up in hospital patients artificially fed by total parenteral nutrition (TPN), a formula of protein, calories and water, after surgery. Surgery not only depletes body stores of selenium—already low in New Zealanders—but TPN is totally lacking in selenium. Not only did blood levels of selenium nosedive in those patients, muscles ached torturously.

One case involving a woman particularly illustrates the problem. She "lived in [an area of New Zealand] from where many anecdotal reports were received of improvement in muscular aches by residents after self-medication [with selenium]," explains Marion F. Robinson, Ph.D., one of the world's most eminent authorities on the effects of low-selenium diets. After surgery and TPN, the woman's blood selenium dropped. She suffered muscle aches and pains, tender thighs, and discomfort so aggravated by walking that she became practically immobile.

Aware of the unofficial reports of selenium's relief of muscle aches, Dr. Robinson and her staff supplemented the woman's diet with 100 micrograms of selenium a day, given intravenously. Within a week, the woman was able to walk again without pain.

If that were an isolated case, Dr. Robinson and her staff may have been skeptical. But they mention that in a separate double-blind study, 7 out of 12 people who received 100 micrograms of selenium a day were also relieved of those symptoms under similar circumstances.

"This could be the first clinical report supporting the essential role of selenium in human nutrition," write the investigators. Furthermore, they point out that people who live in areas of low soil selenium, and then undergo surgery or subsist on TPN—or both—are especially likely to develop selenium deficiency severe enough to produce aches and pains. Other factors which may lower selenium status are the stress of injury or infection, blood loss, or even advancing age (*American Journal of Clinical Nutrition,* October, 1979).

In a more recent report Dr. Robinson says, "Selenium is unlikely to have the same dramatic effect in [people] as it has had in animal nutrition and severe deficiencies are not expected. However, marginal deficiencies might have long-term effects that would be hard to detect and [measure] and might be aggravated under conditions of stress in some vulnerable groups" (*American Journal of Clinical Nutrition,* February, 1980).

Fighting Two Major Health Problems

Those long-term effects may include some common forms of cancer and heart disease. Over and above selenium's basic essentiality, evidence is accumulating that this trace mineral may go a long way toward fighting our two most serious health robbers, cancer and heart disease.

Heart Health Tied to Selenium

The lowest selenium content in water, soil and crops is found in Finland. Finland also has the highest heart attack rate in the world. In central and eastern Finland, where the heart disease rate is the highest in the country, blood selenium levels are the lowest. Taking an even closer look, farming families have the lowest selenium levels of all, as well as the highest rates of heart disease. Dietary intake of selenium overall in Finland is about 20 to 30 micrograms—consistently short of the 50 to 200 micrograms a day needed for basic good health.

In the United States, sections of the southeastern coastal plains of Georgia have the highest stroke rate in the country. And it's a low-selenium area (see map). In northwestern Georgia, by contrast, heart disease is lower and blood selenium levels are higher.

Of course, there are many other factors that enter into heart health, but selenium appears to play a key role.

In certain sections of China, low soil selenium means low dietary and body levels of the mineral—and a high rate of Keshan disease, a rare form of heart muscle disease due to unknown causes. Keshan disease strikes during childhood. In areas where selenium is low, Keshan disease is common. In high-selenium areas, Keshan disease is nowhere to be found. Supplementing the diet with selenium in affected areas has practically wiped out Keshan disease in that country.

If and when similar large-scale studies are carried out in low-selenium countries like Finland, selenium may become an officially recognized part of heart disease prevention in other countries.

A Big Role in Cancer Protection

The whole problem of cancer—in animals and more so in humans, is very complex. Cancer grows in stages and at varying rates. There are many types and many possible causes, like the many roads leading to Rome. Selenium may, evidently, block many of those roads.

"Considerable evidence does suggest that selenium is an anticarcinogen," says John A. Milner, Ph.D., professor of food science at the University of Illinois, Urbana-Champaign. National and international data indicate that high selenium consumption and low incidence of cancer go hand in hand. Reporting to colleagues at the Second International

Symposium on Selenium in Biology and Medicine at Texas Tech University in May, 1980, Dr. Milner stated, "Epidemiologically, there's an association between selenium intake and reduced incidence of tumor formation and deaths.

"And apparently, selenium will work against a number of tumors," added Dr. Milner. "In animal experiments, we've seen a significant inhibition of tumor development in transplanted and certain chemically induced tumors." Tumors disappear or subside significantly after the animals are injected with selenium, said Dr. Milner.

What does that mean for people with cancer?

"Selenium certainly has an important enough role to at least be considered as a therapeutic agent. And this work suggests that selenium may have a preventive role in altering one's susceptibility to tumors in the first place," Dr. Milner told the assembly. In other words, selenium has a role in both prevention and treatment of cancer.

Part of selenium's anticancer effect may lie in the way our immune

Selenium Levels in the U.S.

■ Low — most forage and grain contains low levels

▨ Variable — about half the forage and grain contains moderate levels of selenium

☐ Adequate — most forage and grain contains ample selenium

∵ Local areas where selenium accumulator plants contain unusually high amounts of selenium

Parts of the Northwest, southern coastal plains and most of the Northeast are low-selenium areas, as reflected in plant concentrations.

SOURCE: Adapted from *Micronutrients in Agriculture*, 1972, p. 542, by permission of the Soil Science Society of America, Inc., 677 S. Segoe Rd., Madison, WI 53711.

system responds to disease. Both selenium and vitamin E are known to independently stimulate the formation of antibodies, special proteins that act as the body's defense system. Antibodies charge after invading bacteria, viruses and cancer cells (collectively called antigens) like a posse after a band of cattle thieves. Antibodies only win out, however, when properly armed with selenium and vitamin E.

Aiming for the Selenium-Rich Diet

When it comes to diet, some say we get plenty of selenium; others say we get too little. The people at the selenium symposium—scientists in biochemistry, food and nutrition, animal science and various other disciplines—have been studying selenium for years. What worries many are the possible long-range effects on health of undetected, marginally low intakes.

"Whether human food contains enough selenium for optimum health or to minimize certain diseases is still a critical question," said Ingrid Lombeck, Ph.D., of University Children's Hospital in Düsseldorf, West Germany.

Gerhard N. Schrauzer, Ph.D., one of the pioneers of selenium research, is even more doubtful as to just how much selenium Americans are getting. "We hear all the time that as long as we eat a well-balanced diet, we get as much as we possibly need, if not more. That's the official view.

"Yet," he writes, "compared to the average selenium intake in 27 countries surveyed, based on food consumption data, the U.S. placed toward the end of the list" (*Bioinorganic Chemistry*, April, 1978).

The elderly may be the most likely to fall short. "It's not unusual for elderly Americans to consume less than the recommended levels for many nutrients due to poor selection of food or reduced intakes. Such habits could lead to low selenium blood levels," cautioned Victoria J. K. Liu, Ph.D., of the department of food and nutrition, Purdue University, in a report submitted to the selenium symposium in 1980.

Exact values for selenium content of food are hard to compile—content varies depending on the method of analysis and where the food was grown or raised. But in general, certain food groups are known to run consistently high—or low—in selenium.

Fish and Whole Grains
Boost Selenium Intake

If you relish fish, you're probably getting your fair share of selenium. Fish is the richest source of selenium. In one dietary survey, people who ate fish two or three times a week had the highest selenium intake. Those who ate fish once a month or less had the lowest intake. If you've been neglecting fish in your diet, now's the time to make it a leading item on your weekly grocery list.

Fish is closely followed by meat, especially organ meats like liver and kidney. With the exception of processed meats and dairy products, protein foods tend to provide selenium. In one analysis, tuna, salmon and chicken liver showed ample amounts of selenium. Brazil nuts, which are grown on selenium-rich soil in South America also tend to be high. Fruits and vegetables are low.

Whole grain bread and cereals are also excellent—they retain far more selenium than the refined versions. "Removing the germ of the wheat in cereal is less than desirable from a selenium point of view," says Duane E. Ullman, Ph.D., who addressed the symposium on the subject of selenium in the food chain. In another dietary survey, people who had the lowest blood selenium values ate very little fish and whole grain products.

Processed, sugarcoated cereals are also robbed of selenium. Presweetened breakfast cereals contain 40 to 65 percent less selenium than the original grain.

High Fat Equals Low Selenium

High-fat foods tend to be low in selenium. In many respects, in fact, a high-selenium diet—more fish, whole grain foods, less fat—jibes with the well-known Dietary Goals for the U.S. set forth in 1977.

"I think that it's rather interesting that the high-selenium diet comes closer to the dietary goals than a low-selenium diet, particularly in regard to fat intake," says Orville Levander, Ph.D. Dr. Levander is a research chemist with the USDA Human Nutrition Research Center in Beltsville, Maryland. "So it seems as though if you aspire to match these dietary goals for protein (especially fish), more complex carbohydrates and lower total fat intake, you will at the same time help to improve your selenium status."

Selenium supplements are available to help take the guesswork out of intake. About half the scientists at the symposium indicated by a show of hands that they took selenium supplements.

"The wonderful thing about selenium is that a little bit goes a long way," says James E. Oldfield, Ph.D., former chairman of the subcommittee on selenium for the National Academy of Sciences. "I don't take selenium supplements, because I eat a good diet, with plenty of fish. But I know a lot of my colleagues who do take it," he added.

From time to time, Dr. Schrauzer has suggested that the best way to add selenium to the diet is the "combination of a selenium supplement and a high-selenium diet." He recommends from 150 to 200 micrograms of supplemental selenium a day. "The supplement must be of the highest quality," he adds. Selenium yeast fits that description.

CHAPTER

11

Chromium

Glucose is an all-purpose fuel that powers the body. Part of whatever we eat, whether it's bread, rice, or beans, turns into this simple sugar. To keep blood saturation of glucose at the level cells require, the hormone insulin regulates the rate at which glucose is used by the body. Insulin can't do its job, however, without the help of chromium.

Here's what happens: after we eat a meal, insulin is released to direct the traffic of sugar and carbohydrates. Broken down into the simple sugar glucose, carbohydrates are either ushered along to provide immediate energy or told to pull over to a storage cell and await further instruction. That ability of the body to regulate use of glucose is referred to as glucose tolerance.

Unfortunately, if our bodies aren't producing enough insulin or if the effectiveness of insulin is low—as is the case with maturity-onset (adult-onset) diabetes—we don't have sufficient policing action to pull those extra sugar molecules out of the system and tell them to wait their turn. As a result, the sugar molecules all hit the road at the same time and cause a bumper-to-bumper traffic jam in the bloodstream.

Or the opposite can occur: *too much* insulin means sugar molecules are held back from the system entirely. That's called hypoglycemia—literally, low blood sugar. Both diabetes and hypoglycemia involve an inability to properly handle the sugar that's dumped into the bloodstream.

Chromium Fends Off Blood Sugar Problems and Heart Disease

That's where chromium can help. It may help people with low blood sugar—hypoglycemics—and those with too much blood sugar—diabetics—to handle glucose adequately with less insulin. Chromium may, in fact, act as a "normalizer" of some blood sugar problems.

Chromium—not the inorganic kind that boosts the price tag on new cars, but organic chromium in food—is the active ingredient in a substance called GTF: glucose tolerance factor. GTF is a specific combination of chromium, niacin and amino acids. But for all intents and purposes, chromium is GTF.

Chromium goes hand in hand with insulin to keep our glucose levels balanced. Chromium does that, not by increasing the amount of insulin produced, but by latching on to the insulin that is available and making it more effective.

Without sufficient chromium, blood sugar levels bounce up and down like a seesaw. For the diabetic, the long-term results are often more than merely dizzying: kidney disease, stroke, heart attack, gangrene and blindness.

Disturbances of carbohydrate metabolism are characteristic of other disorders. An added bonus from chromium—as combined in the glucose tolerance factor—is its action in reducing high blood levels of cholesterol and triglycerides, fats that accumulate in the arteries and often lead to heart attack or stroke. According to a study first presented to the American College of Cardiology by Finnish researcher Kalevi Pyörälä, high levels of insulin in the blood should be considered a risk factor for heart disease. In a group of 1,040 men between 35 and 64 years of age, high levels of the hormone were associated with a two- to threefold increase in the incidence of heart attacks (*Family Practice News,* June 1, 1979).

The link between chromium, insulin and heart disease helps to explain why the major cause of death among diabetics is heart disease. The connection is summed up by Walter Mertz, M.D., who discovered chromium in 1955, and is chairman of the USDA Human Nutrition Research Center in Beltsville, Maryland. "The most consistent effect of marginal chromium deficiency is elevated insulin response, and the first effect of chromium supplementation is the restoration of a normal response. It appears . . . that if we improve glucose tolerance, restore normal insulin levels and at the same time lower cholesterol levels—particularly [LDL cholesterol—the undesirable cholesterol]—we may reduce risk for cardiovascular disease."

Chromium Needs Go Up As We Get Older

The possibility that chromium may be the missing link in the prevention of maturity-onset diabetes and heart disease in diabetics isn't farfetched. For one thing, body chromium is known to decline with age. That would leave a person more vulnerable to a deficiency during his middle or later years—which is the case in maturity-onset diabetes. In addition, it's been noticed that insulin-dependent diabetics excrete abnormally large quantities of chromium in their urine.

Older folks aren't the only ones at risk. In one study, Richard J. Doisy, Ph.D., then professor of biochemistry at the State University of New York, Upstate Medical Center, tested the effect of chromium on people between the ages of 20 and 25. Interestingly enough, he found that when those healthy young subjects were given a brewer's yeast supplement every day, their bodies didn't have to produce as much insulin in order to keep their blood sugar levels within bounds.

"This could be interpreted that even in 'normal' subjects the dietary intake of chromium or GTF is marginal," Dr. Doisy concluded. "My contention is that probably one-fourth to one-half the people in this nation are deficient in chromium. . . . We have relatively high tissue chromium levels at birth and it's downhill from there on in. And the result for the health of Americans is that millions have maturity-onset diabetes. And millions suffer from vascular [blood vessel] disease," he told us.

Dr. Doisy also told us that pregnant women run a great risk of developing chromium deficiency. "The fetus concentrates [saps] chromium from the mother," Dr. Doisy explained. "That is why the newborn has what I would consider a relatively high chromium level. And it's well known that the number of children borne by a woman predisposes her to an increased chance of becoming diabetic. I think this is nothing more than an induced chromium deficiency by repeated pregnancies."

A Plan for Protection

Because marginally low chromium intake could mean big health problems, the committee on Recommended Dietary Allowances (RDA) of the National Research Council agrees that chromium should have a place on the charts. Estimated adequate and safe intakes for chromium were established in 1977 and advise that to stay in reasonably good health, intake should range from 50 to 200 micrograms a day. (A microgram is one-thousandth of a milligram.)

While exact chromium values are hard to come by—amounts in food vary from analysis to analysis—a general pattern has emerged: the typical American diet is not providing sufficient chromium, partly because of losses of chromium in food, particularly flour and sugar. White bread contains less than one-tenth the chromium of whole wheat bread. Refined white sugar contains less than one-tenth the concentration of chromium in molasses.

That wouldn't be so bad if we didn't eat so much refined flour and sugar. High intake of refined carbohydrates could actually steal chromium from the body. "The high intake of refined carbohydrates requires greater production of insulin," explained Dr. Doisy. Insulin, when it's released, apparently reacts with GTF, and this GTF is transported in the blood to be used by the muscles and fatty tissue and then excreted.

"You tend to increase your chromium excretion when you're eating excessive amounts of carbohydrates," said Dr. Doisy. "And if the diet is not providing sufficient chromium, then you're going to be in negative balance."

For many Americans, day begins with French toast or an English muffin and an eye-opening brew of Brazilian coffee accented with an olé of cream and sugar. Lunch is a little more mundane: a ham sandwich and a couple of cupcakes. And for dinner, nothing less than a juicy pork roast with deep fried potatoes followed by lemon meringue pie.

Sounds dangerously high in sugar and fat. What it *doesn't* contain—chromium—may be even more critical. Sugar added to fat in the diet increases our chromium liabilities. Americans, with their insatiable cravings for Twinkies, Big Macs and Doritos, could be chalking up big chromium losses.

To see if people's chromium intake satisfied the recommended levels—50 to 200 micrograms a day—Dr. Mertz and three colleagues studied 28 selected daily diets divided into low- and high-fat groups. The food was scientifically designed to meet all nutrient and calorie allowances. The 2,800-calorie, 43 percent high-fat diet contained such dishes as spaghetti, French bread, lima beans, an iced cupcake, Jell-O with whipped cream, roast turkey breast, meat loaf, a soft-boiled egg, a corn muffin and whole milk. The other meal plan contained only 25 percent calories from fat.

The typical high-fat diet was found to have less chromium than the lower-fat diets. In the high-fat group, 8 of the 14 diets were at or fell short of the lowest RDA standards. In the low-fat group, only 3 of the 14 diets were below this level.

If the typical diet did so poorly, imagine what feasts of salami sandwiches, potato chips and soda pop could do to chromium levels. "They'd be much worse," warns Dr. Mertz, who advises people to cut back on their fat and sugar consumption and eat more complex carbohydrates. In other words, plenty of whole grains, beans, and fresh fruits and vegetables, instead of processed foods (see table 25).

To insure that you won't be among those with marginal chromium deficiency, here's what you can do.

• Avoid all refined sugar in any form. Throw out all the sodas, cookies, candies, jams and jellies that harbor the white bandit. Sugar is added to virtually all processed foods, so read labels and avoid products containing it.

• Avoid white flour and everything made of it. Use whole wheat bread, wheat germ and other whole wheat products instead. Chromium is found in the greatest amounts in the hulls and coarse outer portions of grains. White bread, for example, offers 14 micrograms of chromium per 100 grams (about three slices). Whole wheat bread contains 49 micrograms— just shy of the 50 micrograms thought to meet minimum daily need for chromium for most of us.

• Eat whole foods—fruits, vegetables, beans, potatoes, rice and corn. Rebecca Riales, Ph.D., a West Virginia nutritionist, advocates "a basic natural diet offering a variety of foods, especially ones rich in complex carbohydrates and fiber."

TABLE 25 **Food Sources of Chromium**

Excellent	Brewer's yeast	
	Liver	
Good	Potatoes with skin	Whole grain bread
	Beef	Cheese
	Fresh vegetables	Chicken legs
Fair	Fresh fruit	
	Chicken breast	
	Fish and seafood	
Poor	Spaghetti, white	Butter
	Corn flakes	Margarine
	Skim milk	Sugar

SOURCE: Adapted from "Mineral Elements: New Perspectives," by Walter Mertz, *Journal of the American Dietetic Association,* September, 1980.

• Add chromium-rich foods to your menus. Fill up your shopping cart with cheeses, spices (especially chili pepper), mushrooms and liver—all rich in chromium.

• Use brewer's yeast creatively. It's a rich dietary source of chromium with high availability. If used imaginatively, brewer's yeast may not only spice up your soups and stews but add extra oomph to your morning cereal and juice.

"Everybody in the country should be supplementing their diets with brewer's yeast," Dr. Doisy told us. He suggests that 10 grams of brewer's yeast would probably be sufficient to meet the daily requirement. That's a little over one tablespoon.

Some companies add chromium to brewer's yeast to boost its level. In that case, it's usually mentioned on the label. According to Richard Anderson, Ph.D., a chromium researcher at the U.S. Department of Agriculture who has done extensive analysis of brewer's yeast, the form that is added is inorganic, but it's absorbed well by most people because most of us can convert the inorganic to the organic, GTF form of chromium.

12

Silicon

Why do people who live in hard water areas have less risk of heart attack than those who drink soft water? And why do some kinds of fiber (like that in alfalfa) reduce the cholesterol level in blood, while others (like cellulose) do not?

Both answers may involve silicon, the second most common element on earth.

The importance of silicon on our roster of protective minerals is not too surprising when we consider that it's found in connective tissues such as cartilage, tendons, blood vessels (including the aorta of the heart) and similar structures throughout the body. Silicon, researchers think, may play an essential role in making all those tissues strong and resilient.

Bones, to begin with, may depend on silicon as a helpmate to calcium in growth. Bone growth involves two processes: adding more calcium for hardness, plus increasing collagen, the tough connective tissue that binds everything together and gives bones flexibility. Silicon helps with both. Edith M. Carlisle, Ph.D., researcher and adjunct professor at the School of Public Health at the University of California, Los Angeles (UCLA), studied growth and metabolism of bones of chicks grown with and without silicon. She found that silicon-supplemented bones showed a 100 percent increase in collagen over low-silicon bones. Silicon-supplemented bones also showed a slow but significant rise in calcium content, while low-silicon bones did not. The net effect was more and faster bone growth in the presence of silicon.

Crucial for a Healthy Heart

Dr. Carlisle feels that silicon's role is not only important in understanding osteoporosis, but may have implications for the soft tissue calcification that often accompanies heart disease.

Studies of human skin and aortas (the heart's main blood vessel) show that as connective tissue in those organs deteriorates with age, some silicon is lost. More important, it's been found that silicon in arterial walls decreases with the development of atherosclerosis (buildup of waxy deposits in the arteries).

With silicon disappearing from artery walls as atherosclerosis creeps in, it seems logical to wonder whether low intake of silicon isn't the problem. Because drinking water and plant fiber are two primary sources of silicon, a number of studies zeroed in on those two factors.

Klaus Schwarz, M.D., who was with the department of biological chemistry at the UCLA School of Medicine for many years, probably did the most to illuminate the connection between silicon and heart disease. In one study, Dr. Schwarz noted the results of a well-known survey of heart disease deaths in Finland. Between 1959 and 1974, men in an area of eastern Finland died of coronary heart disease at a rate twice as high as a group of men in western Finland. The usual risk factors, like smoking and obesity, couldn't explain the difference.

When a team of investigators led by Dr. Schwarz tested the water in the two areas, they made an important discovery: in the area where the risk of heart disease was high, the level of silicon in the water was extremely low. In western Finland, where the death rate was lower, the level of silicon was significantly higher.

Noting that many other studies have shown hard water—which is high in minerals—to protect against heart disease (and that no one had successfully explained why), Dr. Schwarz proposed that the "water factor" (i.e., the element in hard water that seems to help prevent heart disease) "may be related to the amount of silicon supplied by water in different geological environments" (*Lancet,* March 5, 1977).

The hypothesis that silicon helps protect against heart disease fits in well with the observation that in hard water areas fewer people die of heart disease. While other minerals—calcium, magnesium, copper, selenium and chromium—are also given credit for their protective effect, it just might turn out that silicon, too, makes a difference.

The Saving Ingredient in Fiber

Dr. Schwarz's investigations into silicon didn't end with hard water. When he looked closely at dietary fiber, he found the mineral there, too—in amounts that varied significantly.

Many studies have suggested that a high intake of fiber may lower blood cholesterol levels and reduce the risk of heart disease. In particular, a British study followed a group of 337 men for ten years and found that those who consumed the most cereal fiber suffered far less coronary heart disease than those who ate the least: there were 5 cases of heart disease in the first group and 25 in the second (*British Medical Journal,* November 19, 1977).

In less developed countries in Africa, Asia and parts of Europe where meat is scarcer than it is here, people eat the parts of the animal that we throw away, such as cartilage, gristle and skin. And they eat large amounts of plant fiber. All those foods are rich in silicon, and the people who eat them, for the most part, suffer far less atherosclerosis (the underlying disease of heart attacks and stroke) than we do.

But the link between fiber and heart disease isn't simple. Some kinds of fiber, like cellulose, neither lower cholesterol nor decrease heart attack. And tests with bran are contradictory—some studies say that it lowers cholesterol; some suggest that it doesn't.

When Dr. Schwarz analyzed the silicon content of many forms of fiber, he found a revealing pattern. Sources of fiber with the demonstrated ability to prevent atherosclerosis—like alfalfa, rice hulls, pectin and soybean meal—tested high in silicon. Cellulose, which has no protective effect, tested low. And in wheat bran, where the results are uneven, he found uneven amounts of silicon: three different readings from three different samples.

"Since a high silicon content is characteristic of the active products, silicate-silicon may be the crucial ingredient in these materials," Dr. Schwarz concluded (*Lancet,* February 26, 1977).

But does silicon effectively make its way into the bodies of people who eat fiber? Evidently it does. When Thomas Bassler, M.D., of Centinela Hospital, Englewood, California, had hair samples of patients in a cardiac rehabilitation program analyzed, he found well-elevated silicon levels in those on a high-fiber diet. "Silicon is the index of fiber intake," he told us, "the best index of its *quality.*" Dr. Bassler now advises large quantities of fiber for *all* his cardiac patients, he said.

Is the evidence strong enough to justify taking positive steps to get more silicon into your life? As it happens, the possible benefits of silicon simply provide another reason to follow a natural, unprocessed diet. Many plants are naturally high in silicon—largely contained in the fibrous portions. When food is processed, fiber is usually the first to go—and along with it goes silicon. When whole wheat flour is refined, for example, the final product—flour, bread, cereal, muffins and so on—may have less than one-tenth the silicon of the bran that is left behind. So a diet that leans toward whole foods, like fresh fruits, vegetables and whole grains, will be naturally high in silicon (see table 26).

TABLE 26 **Foods High in Fiber**

Food	Portion	Total Fiber (grams)
Prunes	5 medium	8.2
Sweet potato	1 medium	7.2
Apple	1 medium	6.8
Spinach, cooked	½ cup	5.7
Potato	1 medium	5.3
Almonds	¼ cup	5.1
Plums	4 medium	4.6
Kidney beans	½ cup	4.5
White beans	½ cup	4.2
Corn	½ cup	3.9
Peas, fresh	½ cup	3.8
Blackberries	½ cup	3.7
Lentils	½ cup	3.7
Pear	1 medium	3.5
Banana	1 medium	3.2
Pinto beans	½ cup	3.1
Peanuts, chopped	¼ cup	3.0
Orange	1 medium	2.9
Coconut	¼ cup, shredded	2.7
Whole wheat bread	1 slice	2.7
Apricots	4 medium	2.6
Broccoli, cooked	½ cup	2.6
Raisins	¼ cup	2.5
Zucchini	½ cup	2.5
Celery	2 stalks	2.4
Carrots, cooked	½ cup	2.2
Barley	½ cup	2.2
Summer squash	½ cup	2.2
Brussels sprouts	½ cup	1.8
Tangerine	1 medium	1.8

(continued on next page)

TABLE 26 (continued)

Food	Portion	Total Fiber (grams)
String beans	½ cup	1.7
Onions, cooked	½ cup	1.6
Strawberries	½ cup	1.6
Walnuts, chopped	¼ cup	1.6
Beets	½ cup	1.5
Kale, cooked	½ cup	1.4
Lima beans, dried, cooked	½ cup	1.4
Rolled oats	¼ cup	1.4
Tomato	1 medium	1.4
Brown rice	½ cup	1.3
Asparagus, chopped	½ cup	1.2
Cabbage, raw, shredded	½ cup	1.1
Cucumbers, sliced	½ cup	1.1
Peach	1 medium	1.0

SOURCES: Adapted from
"Composition of Foods Commonly Used in Diets for Persons with Diabetes," by James W. Anderson, et al., *Diabetes Care,* September/October, 1978.
McCance and Widdowson's The Composition of Foods, 4th ed., by A. A. Paul and D. A. T. Southgate (New York: Elsevier/North-Holland Biomedical, 1978).

CHAPTER

13

Manganese

Manganese is a lot like the magician who pulls a rabbit out of a hat. No one can quite figure out how it's done. As for manganese, we know what it does—we aren't quite sure how, though. Growth, bone formation, reproduction, muscle coordination, and fat and carbohydrate metabolism all suffer without manganese, but we have only a few clues as to why it's required.

Nerves, Muscles and Enzymes All Need Manganese

Some of those functions seem to rely on the presence of manganese in enzymes that synthesize substances called mucopolysaccharides. Those are simply intermediate forms of the proteins which make up the supportive and connective tissues of the body—muscles, tendons, skin, cartilage and bone. With low manganese, bones bow. Cartilage develops poorly.

Muscle coordination is poor with low manganese. Muscles can do only what nerves tell them to do. To receive those instructions, each muscle contains bundles of tiny nerve fibers which receive messages delivered every thousandth of a second by special couriers called neurotransmitters, or "nerve messengers." With no conscious prodding on our part, neurotransmitters help us to speak, type, tie our shoes, ride a bike, play racquetball or fix a porch screen—anything that requires finely tuned coordination between brain and body. Neurotransmitters also help us keep our balance, so we don't fall down in the middle of the supermarket or while changing a light bulb.

The part of the brain directing all that (the extrapyramidal system) is normally endowed with a rich supply of manganese. Too little manganese results in abnormal muscular movements. Without clear instructions from the brain and nerves, muscles twitch every which way. Or the musculoskeletal system goes limp without warning. Or holds us too unsteady to ride a bike. The precision between mind and body is lost.

Manganese May Hold Promise for Epilepsy

Manganese's special power to modulate neurotransmitter activity holds forth hope for control of certain nerve-muscle disorders.

Low manganese may trigger epilepsy, according to Yukio Tanaka, Ph.D., at St. Mary's Hospital in Montreal, and Claire DuPont, M.D., Ph.D., of the department of biochemistry at Montreal Children's Hospital in Quebec, Canada. Epilepsy is characterized by episodes of uncontrollable muscular convulsions or lapses in mental function or both. Nerve-muscle communication is not quite right. Both manganese and choline (a B vitamin) deficiencies are believed to interfere with nerve cell membrane stability, and that could be responsible for setting off seizures in some people. Raising blood manganese to normal could possibly control the seizures, suggest Drs. Tanaka and DuPont. Their work with epilepsy in people stems from the observation that manganese deficiency results in loss of muscle control in animals, and seizures in rats born to manganese-deficient mothers.

Another neuromuscular disease, tardive dyskinesia, is often caused by tranquilizers, which raise requirements for manganese as well as for choline and another B vitamin, niacin. Doctors believe the uncontrollable twitching of the tongue, lips and jaws in tardive dyskinesia is caused by an imbalance of brain chemicals. Restoring manganese and the B vitamins could restore balance and reduce the symptoms.

Manganese is necessary for the production of prothrombin, a protein that prompts blood to clot when it's supposed to, preventing us from bleeding to death when cut or bruised. Vitamin K is the prominent factor in prothrombin formation and proper clotting. It now appears that manganese, too, has some influence.

Plants Are Storehouses of Manganese

Although there's no established Recommended Dietary Allowance per se for manganese, 2.5 to 5 milligrams are judged to be adequate.

When it comes to manganese, nuts and whole grain cereals are a silo of nutrition. White flour—and foods made from it—are manganese-poor. One study showed that the germ and bran of wheat (the parts usually removed by milling) contain a generous concentration of 160 parts per million (ppm) and 119 ppm respectively. White flour, stripped of germ and bran, contains a scant 5 ppm. Oatmeal, rice, beans and corn are good; so are roots and tubers like sweet potatoes, and greens (spinach, lettuce and kale, for example). Fresh fruits and other vegetables contain moderate amounts. Except for liver, which is high (see table 27), meat, poultry, fish and dairy products are low.

TABLE 27 Food Sources of Manganese

Food	Portion	Manganese (micrograms)
Oatmeal	1 cup	11,868
Rye, whole grain	½ cup	2,607
Whole wheat flour	½ cup	2,580
Peas, dried, cooked	½ cup	1,990
Brown rice, raw	¼ cup	1,850
Banana	1 medium	1,120
Spinach, cooked	½ cup	745
Beans, dried	½ cup	694
Lettuce, shredded	1 cup	682
Sweet potato	1 medium	594
Corn	½ cup	561
Beets, diced	½ cup	489
Liver	4 ounces	443
Kale, cooked	½ cup	325
Snap beans	½ cup	203
Prunes	5 medium	164

SOURCES: Adapted from
   Human Nutrition, by Benjamin T. Burton (New York: McGraw-Hill, 1976).
   Nutritive Value of American Foods in Common Units, Agriculture Handbook No. 456, by Catherine F. Adams (Washington, D.C.: Agricultural Research Service, U.S. Department of Agriculture, 1975).

How much manganese we get depends on what we eat. Most estimates presume that American diets provide between 2.5 and 7 milligrams a day per person. In a study of military personnel eating freely selected cafeteria meals, about 70 percent of the individual daily intakes were below 2.5 milligrams. Those who did best ate manganese-rich foods: cereal and grain products (notably rice and whole wheat bread), baked beans and other legumes.

14

Iodine

Iodine was almost completely forgotten until recently. In the 1920s, iodine was added to salt to prevent goiter—enlargement of the thyroid gland. Not much more was heard about iodine or goiter again until 1972.

Then, two surprising facts popped up. Goiter is once again on the rise in some parts of the United States. The real puzzle is, iodine deficiency—long assumed to be the single major cause of goiter—is absent. That discrepancy leads scientists to believe that some other, as yet unidentified, factors are at work to thwart iodine's uptake and rekindle goiter.

What's more, iodized salt seems to have outlived its useful purpose as a goiter preventive. Although iodine intake is still regarded as the principal guardian against goiter, it's possible that we're actually up to our necks in iodine—even without iodized salt. Drugs and food additives often contain iodine. Dairy equipment is cleaned with solutions that often contain iodine. Many commercial bakers use iodine-containing dough conditioners. As fossil fuels—coal and oil—burn, they give off iodine, some of which we absorb. And tons of iodine are sprayed into the air and onto soil, water and crops when clouds are seeded with silver iodide to induce rainfall. We're living in a world much different from the one that produced iodine-deficiency goiter 75 years ago.

Iodine for a Healthy Thyroid Gland

Just about all the iodine we take in goes to the thyroid gland to manufacture thyroxine, a hormone vital to growth and metabolism. Thyroxine also helps to convert carotene in food to vitamin A, to synthesize body protein, and to absorb carbohydrates needed for energy.

Located in the neck on either side of the windpipe, the two lobes of the thyroid gland trap iodine as it passes through by way of the bloodstream. In the gland, most of the iodine is bound to protein to form thyroxine; the rest is excreted.

The gland releases thyroxine back into the bloodstream as needed to keep metabolism humming along at a proper, smooth speed. Thyroxine is potent stuff. A single shot into the system by the thyroid gland keeps metabolism in good working order for up to six days—provided, that is, that enough iodine is available as the raw material. Thyroxine is 65 percent iodine.

Our body metabolism hustles along at a relatively constant rate—a little faster after meals and during exercise, somewhat slower while we sleep or rest. But normally, there's no great change. Too little iodine reaching the gland means a sluggish thyroid, a drop in thyroxine output, and an idled metabolism: hypothyroidism. The gland swells, forming a goiter, or bulge in the neck, as its cells multiply in size and number in a corporate attempt to compensate for lack of iodine.

The swelling is painless but unpleasant at best, and can block the windpipe, making breathing difficult. In severe cases, the whole body slows down as a result of stalled metabolism. Weight goes up. Skin thickens. Thought and movement become lethargic. Hair falls out. Women, particularly teenagers and young adults, are especially susceptible, for reasons unknown. If a pregnant woman is iodine deficient, her child can be born with cretinism, a form of mental retardation due to hypothyroidism.

Simple goiter can be surgically removed or treated with drugs and iodine supplements. Adding iodine to the diet will probably halt progress of the disease, but won't cure it. Medication is only partially effective. Surgery is tricky because another important gland, the parathyroid, rides piggyback on the thyroid and controls calcium metabolism.

Goiter was the classic deficiency disease at the turn of the century, prevailing in areas far from the ocean, the earth's prime source of iodine.

Where streams, lakes and croplands were wafted with moist, iodine-rich ocean winds, drinking water and vegetables soaked up iodine—and goiter was absent. In areas far removed or shielded from ocean breezes, goiter was common, affecting up to 70 percent of the children—ostensibly due to low iodine.

Adding iodine to the diet to combat goiter became a priority public health measure. Salt was chosen as a means of supplementation because it was cheap and universally used. Not all salt is iodized, however. In the form of potassium iodide, supplementation is done on a voluntary basis. The Food and Drug Administration requires that manufacturers state, one way or the other, whether or not their salt contains iodine.

Iodized salt is credited with reducing goiter to less than 5 percent by the 1950s. Based on iodine's apparent role in prevention of goiter, the National Research Council recommends daily intake of 150 micrograms a day for teenagers and adults. Pregnant women need a little more—175 micrograms a day—to prevent cretinism in newborns. Breastfeeding mothers should have 200 micrograms a day.

We Can Get All the Iodine We Need without Salt

Iodized salt no longer deserves any laurels. Our food supply is assembled from all over the country and the world, where most soil is rich in iodine. So our dietary supply of iodine is more uniform and adequate than it was 75 years ago, regardless of where we live. And now that we know that salt is likely to raise blood pressure in many people, predisposing them to heart attack and stroke, salt can no longer be justified as a desirable avenue for iodine supplementation.

Other foods, notably ocean fish, provide plenty of iodine. Ocean fish have an exceptionally strong tendency to concentrate iodine in their tissues from the iodine-rich sea in which they swim, making haddock, cod, perch, sea bass and so forth excellent sources of iodine. A six-ounce serving of ocean fish alone provides up to 500 micrograms of iodine— more than in a teaspoon of iodized salt, without the attendant 2,000 milligrams of unwanted sodium. That makes fish an ideal source of iodine for people on sodium-restricted diets or those who want to head off high blood pressure.

Iodine in eggs, milk and other dairy products can be considerable—up to 450 micrograms a quart for milk. That varies with whether the animals' feed was supplemented with iodine, whether the cows were given iodized salt or iodine-containing drugs, and whether or not milking machines were cleaned with iodine-containing disinfectants. All that was yet to come in our grandparents' days, when goiter was prevalent.

Bread sometimes contains iodine from dough conditioners and may contain up to 250 micrograms per slice. Frozen vegetables are often prepared in an iodized brine. Some fast foods contain up to 30 times the recommended levels for iodine, according to one study. Next-door neighbors, living in the same iodine-rich or iodine-poor area, may have quite different intakes, then, depending on what they put into their grocery carts and how often they eat at fast-food restaurants.

Table 28 gives averages of iodine content of some foods, including ocean fish—the most reliable food source of iodine.

TABLE 28   Food Sources of Iodine

Food	Iodine (micrograms per 4 ounces unless specified)
Kelp powder	3,400 per 1 teaspoon
Haddock	454
Cod	209
Shrimp	186
Sea perch	106
Halibut	74
Herring	74
Mackerel	53
Sardines	40
Bluefish	37
Sea bass	35

SOURCES: Adapted from
Nutritive Value of American Foods in Common Units, Agriculture Handbook No. 456, by Catherine F. Adams (Washington, D.C.: Agricultural Research Service, U.S. Department of Agriculture, 1975).
Iodine Content of Foods, by Chilean Iodine Educational Bureau (London: Stone House Bishopsgate, 1952).
NOTE: Other seafood, such as salmon, are also good sources of iodine. However, exact values vary or are not available.

Kelp, made from powdered seaweed, is rich in iodine by virtue of the fact that, like ocean fish, it grows in the sea. Kelp also contains various amounts of other minerals and vitamins and is often used as a food seasoning. Sodium in one teaspoon of kelp is only 91 milligrams, compared to a whopping 2,000 for salt. Still, it's not entirely sodium-free, which should be taken into consideration by people on extremely low-sodium diets.

For most people, kelp provides a nutritional way to season food. Some caution is necessary before reaching out to kelp powder or tablets as an iodine supplement, however. One teaspoon of kelp contains 3,400 micrograms of iodine—more than in 2½ pounds of fish—and over ten times our daily recommended level. Most people can handle some excess iodine. Using kelp every day, however, totaled in with other sources, could pose problems for people who are iodine-sensitive. From 1 to 3 percent of the population may react to high levels of iodine taken in over a period of time. Some dermatologists report cases of acne, eczema and other skin reactions brought on or aggravated by too much iodine. Some trace the cause to kelp, others to overindulgence in fast foods. Eliminating one or the other usually solves the problem.

Overzealous use of iodine-rich kelp could also overactivate the thyroid in some people. Most cases of hyperthyroidism stem from inborn errors of metabolism; moderate cases, however, may be aggravated by too much iodine. Should the thyroid become overactive, flooding the system with too much thyroxine, metabolism speeds up like a runaway locomotive.

While too much iodine isn't the cause of most overactive thyroids, people who have reason to believe they have a mildly overactive thyroid should probably stay away from concentrated sources of iodine like kelp.

CHAPTER

15

Cobalt

The Vitamin B_{12} Mineral

Cobalt is the mineral that thinks it's a vitamin—for good reason. Cobalt is an integral part of vitamin B_{12}—so integral, in fact, that the byword for that vitamin is cobalamin: *cobalt* + vit*amin.*

Cobalamin is vital to all body cells, but its effect is most pronounced on healthy growth of red blood cells because they develop at a rate of at least 200 million a minute. In our bone marrow, which is a nursery for erythroblasts (immature red blood cells), cobalamin nurtures young red blood cells into normal, mature erythrocytes. Without cobalamin, red blood cells grow abnormally large, yet incompletely developed, and too few in number, resulting in a condition called pernicious anemia. Milder symptoms are paleness, fatigue, diarrhea, heart palpitations, and numbness in fingers and toes. Untreated, pernicious anemia can be fatal.

Until 1926, pernicious anemia was *always* fatal, its cause unknown and no cure in sight. The discovery of a cure teaches us a few main points about food sources of cobalamin and why it's essential to healthy blood and nerves.

Researchers discovered that pernicious anemia could be cured if a patient was fed ¾ pound of raw liver a day—a cure about as delightful as the disease itself. Some special substance in the liver (called extrinsic or animal protein factor) seemed to combine with something equally special in gastric juice of the stomach (called intrinsic factor) to restore orderly growth of red blood cells and cure the disease. As it turned out, after another 20 years of research, the first substance was found to be cobalamin. The second was a normal part of gastric juice that prompts absorption of cobalamin and is lacking in people with pernicious anemia. The reason liver worked is that in high enough amounts (1,000 times what is normally required), enough cobalamin eventually trickles through to overcome the absence of the intrinsic factor in susceptible people.

Previously, cobalt in any form was thought to be essential only to sheep and cattle, but not to people. Plants have some cobalt, but don't need it in vitamin form and don't make cobalamin. Animals need cobalamin to grow and survive, but can't manufacture it themselves. Instead, stomachs of healthy animals serve as internal fermentation vats in which bacteria convert the cobalt obtained from plants into cobalamin, and turn the vitamin over to their hosts. From the stomach, cobalamin is absorbed and finds its way into organs, muscles, milk (and sometimes eggs) of the animal.

Bacteria in the digestive tracts of people also change cobalt into cobalamin. By some trick of nature, however, the transformation takes place so far down in the colon (the tail end of the intestine) that it's generally believed cobalamin passes out of the system without being absorbed. So animal proteins—liver, other organ meats, muscle meats and dairy products—are the most reliable dietary sources for people.

Under the influence of gastric juice in our stomachs, cobalamin is primed for active duty by many nutrients, including niacin and riboflavin (two B vitamins) and manganese, another mineral. As food passes through the digestive tract, gastric acid releases cobalamin from tight protein bonds in food and ushers it to receptor sites in the intestine. (That action, incidentally, is helped along by calcium.)

Failure at any stage along the way can render even the best dietary cobalamin unavailable. A severe deficiency is most often the result of poor absorption rather than poor diet. Lack of intrinsic factor in gastric acid completely blocks uptake of the nutrient, as in pernicious anemia. Efficiency of absorption also goes down as we age, and when intake of vitamin B_6 (pyridoxine) or iron is low.

Once absorbed into the bloodstream, cobalamin circulates to various tissues. We've already shown what happens to red blood cells without it. The numbness and tingling in fingers and toes in pernicious anemia reflects the role of cobalamin in a healthy nervous system as well. The mineral-turned-vitamin keeps glutathione, an essential part of several enzymes involved in carbohydrate metabolism, biologically active. Because the nervous system relies almost entirely on carbohydrates as fuel, anything that disrupts carbohydrate metabolism cuts off the energy supply to the brain, spinal cord and nerves. When cobalamin is low or poorly absorbed, nerves are deprived of energy, and the result is a sensory motor system that's kaput. Skin tingles. Gait is unsteady. The mind starts to lose its sharpness. If the condition drags out for months or years, damage to the brain is irreversible.

Cobalamin may help metabolize proteins and essential fats vital to healthy nerve fibers. Myelin, the protective sheath of protein and fat that coats nerve fibers, wears thin in cases of cobalamin deficiency.

Cobalamin is also necessary for the metabolism of folic acid, another B vitamin, which teams up with it to prevent pernicious anemia.

Red-Blooded Vegetarians Need Cobalt

Because the body tends to hoard cobalamin, deficiencies take a long time, often years, to develop. The body jealously guards what precious cobalamin it takes in, stocking its larder for times when animal protein is out of range of the spear, rifle or pocketbook. Beyond what is needed for immediate feeding of nerves and blood cells, excess cobalamin is stored in the liver. Uptake of cobalamin by the liver is facilitated by vitamin C. The average amount of cobalamin stored is 2 milligrams (2,000 micrograms)— enough to last about six years.

We need a small amount of cobalamin—3 micrograms a day—to keep nerves running smoothly and red blood cells healthy. Most people eating meat or dairy products take in from 7 to 30 micrograms a day. Liver is the richest source, reflecting the fact that in animals, as in people, that organ is the main storehouse of the nutrient. Kidney, lean beef, lamb, veal, poultry, ocean fish, milk, cheese and eggs are also good sources (see table 29 for some representative values).

Some vegetarian foods acted on by bacteria or fungi seem to contain some cobalamin, the result of a fermentation process similar to what takes place in an animal's stomach. While there's some question as to just how reliable those sources may be, they may explain why pernicious anemia is not as high as expected among vegans—vegetarians who eat no animal products at all. Tempeh, a fermented soybean food originating in Indonesia, is eaten by many vegans, as well as other people, in North America. Soy sauce may also provide some cobalamin. Nutritional supplements containing cobalamin (vitamin B_{12}) seem to be the most reliable way to add cobalamin to a strict vegetarian diet.

TABLE 29 **Food Sources of Cobalamin (Vitamin B₁₂)**

Food	Portion	Cobalamin (micrograms)
Beef liver	4 ounces	124.7
Lamb	4 ounces	3.4
Beef, lean	4 ounces	2.6
Tuna, drained solids	4 ounces	2.4
Haddock	4 ounces	1.8
Egg	1 large	1.1
Swiss cheese	2 ounces	1.0
Milk, whole	1 cup	0.9
Cottage cheese	½ cup	0.7
Chicken, light meat	4 ounces	0.5
Cheddar cheese	2 ounces	0.4
Yogurt	1 cup	0.2

SOURCE: Adapted from *Pantothenic Acid, Vitamin B₆ and Vitamin B₁₂ in Foods,* Home Economics Research Report No. 36, by Martha Louise Orr (Washington, D.C.: Agricultural Research Service, U.S. Department of Agriculture, 1969).

Whether vegans can do without animal foods and escape pernicious anemia is a sensitive subject. Some vegans argue that in countries where people are strict vegetarians, usually for religious reasons, whole populations have shunned animal foods for generations without suffering symptoms of severe nutritional deficiency. Among the largely vegetarian population of India, pernicious anemia is uncommon. One possible reason, however, is that the water is slightly contaminated with vitamin B_{12}-containing animal wastes, supplying the diet with cobalamin. In this country, many vegans take some sort of B_{12} supplement just to be sure.

Compounding the issue is the fact that some meat-eaters get pernicious anemia and many vegans don't. But the fact remains that children born to vegan mothers in this country who don't choose a careful diet and who feed their newborns breast milk alone, have shown up with pernicious anemia. Children are particularly vulnerable, perhaps because they lack the savings account of cobalamin in adults who switch from meat to vegetable proteins. The result in such children may be irreversible brain damage or poor growth and mental development. Keeping that in mind, vegans — especially vegan mothers of young children — would be wise to include either a high-vitamin B_{12} yeast or B complex supplement in their daily diet.

16

Fluorine

In 1902, a dentist in Colorado Springs noticed that many of his patients who had no cavities also had a curious brown stain on their teeth. The cause of the brown mottling—and perhaps of the cavity protection— turned out to be an excess of fluorine in their drinking water. Communities with too little fluorine in their water considered adding some in order to reduce tooth decay. And the rest, as they say, is history.

Fluorine and Our Teeth

To understand the present controversy behind community fluori- dation programs, we first must recognize exactly what fluorine does for the health of our teeth and bones. For the most part, teeth are composed of fine masonry work of calcium crystals called hydroxyapatite. When fluorine is plentiful, it substitutes for some of the calcium, forming larger, more perfect crystals of fluoroapatite. Those fluorine-rich crystals are more resistant to the strong acids in saliva that, along with digesting

140

our food, eat away at teeth and form cavities. Even small differences in the pH (level of acidity) in the mouth influence the extent to which enamel dissolves. It doesn't take much fluorine to reduce cavities.

Fluorine in saliva is absorbed directly by the teeth, adding strength and rigidity. In addition, it seems that fluorine draws calcium phosphate from the saliva and may enhance renewal of tooth structure once decay has begun. So fluorine acts as a preventive as well as a repair mechanism.

On a larger scale, fluorine adds to the strength and rigidity given bones by calcium. And as an added bonus, fluorine has been shown to protect against the overall effects of magnesium deficiency.

Our average intake of fluorine from food ranges from 1.3 to 1.8 milligrams a day. Table 30 shows the fluorine content of many foods. Tea is an exceptionally high source of fluorine, but, like coffee, acts as a stimulant

TABLE 30   Food Sources of Fluorine

Food	Portion	Fluorine (micrograms)
Mackerel	4 ounces	3,062
Sardines, canned	4 ounces	828–1,814
Mackerel, canned	4 ounces	1,361
Salmon, canned	4 ounces	510–1,021
Potato	1 medium	11–960
Cod	4 ounces	794
Shrimp, canned	4 ounces	454
Crab meat, canned	4 ounces	227
Beef	4 ounces	33–227
Apple	1 medium	8–195
Kale, cooked	½ cup	9–165
Spinach, cooked	½ cup	18–162
Chicken	4 ounces	159
Round steak	4 ounces	147
Milk, whole	1 cup	25–134
Soybeans	½ cup	117
Beef liver	4 ounces	112
Wheat germ, toasted	¼ cup	21–96
Egg	1 large	68
Grapefruit	½	66
Oatmeal	1 cup	60
Brown rice, raw	¼ cup	55
Corn	½ cup	51

SOURCES: Adapted from
    Nutritive Value of American Foods in Common Units, Agriculture Handbook No. 456, by Catherine F. Adams (Washington, D.C.: Agricultural Research Service, U.S. Department of Agriculture, 1975).
    Human Nutrition, by Benjamin T. Burton (New York: McGraw-Hill, 1976).

and for that reason is not an acceptable source of fluorine, especially for children. Fish, on the other hand, is an excellent source.

Fluoridation of drinking water adds from 0.4 to 1.1 milligrams to daily intake of fluorine by children and from 1.0 to 1.5 milligrams to that by adults, over and above what's in food. All water contains some fluorine naturally: how much varies from area to area. The rate of tooth decay in various communities was measured after the findings in Colorado Springs. In areas where the water supply contained one part per million (ppm) or more of fluorine (about one milligram per quart), children had 50 to 60 percent fewer dental cavities than children in low-fluorine areas. As a public health measure, many states have since required that communities of 20,000 or more in low-fluorine areas meet the one ppm level by adding fluoride (a compound of fluorine) to the drinking water.

Should the fluorine content of the water unintentionally reach 2.5 ppm, the unsightly brown mottling of teeth (fluorosis) seen in Colorado Springs will show up—a result of too much fluorine. At 8 to 20 ppm, osteosclerosis, or excess buildup of fluorine in teeth and bones, with abnormal hardening of soft tissues, can develop. The back is most likely to be affected. Spinal vertebrae may fuse, making it difficult to walk. High levels of fluorine interfere with formation of collagen, the body's connective tissue. At 50 ppm, growth is depressed, and at 2,500 times recommended levels (an unlikely concentration in water), poisoning is fatal.

But even at one ppm of fluorine added to drinking water, there can be problems. George L. Waldbott, M.D., a clinician in Warren, Michigan, reports the following incidents:

A 40-year-old woman suffered painful spastic bowels, nausea, vomiting, bloating of the abdomen, frequent urination and headaches. Strangely, when away from the city her condition improved, only to recur upon her return. She was not aware that fluoride was being added to her water.

A 35-year-old woman suffered more severe symptoms, to the point where she became incoherent, drowsy and forgetful. Urine tests showed high levels of fluoride. Within two days after she began using nonfluoridated water, says the author, her symptoms began to clear up. She recovered completely after avoiding fluoridated water for drinking and cooking.

A 13-year-old girl with stomach upset and loss of mental alertness was suspected of having a brain tumor. The symptoms showed up only on Mondays and Thursdays, however—when she quenched her thirst with a long drink of fluoridated water after gym class. Symptoms cleared up completely when she switched to drinking distilled water only.

Thirty people in Saginaw, Michigan, came down with an unusual illness. Nine cases resembled that of the 35-year-old woman above; the others had stomach upsets and bladder problems. Most were unaware that they were drinking fluoridated water at the time. Their troubles gradually cleared up when fluoridation was discontinued.

Those cases highlight Dr. Waldbott's experience with chronic, nonskeletal effects of artificially fluoridated water—and prompt him to raise some important questions.

"During recent decades the great expansion of the use of fluoride, especially in the smelting, glass, enamel, oil, and numerous other industries, has paralleled its increase in our daily diet, in our water supplies, and in the air we breathe. Would it not be desirable, therefore, to explore to what extent this highly reactive ion present in everybody's bloodstream contributes in a given population to the [development] of certain kinds of arthritis, gastritis, colitis, lower urinary tract disease, chronic headache, and other neurologic symptoms which in the past have defied a satisfactory explanation?" (*Southern Medical Journal*, March, 1980).

The possible hazards of fluoridation raise questions about its desirability. As a result, some communities have rejected fluoridation. Advocates of fluoridation insist that the health risks are small compared to the gains, and that our kidneys are able to remove excess fluorine, flushing it out before harm is done. Critics aren't so confident. In addition to possible health hazards, many question the ethical considerations of what amounts to compulsory medication, especially when other channels are open—methods that leave individual families free to choose how they get their fluorine.

Fluoride tablets are available for people whose water isn't hooked up to a community supply or who live in an unfluoridated area. Couldn't tablets be used by people in all low-fluorine areas, if they so chose?

Prevention of tooth decay is especially important in children, and many infant vitamin supplements have fluoride added. (In areas where water is fluoridated, sale is by prescription only.) Couldn't parents take the responsibility of seeing that their children are getting enough fluoride, in water or tablets, as part of a family dental plan? Critics say parents won't follow through, and that people with low incomes don't always have a regular dental program. Tablets run the risk of overdose, a serious potential problem, they add.

Switching the mode of fluoridation from water to an alternate staple, such as bread, has been considered. The value of fluoridated toothpaste is a possibility, but needs further evaluation.

In any event, fluoridation of water is one answer—but certainly not the *only* answer—to cavity prevention.

17

Chlorine

Chlorine and Good Digestion

Chlorine's intended mission on earth was not to disinfect swimming pools, but to help us digest our food.

As part of hydrochloric acid, chlorine rallies the digestive juices of the stomach. A combination of hydrochloric acid and powerful digestive enzymes gobbles up food particles, mashing them into a semiliquid pulp called chyme, which is then squirted into the upper intestine for final digestive breakdown.

Hydrochloric acid is one of the most corrosive acids. Outside the body, it will corrode metal and must be stored in glass or ceramic containers in the lab. Sheets of fat prevent it from burning a hole in our stomach lining when it's done making mush of our dinner. Secretion of too much acid, sparked by the hormone gastrin, is held responsible for stomach ulcers. Too little hydrochloric acid impedes proper digestion of food and absorption of minerals, and can even cause anemia. Indigestion caused by too little hydrochloric acid can often be relieved with hydrochloric acid tablets, which take up where nature reneges.

Chlorine is also found (as chloride) in the bath of cerebrospinal fluid that protectively surrounds the brain and spinal cord. And chlorine works with two other minerals, potassium and sodium, to maintain body water balance and to keep the necessary proportion of minerals in and out of cells in equilibrium.

We're most familiar with dietary chlorine as part of ordinary table salt, sodium chloride. Almost all food contains some form of chlorine, though, depending on the soil on which it was grown or raised. Animal foods are the richest source. In addition to what's naturally present, chlorine compounds are sometimes used in the processing of meat, poultry, bread and vegetables. So people on sodium-restricted diets need not worry that they'll miss out on chlorine for lack of added salt in their diets.

Why Chlorinated Water May Cause Problems

Chlorine in water is an entirely different matter from chlorine in food. Chlorine used to disinfect swimming pools and protect against the spread of water-borne diseases like cholera and typhoid in public water supplies is an activated form of chloride, with no nutritional value. Chlorination may, in fact, *cause* some serious health problems. (For details on problems associated with chlorination and how you can dechlorinate the water you consume, see chapter 25, Canceling Out Lead and Other Harmful Substances.)

18

Sulfur

Fire and brimstone.

We all know what fire is. But brimstone? It's another word for sulfur. As a dietary component, it's invaluable.

At least three vitamins, all B's, contain sulfur: thiamine (B_1), biotin and pantothenate.

The Protein Builder

In its larger role, sulfur is a key ingredient in protein, the building and maintenance material of our bodies. Carbohydrates and fat supply us with fuel, just as gasoline fuels a car. When we need to replace the spark plugs, fix a dent, or rebuild the car's transmission, however, fuel is of no use. And when it comes to maintenance and repair (and growth of our bodies) only protein will do.

Protein in our food—meat, chicken, fish, milk, eggs, beans, nuts and grains—is broken down in the stomach (and duodenum—part of the small intestine—just below) into its basic individual parts, called amino acids. Those pass into the bloodstream and are taken up by cells and tissues throughout the body, where they're reconstructed into hundreds of new protein structures. Muscles, tendons, cartilage, hair, nails, eyes, brain and other organs all contain protein.

Sulfur-containing proteins work behind the scenes, too, as the basic ingredients in many vital compounds.

• Hemoglobin, the oxygen-carrying substance in blood, contains protein—and sulfur.

• Many hormones—the substances secreted by glands to regulate important body functions—contain protein. Insulin, the hormone which regulates carbohydrate metabolism, is basically a protein. So are adrenaline and thyroxine. Sulfur is indispensable to all of them.

• All enzymes have protein as their basic unit, often coupled with either a vitamin or a mineral. The liver alone contains about 1,000 enzymes, many of which are sulfur-containing proteins.

• The antibodies that combat infection and stave off disease are sulfur-containing proteins.

Sulfur-containing proteins also serve as "toxin bouncers," helping to protect us against harmful contaminants by linking up with undesirables and escorting them out of the body. In protein depletion, ability to tolerate the effect of chemicals is reduced, rendering us less resistant to poisons or to the side effects of drugs.

Protein-rich food is the key route for sulfur entering our systems. Some fruits and canned vegetables are artificially sulfurized by food processors to retain color and taste during storage, but that sulfur has no nutritional value. Neither does sulfur emitted into the air by heavy industry.

A diet containing 100 grams of protein a day will provide 0.6 to 1.6 grams of sulfur, depending on what protein we choose. The quality of protein is as important to health as the quantity. While animal proteins—meat, fish, eggs, cheese and milk—contain all of the amino acids essential for growth and repair, plant proteins are not as complete, being relatively short on essential amino acids. As it happens, amino acids lacking in one group of plant proteins, like legumes (beans and peas), will be provided by either of the other two: grains (wheat, rice, barley and corn) or nuts. By combining two or three types of plant protein at the same meal, a protein balance as complete as meat or other animal food can be achieved. Adding a small amount of animal protein to plant proteins does the same thing. In that way, traditional combinations such as beans and corn, rice and chili, peanut butter and wheat bread, cereal and milk, and macaroni and cheese strike a good balance of usable protein.

19

Molybdenum

A Little-Known Mineral, Hard at Work

Small amounts of molybdenum hide out in every cell and tissue of our bodies. For reasons that escaped earlier notice, this obscure mineral is now coming into its own as an essential nutrient, as important to health as some better-known nutrients.

Molybdenum (pronounced "mo-LIB-deh-num") works as part of a special enzyme, xanthine oxidase, which performs two basic but very important tasks. First, the enzyme mobilizes iron from the liver, where most body iron is stored. All the iron in the world does us no good if it remains locked away in the liver, shut off from the circulating bloodstream. Molybdenum-containing xanthine oxidase frees iron so that it can help blood carry life-sustaining oxygen to cells and tissues.

In another part of the body, xanthine oxidase gathers up traces of nitrogen left over from the digestive breakdown of protein in food and turns it into uric acid. Along with urea, another major waste product, uric acid is then whisked out of the body as urine by the kidneys. That's important, because nitrogen wastes are extremely toxic. Even smidgens of uric acid left to accumulate in the blood will poison us.

Dental enamel is rich in molybdenum. Some research indicates that molybdenum may enhance the effect of fluorine in prevention of tooth decay, possibly by promoting retention of fluorine.

Primarily because of its role in xanthine oxidase, molybdenum is recognized as an essential trace mineral. Adults need a tiny amount—150 to 500 micrograms (that's 0.15 to 0.5 milligrams) a day, according to the government's Recommended Dietary Allowance. Molybdenum is readily and rapidly absorbed, perhaps to compensate for the trace amounts we take in.

Meats, grains, legumes (beans and peas) and dark green leafy vegetables are the richest sources of molybdenum. Because the amounts in plants vary greatly with the molybdenum content of the soil, exact levels are not given in tables of food composition.

As with other minerals, refining takes its toll on molybdenum in food. In a study of the mineral content of North American wheats and flours, wheat had twice as much molybdenum as white flour made from it. Because no deficiencies of molybdenum have been reported in people (although they do occur in animals), authors of standard nutrition texts usually assume that even the most marginal diets provide the little molybdenum we need. Estimates of molybdenum intake in the United States range from 100 micrograms to 350 micrograms. Poor food choices—notably too much refined sugar and white flour—could push molybdenum levels to the lower end of the scale. "Deficiency is theoretically possible because refined sugar and grain retain little of their original molybdenum," writes Robert A. Shakman, M.D. (*Archives of Environmental Health*, February, 1974).

Molybdenum supplements are not recommended. Too much molybdenum—far beyond what is normally present in food—can trigger a copper deficiency, because of an antagonistic relationship between the two minerals. The best way to assure ourselves of a healthy supply of molybdenum is simply to choose whole foods over refined.

20

Vanadium

Vanadium is relatively new to the vocabulary of nutrition. Years of painstaking work with animals showed, by the early 1970s, that vanadium is needed in amounts almost too small to measure, and influences several body processes. That basic need for vanadium, we're told, probably also applies to people.

Our animal counterparts in the lab show a drop in red blood cells on low-vanadium diets, for certain phases of iron metabolism and red blood cell growth depend on it. Bones, cartilage and teeth require minute amounts of vanadium for proper growth. There's some evidence, too, that vanadium may be exchanged for phosphorus in the mineral crystals of tooth enamel, contributing to resistance to tooth decay.

Vanadium at Work in Our Arteries

Most fascinating, however, is vanadium's effect on changes in fatty substances such as cholesterol and triglycerides in the blood. Animals fed low-vanadium diets show a change in blood fats. Studies of chicks have established that higher levels of vanadium can lower tissue levels of cholesterol, probably by action of one or two enzymes. The implications for a similar protective role in people is exciting. Assuming we are healthier with lower blood lipids (fats) than with higher levels, vanadium may turn out to be one more mineral pulling for the good health of our hearts and arteries, by warding off accumulation of fatty atherosclerotic plaques that can block the flow of blood.

It is estimated that we need from 100 to 300 micrograms of vanadium a day. Once absorbed, vanadium acts quickly. Most passes through the system within 24 hours. Little is stored, usually in bone and liver. After that, mobilization is slow.

Not much has been done to measure vanadium in food. Duane R. Myron, Ph.D., and colleagues at the USDA Human Nutrition Laboratory in Grand Forks, North Dakota, found that whole grains, seafood, and meats such as liver were good sources. Prepared foods, surprisingly, were even higher (*Journal of Agricultural and Food Chemistry,* March/April, 1977). However, vanadium in prepared foods is probably picked up from stainless steel processing equipment and may be of little use to people.

"I question whether vanadium picked up during processing is available to people," says Leon Hopkins, Ph.D., trace mineral researcher and chairman of the department of food and nutrition at Texas Tech University.

Better, instead, to eat those foods judged to be naturally adequate in vanadium.

21

Tin

A great burst in protein synthesis occurs immediately after birth. Quite possibly, tin acts as one of the messengers that spark that process and stimulate growth.

Before tin's role in growth was detected, its presence in the body was simply considered to be residue from the world around us, of no particular nutritional significance. Now, it's tentatively been added to the growing list of essential trace minerals.

Exactly how tin works is still anyone's guess. "The biochemistry of tin is completely unexplored territory," Klaus Schwarz, M.D., a leading trace mineral researcher, said in 1974. That remains true today. (*Trace Element Metabolism in Animals,* University Park Press, 1974).

Consequently, very little information exists on the tin content of food. Lacquer coating has greatly cut down on the amount of tin that leaches into our food from metal containers, so getting too much is not the problem it used to be. Estimates of intake range from 3 to 17 milligrams a day. Needs are estimated at 3.6 milligrams or so. Right now, deficiency of tin is unknown in animals or man.

22

Nickel

Nickel is very much a two-sided coin. As a nutrient in food, there's a good chance it's essential to health. Inhaled in large doses as a gaseous by-product of industry, heating fuel, cigarette smoke and car exhaust, nickel is a harmful contaminant. For simplicity's sake, we'll discuss nickel's role as a normal food component here and address exposure to nickel compounds in the air in the next section (see chapter 25, Canceling Out Lead and Other Harmful Substances).

Many foods we eat and many tissues in our bodies contain trace amounts of nickel. At first, nickel—like tin—was thought of only as a contaminant, with no nutritional value. Based on animal experiments showing that nickel is necessary for several body processes, it has graduated to the status of an essential nutrient for people, too.

Nickel reacts with vitamin B_6 to set off certain important changes in body protein. Nickel activates certain enzymes, some of which may be involved in breakdown and utilization of glucose, the fuel of life.

Whether true nickel deficiencies occur is not known. Heavy sweating may increase the need for nickel. People with diseases that interfere with intestinal absorption or who are under extreme physiological stress (prolonged heat or cold, surgical trauma, infection) may wear down nickel stores. Uncorrected uremia (a kidney disorder) or cirrhosis of the liver can deplete nickel stores. Iron deficiency anemia symptoms may be aggravated by low nickel.

Dietary intake varies from just a few micrograms to several hundred micrograms of nickel a day, depending on what we eat. All fats and animal products are low in nickel, since it doesn't generally accumulate in animals. Seafood is an exception. Cereals, grains, seeds, and certain beans and vegetables are also good sources of dietary nickel. (Table 31 gives a more detailed list.)

Estimates are not precise, because actual amounts depend on the nickel content of soil. Over and above nickel that's naturally present, small amounts leach into food from a couple of other sources. Some fungicides commonly sprayed on crops contain nickel. Stainless steel food processing equipment (including ordinary pots and pans) add some nickel, especially if the food cooked is acidic. Those incidental extras are not judged to be a problem, according to the National Academy of Sciences.

We eat about 500 micrograms of nickel a day in our food. Some of us eat much less—and some more. Henry A. Schroeder, M.D., and co-workers calculated that a diet composed of meat, milk, fruit, refined white bread, Wheatena, butter and corn oil would supply 3 to 10 micrograms of nickel per day. A diet providing the same amount of calories, protein, carbohydrates and fat from meat, milk, oysters, oats, whole wheat or rye bread, some vegetables, potatoes and legumes, with little added fat, might contain 700 to 900 micrograms of nickel (*Nickel,* National Academy of Sciences, 1975).

Very little of the nickel we eat is actually absorbed. The intestine seems to stubbornly limit how much will pass into the system, perhaps in deference to nickel's potential for harm. Most of it passes through in urine or feces. To be sure we retain enough, the kidneys keep track of nickel. If we eat only a little (as in the first diet described above), our kidneys excrete very little, to keep the body pool adequate. If we eat larger amounts (as in the second diet), the kidneys excrete nickel more freely. That system of checks and balances—called a homeostatic mechanism—helps to insure a relatively constant level of nutrition.

TABLE 31   Food Sources of Nickel

Food	Portion	Nickel (micrograms)
Beet greens, cooked	½ cup	141
Cider	1 cup	136
Kidney beans, dried	¼ cup	120
Peas, split, dried	¼ cup	83
Navy beans, dried	¼ cup	82
Lentils, dried	¼ cup	76
Clams, uncooked	4 ounces	66
Kale, cooked	½ cup	62
Banana	1 medium	60
Swiss chard, cooked	½ cup	52
Chicory	1 cup	50
Green beans, cooked	½ cup	41
Pear	1 medium	37
Lettuce, looseleaf variety	½ cup	31
Broccoli	½ cup	26
Apricot halves, dried	¼ cup	25
Peas	½ cup	24
Sardines, drained solids	4 ounces	24
Celery, chopped	½ cup	22
Whole wheat bread	1 slice	21
Spinach, raw	1 cup	19
Lettuce, crisphead variety	1 wedge	19
Escarole	1 cup	14
Bread, white	1 slice	14
Tomato juice	1 cup	12
Tomato	1 medium	4
Crab meat, canned	4 ounces	3
Egg	1 medium	2

SOURCES: Adapted from
   Nickel, by Committee on Medical and Biologic Effects of Environmental Pollutants (Washington, D.C.: National Academy of Sciences, 1975).
   Nutritive Value of American Foods in Common Units, Agriculture Handbook No. 456, by Catherine F. Adams (Washington, D.C.: Agricultural Research Service, U.S. Department of Agriculture, 1975).

23

Strontium

In the future, scientists might add another element to the list of sparse but essential trace minerals—strontium.

That's the opinion of Stanley Skoryna, M.D., director of medical research at St. Mary's Hospital in Montreal. Dr. Skoryna, who has conducted more research on strontium than any other scientist, recently talked with us about the mineral.

The Bone and Tooth Aid

Strontium, Dr. Skoryna explained, is chemically similar to calcium and can perform some of the same functions in bone structure. Researchers in the United States have found, for example, that in areas where strontium levels in the water are high, the rate of tooth decay is low. And one study suggests that the mineral may be helpful in the treatment of osteoporosis, the bone loss that often accompanies old age.

Dr. Skoryna's most recent studies focus on the role of strontium in cell metabolism. "Strontium may be effective in protecting the mitochondria, tiny structures within the cell that are important in energy production," he says. "Various kinds of cell injury, such as that caused by toxins, can damage mitochondria."

One reason why strontium research has been neglected, Dr. Skoryna says, was the scare over strontium 90 some years back. Strontium 90, a radioactive isotope of strontium, is produced by nuclear reactions, and it can be absorbed into the skeleton and cause lasting damage. Dr. Skoryna emphasizes that stable strontium, the form that occurs in nature, is not radioactive. In fact, stable strontium is one of the least toxic of trace minerals—it is far less toxic than fluorine, for example. This means, he says, that supplements of strontium well beyond the normal intake may be given with no fear of side effects.

Dr. Skoryna told us that the normal American intake of strontium is probably well below the optimal level. So, given its low toxicity and ostensible medical value, Dr. Skoryna believes that strontium should be a food supplement of the future. "Strontium does no harm. It may be useful in specific conditions where it should be given in higher amounts. And, I think, it might have a generally beneficial effect as a dietary supplement."

24

Adding to the List: Tomorrow's Health Builders

Reporting on the state of mineral research is like shooting at a moving target. The study of minerals is a rapidly advancing science. Most likely, more minerals will be added to the list of nutrients essential to health as more sophisticated techniques of studying body tissues and food components develop.

About 20 trace minerals are now under investigation. And, who knows, many of those now being studied may prove essential to human health. The new candidates share certain properties of recognized nutrients: they occur in normal cells and tissues, are available in our diet, and flow through our blood at constant levels. These minerals include:

Barium	Beryllium
Bromine	Cesium
Gold	Germanium
Aluminum	Rubidium
Antimony	Titanium
Boron	Tungsten
Lithium	

PART
III

WINNING AGAINST HIDDEN HAZARDS

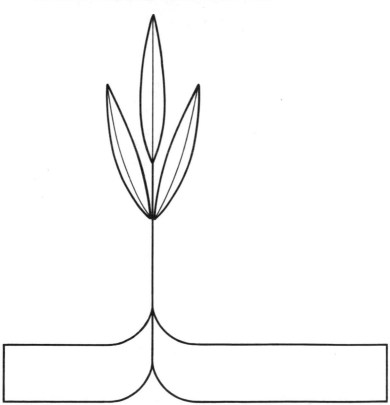

25

Canceling Out Lead and Other Harmful Substances

Minerals aren't always good for us. A few — like lead and cadmium — cause serious health problems at all but the lowest levels. Others — copper and nickel, for instance — are good at levels normally encountered in food, but at higher levels, as industrial pollutants, act as poisons. And along with others, like chromium and strontium, they are good in one chemical form but bad in another.

The so-called heavy metals — lead, cadmium, mercury, nickel and so on — are bent for harm because of two mulish properties. For one thing, those minerals are a lot like the uninvited party guest who lingers on and on. Once lead and cadmium find their way into bone or nerve cells, they're reluctant to leave, exiting slowly, if at all. And what makes heavy minerals even more pesky is their strong attraction to biological tissues.

Small amounts of lead and cadmium, like other trace minerals, have been around for millions of years. Our bodies are equipped to handle at least some. Above certain levels, though, daily exposure is associated with a variety of serious health effects. Studies show that air pollutants may elevate our blood pressure and lower immunity to infection. They may impair learning in children. Pollutants may even cause cancer and complicate heart disease.

All is not gloom, however. Any glut of heavy minerals in the environment is man-made and therefore preventable.

Workers in certain industries, like metal ore refineries and lead battery plants, suffer the highest exposure to harmful elements. Toxicologists (poison scientists) have no trouble identifying the dynamic body changes that follow massive daily doses. Community exposure to multiple minerals is more complex. Not only is the level of exposure often too small to produce direct symptoms, but the time lag before any symptoms show up can be as long as 30 or 40 years— and then the diagnosis can be tricky. So the implications for the health of millions of people, exposed to lower levels 24 hours a day, 7 days a week over many years, are less clearly understood and of greater concern.

Lead

More has been written about lead than any other mineral, good or bad. Certainly, lead's the most infamous of the harmful minerals, with heavy exposure linked to nerve and reproductive disorders. Lead interferes with copper and iron metabolism, disrupting normal production of hemoglobin in blood. Low levels can also undermine our ability to fight off infection and the effects of other harmful toxic substances.

Hundreds of thousands of years ago, lead was no problem. Small amounts were released into the soil and water as rocks weathered. Still less was released into the air. Skeletons unearthed from preindustrial ruins in Peru and Egypt show that ancient people took in only trace amounts of lead—0.002 parts per million—in food, water and air.

Today, people march to the beat of a different drum—the oil drum. And we take in 500 times as much lead, largely from auto exhaust and heating fuel. Metal refining adds its share, too. Layers of age-old snow in Greenland, examined by cross section, show that lead content has multiplied 400 times over natural concentrations. We breathe lead in—it's sucked through our lungs or swallowed. Airborne lead settles on plant leaves and animal fur. Lead collects in soil humus—the rich, acidic, organic fraction of the earth. Taken up by plant roots, lead is then passed on to human and animal consumers.

We take in about 300 micrograms of lead a day from contaminated food, water and air. That's just shy of the 429-microgram limit set by the World Health Organization, based on the assumptions that lead ingestion is unavoidable and that we can take in a certain amount of lead without harm. We absorb only about 10 percent of lead swallowed with food, more when the stomach is empty. Oral lead is first dissolved by gastric juices in the stomach and absorbed by the small intestine. Airborne lead is more of a direct assault, absorbed rapidly by the lungs.

No level of lead, no matter how small, is truly harmless. Lead's effect is cumulative; it builds up gradually and stays indefinitely. It's a little like eating too much candy and slowly growing overweight. Most lead we take in is shuttled to our long bones, where it rests undisturbed unless stirred up by low calcium intake, healing of fractures or chronic alcoholism. The rest does its dastardly work in the brain, nerve cells and bloodstream, producing anemia, learning problems and other disorders.

"Health problems caused by exposure to low levels of lead are common," says Herbert Needleman, M.D., associate professor of psychiatry at Harvard Medical School and leading spokesman on lead poisoning. "The symptoms of low-level lead poisoning are very general. Lead can produce headache, fatigue, irritability and depression. In many cases, doctors may not think of lead as the cause."

Those at highest risk from lead exposure—the elderly, pregnant women, and young children—breathe it, drink it and eat it every day. So do the rest of us. We're each carrying about 500 times more lead in our bodies than did our preindustrial ancestors. Until the mid-1970s, auto exhaust from cars running on leaded gasoline was responsible for 90 percent of our lead intake. Heavily trafficked streets—on which more than 100 or so cars traveled each day—were burdened with the most. Lead in gasoline is now being phased out to cut down on lead emissions from autos, buses and trucks.

You don't have to be a toll collector at the Lincoln Tunnel to be exposed to lead, though. Rain, wind and snow scour lead from the atmosphere, delivering it to soil and water. Drinking water contains an average of 13 micrograms per liter. The average may be quite a bit higher in older homes, especially where old leaded pipes remain, and the water is soft. Soft water is more acidic, and acid water is more corrosive, dissolving lead from pipes.

Simple household or street dust acts as a catchall for airborne particles of all sorts and is now being given serious attention as a significant source of lead. Colored newsprint and gift wrap contains not only lead, but other toxic metal dyes released into the air as they burn. Tin cans add lead to food. Half the lead in our food—from 50 to 250 micrograms of lead a day—comes from soldered metal cans. "If lead-soldered cans were banned, the average dietary lead intake of most Americans would be reduced by half," say scientists Dorothy M. Settle and Clair C. Patterson, Ph.D., division of geological and planetary sciences, California Institute of Technology (*Science,* March 14, 1980).

Children are particularly susceptible to lead poisoning

For one thing, children absorb five times more lead than adults, because the metabolism of a growing child is so high. Until about age five, children, like puppies, tend to put anything in their mouths—hands, feet, shoes, dust, dirt, paper, plaster, toys and chips of paint. Children suck on furniture, woodwork, fences, windowsills—in general, objects that pose potential harm.

Lead-based paint is by far the most notorious cause of outright, high-level lead poisoning in children. As old paint dries and ages, it peels and chips into tempting, sweet-tasting morsels for small children. It also chalks, contributing to lead in dust on floors and furniture—dust which ends up in toddlers' mouths. Where there's peeling paint, there's often broken linoleum and old putty—two other lead sources. The hand-to-mouth activity of young children provides a steady route for lead into children's stomachs.

The brain is the target organ for lead. High doses bring serious symptoms: clumsiness, poor coordination, weakness, abdominal pain, persistent vomiting, constipation, and sometimes unconsciousness and brain damage. Milder symptoms are often vague: fatigue, sallow complexion, generally poor feeling, loss of appetite, irritability, disturbed sleep and changes in behavior. Untreated, the lead-poisoned child may develop learning disabilities and emotional disturbances.

Using rats fed contaminated drinking water, one scientist was able to show how lead probably affects behavior and learning in children. Ellen Silbergeld, Ph.D., at the National Institutes of Health in Bethesda, Maryland, fed rats low levels of lead in their drinking water for their first 30 days of life—the equivalent of the first five years of childhood. The rats' behavior and learning ability were impaired. Lead gets inside the nerve cells where it tenaciously remains, first affecting the energy metabolism of the cells, but more important, disrupting the release of neurotransmitters, the chemical messengers between nerve cells (*Chemical and Engineering News,* June 23, 1980).

Before 1975, paint contained from 1 to 10 percent lead. The Consumer Product Safety Commission ruled that any paint with lead concentrations higher than 0.06 percent by weight is unsuitable for household use. That includes walls, woodwork, outdoor furniture and toys. And it's only one of eight acts of legislation enforced by six federal agencies setting out to help control lead-based paint hazards to children. Older schools, homes and day-care centers with old, peeling lead-based paint are still a threat, often found in deteriorating buildings in low-income urban areas. The U.S. Public Health Service estimates that each year 400,000 children have increased blood lead levels and 16,000 require treatment for outright lead poisoning. The implications of lead's effect on learning and behavior in children already disenfranchised by low income and minimum educational background are disturbing. What's more, poor children are also prone to nutritional deficiencies of protein, iron, zinc, calcium and vitamin C, which make lead toxicity more severe. So do heat and dehydration. The fact that children are double-dosing—eating lead, plus breathing the same lead-laced air and eating the same canned food as adults—compounds the problem.

More affluent children and their parents aren't immune. The Centers for Disease Control (CDC) in Atlanta, Georgia, tells us that as young couples buy and renovate inner city homes, they and their children are subject to the same dangers. John Gallagher, chief of Program Services Branch, Office of Environmental Health Services Division at CDC, told us it's not unheard of for adults to come down with lead poisoning after a zealous weekend of do-it-yourself scraping and painting. Children creeping along in the rubble are also at risk. (We'll share some tips on how to prevent lead poisoning a little later on.)

A child or adult suspected of having lead poisoning, who lives in or frequently visits an area where lead-based paint is likely to be a problem, should be taken to a doctor for a blood test. Interestingly, signs of lead poisoning in the family dog are a sure warning that the children are at risk. While blood tests do not reflect total body burden, they give some idea of how long the child has been exposed and how much lead has accumulated. If diagnosed and treated quickly, lead poisoning often can be reversed by medical antidotes that remove lead from the soft tissues, but not from the bones. And, of course, continued exposure to lead must be stopped.

What's to be done about large-scale, low-level exposure to lead? One of the more outspoken scientists in the field of lead research—and one of the most concerned—is Clair C. Patterson, Ph.D. In a report to the National Research Council in 1979, Dr. Patterson criticized regulatory bodies for foot-dragging on the lead issue. He feels that public pressure will eventually halt the mining and smelting of lead. There *are* alternatives, he points out. "Important steps have already been taken to reduce lead intakes within the general population. Lead closures in food and drink cans have been replaced on a significant scale by the use of aluminum cans, . . . steel cans, and plastic seals in crimped steel seams. Plastic or aluminum foil covers are being substituted for lead foil covers over cork on wine bottles. Nonleaded paints and putties are available in increasing quantities. Nonleaded glazes are being used on dinnerware. The economic costs of producing these nonleaded alternatives are in many cases demonstrably less than are the costs of producing leaded materials."

Cadmium

A second airborne pollutant, cadmium—like lead—used to be rare. Because industry has mined and used it so widely, cadmium has joined lead as an unwanted addition to our food, air and water supplies. It's associated with lead in paint, solder and auto exhaust. Cigarette smoke insults blood and lungs with cadmium. Once in the body, cadmium is reluctant to leave. Ten to 20 years of stockpiling cadmium can lead to a sudden explosion of poor health: high blood pressure, kidney disease, emphysema and iron deficiency anemia. As a result of environmental contamination, the average American is thought to take in about 70 micrograms of cadmium a day (*Medical Hypotheses,* December, 1979).

Mercury

Mercury is not just a heavy, silvery-white liquid that breaks into wiggly little beads when a thermometer breaks. In nature, rainfall scrubs mercury out of the earth's crust, releasing it into streams, lakes and oceans in small amounts. Manufacture of paints and plastics, use of fungicides and burning of fossil fuels all release additional mercury into air and water in larger quantities.

Large fish at the top of the aquatic food chain—notably tuna, halibut and swordfish—accumulate more mercury than plants or other animals. They also eliminate mercury quite slowly. Outbreaks of mercury poisoning in Japan, the United States and elsewhere from time to time since the 1940s have been traced to unusually high levels of methylmercury—the most toxic kind—in fish from industrially polluted waters.

The most glaring of mercury's harmful effects are on the nervous system: tremors and poor coordination, and in severe cases, brain damage. Low-level contamination with mercury over a long period could disturb liver function, damage kidneys, pancreas and bone marrow, and aggravate hypertension and diabetes.

In 1972, the World Health Organization set 0.3 milligrams (300 micrograms) as the tolerable weekly intake for mercury. Actual tolerance depends on individual sensitivity—many people may be able to tolerate a bit more. A predatory fish from heavily polluted waters may contain up to 4 milligrams per six-ounce serving; the same amount of fish from unpolluted waters may contain as little as 67 micrograms. The actual amount varies with species, size, and locale, among other factors. The Food and Drug Administration has set a limit of 1 microgram of total mercury per gram (168 micrograms per six-ounce serving) for commercial fish sold in this country. Only a fraction of that is methylmercury. So eating fish twice a week doesn't seem to pose any unusual health hazard. People who unknowingly fish heavily contaminated waters and live off their catch are at greatest risk, according to the National Research Council (*An Assessment of Mercury in the Environment,* National Academy of Sciences, 1978).

To head off potential problems, sport and commercial fishing areas in the United States and Canada are closed from time to time due to unacceptable levels of mercury pollution, or health warnings are issued in sport fishing areas. To find out if a prospective fishing spot is safe, call the Fish and Game Commission in the United States or the Ministry of Natural Resources in Canada, in the specific state or province you may plan to fish in.

Samples of prehistoric fish indicate that seafood has always been rather high in mercury, even before industry started spurting it into the environment. And some bodies of water have high concentrations of mercury, with no man-made source of contamination. It's possible that a natural detoxifying mechanism may be at work to protect against mercury's potentially harmful effects, since people have always enjoyed fish as an abundant source of food. Fish also contains selenium, which experiments show blocks some of the effects of mercury, possibly by immobilizing it before it can reach vital organs. Sulfur, too, binds with mercury and may add protection.

Drinking water does not appear to be a significant source of mercury. Just to be sure, federal drinking water standards limit mercury to two micrograms per liter (about a quart) of water.

Chlorine

Used for 70 years to prevent the spread of waterborne disease, chlorination—the "ideal" water treatment method—is now coming under fire.

The heart of the problem is that chlorine combines with many organics to form new compounds, including chloroform—a known carcinogen (cancer-causing substance). Evidence that seems to establish a firm link between heavily chlorinated water and cancer in people drinking that water is being scrutinized by the U.S. Council on Environmental Quality.

First, a research team from the Columbia University School of Public Health began looking into the deaths of housewives in seven New York State counties. The team, headed by Michael Alavanja, D.P.H. (doctor of public health), examined each female death from cancer of the gastrointestinal or urinary organs in the years 1968 to 1970. Because the prime suspect in these cancer deaths was chlorine, the researchers chose to study women: 85 percent of them were housewives, and they likely drank the same water throughout the day. Since the population in these counties was very stable, most of the women had spent their lives in the same locale, drinking from the same source, year in and year out.

The scientists found that women in the study who drank chlorinated water ran a *44 percent greater risk* of dying from cancer of the gastrointestinal or urinary tract than those who drank unchlorinated water

(*Report of Case Control Study of Cancer Deaths in Four Selected New York Counties in Relation to Drinking Water Chlorination,* Columbia University School of Public Health, December, 1976).

"To our knowledge, this is the first time a significant statistical relationship has been demonstrated between human gastrointestinal and urinary tract cancer mortality and chlorinated drinking water," Dr. Alavanja said. He recently completed a second study on men with essentially the same statistical correlation between cancer and drinking water.

After that, a close look at thousands of cancer deaths in North Carolina, Illinois, Wisconsin and Louisiana showed that a significantly higher proportion of lower-gastrointestinal cancer victims had drunk from chlorinated water supplies than individuals who died of other causes. Those studies strongly support current attempts by the Environmental Protection Agency (EPA) to regulate the level of chloroform and other similar cancer-causing substances in drinking water.

In addition to cancer, chlorinated water has also been linked to high blood pressure and anemia. Studies in Russia have shown that men drinking water with 1.4 milligrams of chlorine per liter have higher blood pressure than those drinking water with only 0.3 or 0.4 milligram per liter (*Chemical Abstracts,* vol. 77, 1972, abstract no. 29875).

In this country, John Eaton, Ph.D., professor of medicine at the University of Minnesota, found that a chlorine compound had a deleterious effect on red blood cells. He made this discovery in 1973 while studying patients who had developed severe anemia during treatment at two artificial kidney centers in Minneapolis—both centers used chlorinated water in their kidney dialysis machines. In his laboratory, Dr. Eaton found that these patients' red blood cells had been severely damaged by the chlorinated water. His findings were confirmed at a third artificial kidney center in Minneapolis. This third center had chlorine-free water, and its patients did not develop anemia (*Science,* August 3, 1973). Now, new federal water standards in many states prohibit exposing dialysis patients to chlorine above 0.1 part per million.

Recent EPA studies indicate that the synthetic chemicals formed in the chlorination process are far more dangerous than chlorine itself. Called trihalomethanes (THMs), they are the largest group of synthetic chemicals found in drinking water. "They are found in virtually every drinking water supply that is disinfected with chlorine, and not uncommonly at concentrations of several hundred parts per billion," according to an EPA report (*Federal Register,* February 9, 1978).

One solution may be use of alternative disinfectants that will not lead to formation of chloroform or other harmful compounds. Examples are chlorine dioxide (used in Europe for the past 25 years), bromine chloride, chloramine, and ozone. Some of those may pose unwelcome health effects of their own, however.

Nickel

Because it peppers all natural waters and practically all soil and food, we are unavoidably exposed to oral intake of small amounts of nickel every day. Oral nickel is no problem. We excrete excess nickel in feces. In natural concentrations and forms, nickel is no threat. It may even be helpful.

Inhaled nickel is another story. As we burn petroleum and coal, refine nickel ore, incorporate nickel in making plastics and rubber products, and use it to electroplate a myriad of objects, nickel fumes leak into the atmosphere. Auto exhaust and smoking add even more. The only natural phenomenon that scatters any nickel at all into the air is a volcanic eruption or two every 50 or 100 years. Such fits of nature hardly compare to hefty daily doses from industry and tobacco use.

Breathing in dust and vapors of nickel carbonyl—the most toxic form—is hazardous. Stable in air, breath and body fluids, toxic nickel stays and stays and stays in the body, slow to break down into weaker compounds. Nickel workers throughout the world show up with very high rates of lung and nasal cancer from heavy, direct exposure. Nickel present in asbestos may possibly contribute to the association between inhalation of asbestos fibers and cancer. And animal experiments suggest that nickel may cut down the body's natural antiviral defenses in cells, allowing tumor viruses to flourish unchecked, thereby abetting some forms of cancers.

Few of us work in nickel refineries or electroplating plants. Yet we may be exposed to some of the same risks. Auto exhaust and tobacco smoke—from pipes, cigars and cigarettes—contain volatile forms of nickel. Each cigarette, for example, contains 2 to 6.2 micrograms of nickel per smoke, 10 to 20 percent of which is inhaled. After going through two packs a day, a smoker has sucked in up to 5 milligrams of nickel per year—something the cigarette ads fail to mention.

So far, all that's been established for certain is that nickel workers who smoke heavily are particularly susceptible to respiratory cancers. What about smokers in industrialized cities? Or nonsmokers, city or country? There's no need for alarm yet, says the National Academy of Sciences. But in a comprehensive report on nickel and health, that advisory group expresses concern over the possible effects of further nickel contamination—contamination which seems to be headed up before it comes down—and recommends that close watch be kept on the metal (*Nickel,* National Academy of Sciences, 1975). It wouldn't be surprising to see the same kind of constraints put on nickel that now apply to lead.

Chromium

Trivalent chromium—the kind in food—is harmless. In fact, it's essential to good health. An alternate form, hexavalent chromium, is not so benevolent. Hexavalent chromium produces gastrointestinal hemor-rhage, may cause cancer of the lungs and esophagus, and skin ulcers.

As a pollutant, high levels of hexavalent chromium are found in heavily industrialized areas. It's also a contaminant in some water supplies. Tobacco plants selectively absorb chromium, so cigarette smoke is a heavy carrier.

Vitamin C converts hexavalent chromium to the innocuous form, trivalent chromium.

Strontium 90

This substance is radioactive and harmful, as compared to stable, helpful, nonradioactive strontium. Strontium 90 is a product of nuclear reactions. As more and more nuclear power plants spring up, there's an ever-increasing probability of radioactive strontium being accidentally released into the environment.

Both forms of strontium can masquerade as calcium in bones—the two are chemically similar. The problem is, strontium 90 continues to give off radioactivity inside the body. It also interferes with conversion of vitamin D into a form that enhances calcium absorption. That leads to weak bones.

Getting enough of the bones' prime mineral, calcium, helps to foil strontium 90's masquerade. When dietary calcium is high, strontium 90 heads for the exits. The kidneys intercede and flush it out, reducing the amount retained by the body. If less calcium is available, however, stron-tium 90 will be free as an undesirable substitute.

Copper

Copper doesn't give off metal fumes as readily as lead, cadmium or nickel, so ill effects from industrial use seem to be small. As it occurs naturally in food and water in trace amounts, copper is vital to body functions. However, the copper found naturally in water is often supple-mented with copper from industrial wastes and corroded plumbing—corrosion that increases when water is either chlorinated, soft or acidic. Some water companies introduce copper into reservoirs to control growth of algae. In higher amounts it can become dangerous, causing irritation of the gastrointestinal tract and possibly mental disorders.

A greenish stain just below the faucet is a sign of excessive copper. Details on how to test your water for copper and other minerals appear later in this chapter.

Molybdenum

Frequently used in metallurgy and often a constituent of fertilizers, molybdenum has been found in surface waters and groundwaters at very low concentrations. Although molybdenum aids the body in production of uric acid, excessive amounts have been associated with gout and bone disease.

Beryllium

Generally used in the manufacture of metal alloys, beryllium is harmless in small amounts. But researchers have found some association between beryllium and cancer in laboratory animals. The EPA has not set any limit on beryllium in drinking water.

Silver

Sometimes added to municipal water supplies to act as a disinfectant, silver is also used in certain types of activated carbon water filters, to prevent or slow the growth of bacteria. We are told that it should pose no problem. And in trace amounts it probably doesn't. Large doses, however, can cause anemia and possibly death. Occupational and medical exposure to silver causes a permanent ashen-gray discoloration of the skin, internal organs, and membranes lining the inner surface of the eyelids.

A Personal Strategy against Harmful Minerals

Short of setting up camp at the top of the Andes or taking off for the nearest deserted tropical island, it seems impossible for most of us to totally escape exposure to at least some harmful minerals. Of course, the types of minerals and their concentrations vary from place to place. For example, in areas of heavy rainfall or serious erosion, water concentration of trace minerals tends to be higher. Mining and industrial manufacturing also affect the type and concentration of minerals in a given location. If you live near a steel plant, iron foundry, or zinc mine, for example, your water supply may be burdened with a higher-than-average concentration of copper, zinc, or aluminum, not to mention a potentially deadly dose of cadmium, mercury or lead due to by-products of those industries.

Undesirable minerals from solid waste landfills seep into soil and water. Heating fuels in homes, restaurants and office buildings release particles into the air. Pesticide sprays dribble minerals into air, food and water. All combined with the noxious particles spewed into the air by car, bus and truck exhaust. Even the blue skies over the Rocky Mountains are tainted with polluted air from smoggy California.

We can't revert to a medieval society, where the air was purer but our standard of living less lavish. The next best thing would seem to be to establish and maintain "safe" levels of harmful minerals in the environment.

What's safe, though? Who decides? Recommendations come from

federal agencies like the Environmental Protection Agency and the National Institute for Occupational Safety and Health (NIOSH), established to research and enforce environmental standards in this country. Legislation such as the Clean Air Amendments (1970) and the Safe Drinking Water Act (1974) attempts to keep our exposure to recognized hazards to a realistic minimum. Chemists and chemical engineers are working to help control industrial pollution by designing means of control before a plant is built. That's usually simpler and less expensive to business and, ultimately, to the consumer, than modifying existing factories.

There are some problems. When it comes to carcinogens (cancer-causing substances), it's just about impossible to define safe levels. And the presence of toxic substances, including some potential carcinogens, in commercial products may remain undisclosed as trade secrets.

Many of us feel we'd like more control over what we eat, drink and breathe. We can write to our government representatives and express concern, but somehow, faraway legislation and research don't seem so reassuring when we find ourselves sitting in a traffic jam, nearly gagging on exhaust fumes. Or drinking water in an unfamiliar place and a distant city. Or moving into an apartment building downwind from a smelting plant. Blitzed by unwanted pollution, we welcome any extra protection. A nutritional blockade—combined with a few simple means of side-stepping major sources of pollution—is the strongest line of defense. The following suggestions may be of help.

Build a Nutritional Blockade against Pollution

1. Eat regular meals. Food neutralizes some of the toxic effects of lead, so eating frequent meals is one of the simplest ways to reduce lead toxicity. Relatively little of the lead we ingest with meals—6 to 14 percent—is absorbed, while 70 percent of the lead we take in between meals gets into our bloodstream. When we go without eating, body fat is mobilized to provide needed calories, and bone minerals are freed to maintain blood levels of calcium. Because bone and fat are two major storage sites for lead, it, too, will be released into the system.

2. Cut down on fat intake. Fat soaks up lead like a sponge. Increased dietary fat enhanced absorption of lead in animals studied by researchers at the Centers for Disease Control (*Environmental Health Perspectives,* April, 1979). Butter, oil, fatty meats, cream, desserts and snack foods are the most common sources of dietary fat. Many can be eased out in favor of less fatty foods and condiments.

3. Be sure to get enough calcium. Calcium, along with iron, phosphorus and vitamin D, intercepts lead entering the body and carries it off to the bones or fatty tissues, before it gets a chance to infiltrate organs such as the liver or kidneys, where it could disrupt metabolism. Studies of babies show that as dietary calcium goes down, absorption of lead goes up—*even when calcium is adequate by current standards* (*Environmental Health Perspectives,* April, 1979).

If calcium intake is low, the body starts borrowing minerals from bone to make up for low intake—as it does in many cases of osteoporosis—and lead levels in the kidneys and blood go up dramatically.

Calcium also protects against strontium 90, by making it harder for that mineral to take its toll on bones. When calcium is around, strontium is thwarted.

Calcium may prevent cadmium's toxic effects. A group of rats were fed a diet containing cadmium and low levels of calcium. Another group was also fed a diet containing cadmium, but with high levels of calcium. Compared to the first group, those getting extra calcium absorbed significantly less cadmium (*Third International Symposium on Trace Element Metabolism in Man and Animals,* July, 1977).

4. *Boost your vitamin C* and **5. *Think zinc.*** A study by researchers at the Brain Bio Center in Princeton, New Jersey, shows that vitamin C and zinc protect against lead poisoning. Led by research biochemist Rhoda Papaioannou, the team of researchers studied 22 workers in a battery plant where the air was filled with lead—so much lead that many workers showed signs of lead poisoning. For the study, the workers took 2 grams (2,000 milligrams) of vitamin C and 60 milligrams of zinc daily. Before the study began and 6, 12 and 24 weeks later, the researchers measured the levels of lead in the workers' blood, and other signs that would indicate any decrease in lead poisoning.

After 24 weeks, the workers' average blood levels of lead had dropped 26 percent. Some of the other measurements also showed a decrease in lead poisoning.

"These changes were striking in view of the fact that they were achieved while the workers were on the job and constantly exposed to high levels of lead," write the researchers (*Journal of Orthomolecular Psychiatry,* July, 1978).

How did vitamin C and zinc work to stop lead poisoning? The researchers theorize that they may prevent the absorption of lead from the digestive tract.

But these two nutrients not only stop lead from being absorbed, they may also "protect against lead already absorbed"—cleaning it out of the system—the researchers say. "Vitamin C and zinc might also prevent the symptoms of low-level lead poisoning," Ms. Papaioannou told us. "By increasing zinc and vitamin C, everyone could be better protected against the inevitable lead exposure that is part of modern life," she added. "It would be better to clean up the environment, but in the meantime we can at least protect our bodies."

Vitamin C also protects against other heavy metals, including cadmium and mercury, excess fluoride, and exposure to industrial chromium, cobalt and copper.

Zinc, too, fights cadmium. In one study, scientists fed young quail a diet containing cadmium. When zinc was added to the diet, the level of cadmium in their tissues dropped. "Zinc is an important element in preventing the accretion [accumulation] of low levels of cadmium similar to those present in the diet of man," wrote the scientists (*Federation Proceedings,* March, 1977, abstract no. 4656).

6. Keep up your iron reserves. Eating a diet well supplied with iron helps the body resist the effects of lead. Iron deficiency increases susceptibility to lead toxicity in rats. Getting enough iron tends to reduce uptake of lead by the intestine.

In fact, iron-deficient people may absorb as much as 24 percent of dietary lead instead of the usual 10 percent, say researchers in Scotland who compared lead and iron absorption in experimental diets fed to ten people (*Lancet,* August 2, 1980).

Iron may also shield against cadmium. "Levels of dietary iron that exceed the normal requirement offer almost complete protection against cadmium toxicity in the growing rat," wrote Orville Levander, Ph.D., in *Federation Proceedings* (April, 1977).

And iron may get a helping hand from vitamin C. Researchers fed two groups of rats diets containing cadmium. A few weeks later, the cadmium was taken out of their diets, and one group received iron and vitamin C. Their "recovery rate" from the ill effects of cadmium was much faster than the nonsupplemented group (*Nutrition Reports International,* December, 1977).

7. *Selenium adds another ounce of prevention* against an onslaught of pollution by counteracting cadmium and mercury.

Selenium and cadmium compete for binding sites in the body. If selenium gets there first, cadmium steps aside.

Selenium reduces the toxicity of mercury and reduces its effects on kidneys, although the exact relationship is not clear. "It is clear that organisms with a diet supplemented by selenium or with high natural levels achieve an added degree of protection against methylmercury poisoning," says the Environmental Studies Board of the National Research Council (*An Assessment of Mercury in the Environment,* National Academy of Sciences, 1978).

Fish and seafood are naturally high in selenium. And selenium-rich yeast is one man-made technical achievement that serves good purposes only: helping to keep nutritional status hearty enough to fight off heavy metal toxins.

8. *Vitamin E also chips in* to aid zinc and vitamin C against lead. A team of researchers fed laboratory animals large amounts of lead and varying amounts of vitamin E. The animals with the lowest levels of vitamin E in their diets had the highest levels of lead in their tissues, showing that vitamin E can prevent lead absorption (*Federation Proceedings,* March 1, 1977, abstract no. 4742).

Together, selenium and vitamin E team up to cancel out toxic metals that vitamin E alone cannot counteract—cadmium, mercury and silver.

9. Kelp shields against fallout. Kelp is a seaweed. Several studies have reported that a substance extracted from kelp—alginate—has the remarkable ability to actually inhibit the body's absorption of certain poisonous materials. Among them is strontium 90.

Yukio Tanaka, Ph.D., at St. Mary's Hospital, Montreal, told us of research with two extracts from Pacific brown kelp: alginate and fucoidin. In experiments with mammals, alginate inhibited the absorption of radioactive strontium and cadmium. Fucoidin prevented the absorption of lead. Dr. Tanaka also cited the work of another researcher, Jerry Stara, whose experiments with animals showed that alginate can also remove strontium 90 that has already been absorbed. And a British study reported in *Nature* (December 25, 1965) demonstrated that alginate reduced strontium absorption in humans to one-eighth of what it was without alginate.

Safeguarding Your Food Supply

10. Buy solder-free cans when shopping for groceries. Canned goods with soldered seams—that is, joined together with molten lead—contribute to the lead content of food. Identifying soldered cans is easy. Look for a vertical seam running up and down the side of the can. That seam is often sealed by pouring hot, molten lead solder (pronounced "SAH-der") on the outside of the seam and brushing it into the seam as it cools and solidifies. Solder forms a rough patch of grayish-silver metal of different color and texture from the smooth, shiny, tinned surface of the can. The solder makes an airtight seal, but it comes in contact with food inside. While the individual dose may be small, people who wish to reduce their overall lead intake from food, water and air may wish to choose canned goods carefully.

If the shiny sides of the can come together in a smooth, neat vertical crack that is not smeared and discolored, chances are it's not soldered, according to Dr. Patterson and Dorothy Settle at California Institute of Technology. If the seam is hidden by a paper label, gently pull the label away from the seam for ¼ inch or so for closer inspection. Forged steel or aluminum cans are seam-free and unsoldered.

11. Eat whole grain bread and rice. In wheat and rice, traces of cadmium are found in the starchy endosperm. Zinc, selenium, calcium and vitamin E are concentrated in the germ and bran. Those protective factors are stripped away when grain is milled into white flour, white rice and refined cereal.

12. Wash fresh fruit and vegetables before serving. The surface deposits of heavy metals are removed or diluted by washing produce. Peeling adds further protection, although some fiber and vitamins are lost.

13. Cook vegetables quickly, in little or no water. Steam whenever possible. Experiments conducted at the Gardiner Institute of Medicine and the University of St. Andrews in Scotland showed that carrots, cabbage and peas (representative of root, leaf and seed vegetables) showed a significant uptake of lead from cooking water. The longer the vegetables were cooked, the more lead they absorbed. Meats cooked in water also absorb lead, say the researchers, and other toxic metals, such as cadmium, could behave in a similar way (*International Archives of Occupational and Environmental Health,* vol. 44, no. 2, 1979). You'll probably want to have your drinking and cooking water tested for mineral content, regardless. If your home has old leaded plumbing or you live in a soft water area, you may wish to cook with bottled water, especially for pasta, rice and beans, which require longer cooking in water.

Action Tactics against Pollution

14. Exercise. Antidote Number 14 is, simply, Sweat the Lead Out. Sedentary people, apparently, absorb more lead from the food they eat. Once in the body, it stays there. Runners, on the other hand, breathe in much more airborne lead during their sprints, yet may retain far less. Dr. Patterson, of the division of geological and planetary sciences, California Institute of Technology, theorizes that even though runners are exposed to far more lead, they may fare better than fellow Smog Belt dwellers who are less active. The trained body, says Dr. Patterson, seems to be able to activate some kind of defense mechanism to prevent absorption of ingested lead—possibly due to healthier metabolism of calcium.

15. Quit smoking. If you smoke, now's the time to quit. Smoking reduces vitamin C levels by an average of 40 percent. Not only does smoking drain your body of its power to fight off pollution, but tobacco smoke contains appreciable amounts of cadmium, nickel and toxic chromium, thus adding insult to injury.

If you find that you can quit only by first cutting down, up your intake of vitamin C. Same goes if you're often caught in situations where people around you enjoy creating their own personal smoke screens.

If you're a nonsmoker, give yourself a blue ribbon. You're already practicing nonpollution.

Cleaning Up Your Drinking Water

16. Test your water. Knowing which minerals are present in your home water supply could help you make some important decisions about your health—like considering plumbing remedies or looking for an alternative water source if your water is high in hazardous minerals.

A community water supply survey in 1970 evaluated the condition of water between treatment plant and home (see table 32). What they found was that 30 percent of the samples taken from the tap had mineral concentrations exceeding the government limits in existence at that time. In one case, for example, the cadmium content was 11 times greater than allowed in drinking water. In other samples, iron content was 90 times higher than acceptable; manganese, 26 times higher; and lead, 13 times greater than set limits (*Journal of the American Water Works Association,* November, 1970).

TABLE 32 ## Community Water Supply Study of 2,595 Distribution Samples from 969 Public Water Supply Systems

	Standards		
Mineral	Limit (milligrams per liter)	Maximum Concentration (milligrams per liter)	Percent Exceeding
Cadmium	0.01	0.11	0.2
Chromium	0.05	0.08	0.2
Copper	1.0	8.35	1.6
Iron	0.3	26.0	8.6
Lead	0.05	0.64	1.4
Manganese	0.05	1.32	8.1
Silver	0.05	0.026	0.0
Zinc	5.0	13.0	0.3

Water samples below are not distribution samples, but finished water samples.

Arsenic	0.05	0.10	0.2
Barium	1.0	1.55	⟨0.1[a]
Selenium	0.01	0.07	0.4

SOURCE: Reprinted from "Survey of Community Water Supply Systems," by Leland J. McCabe et al., *Journal of the American Water Works Association,* November, 1970.
NOTE: [a] This constituent was evaluated only on selected samples. The remainder were assumed not to exceed the limit.

Those with individual water supplies such as wells and cisterns are not exempt from this problem, because copper and lead household plumbing also can be a major contributor of metal pollution.

If you live in a hard water area (and do not have a water softener sharing space with your water heater) you may be somewhat exempt from this extra dose of minerals. Calcium and magnesium—good minerals—tend to accumulate inside water pipes, and create a natural lining which protects plumbing from excessive corrosion. On the other hand, if your water is naturally soft, you may have two strikes against you. One, your plumbing lacks any protective shield. Two, naturally soft water tends to be somewhat acidic, and acidic water is more corrosive. In Boston, for example—where the water is both soft and acidic—half the water samples taken from taps on Beacon Hill exceeded the lead limit.

All you need is litmus paper (available in many pharmacies) to check the acidity or pH of your water. Take a look at the pH value of your water and check it against the figures shown in table 33. As you can easily see, the higher the pH of water (or the less acidic), the less metal seems to be present in it. Cadmium, lead and zinc corrosion seem to be slightly higher at the pH range of 7.0 to 7.4, but the corrosion of other metals is greater at lower pH measurements. Copper especially increases when the water measures at or below a pH of 6.9. If you have copper plumbing and your water's pH measures low, you can be fairly certain you have traces of copper in your water.

For safety, then, let your tap water run for about two minutes or so in the morning before drinking it. Because water has been in contact with the pipes overnight, there's likely to be a higher concentration of trace minerals from your plumbing system. But by flushing your water lines, you can rid the system of the night's mineral-laden water.

The best time to take a water sample for testing is also in the morning—mineral concentrations are highest then. After all, if your water is leaching dangerous minerals like cadmium and lead or excessive amounts of copper from your pipes, you ought to know about it. Besides, water is presumably checked for purity before it leaves the municipal treatment plant, but usually not when it comes out of your tap. And that is the water you drink. If your water comes from your own source—a spring or well, for example—the importance of testing its quality is even greater, since it probably hasn't been checked for metals at all before you drink it.

State and local public health offices will often perform water testing, usually for only a select number of minerals. Generally speaking, it's less time-consuming to begin by contacting your local water authority, county health department, or regional Department of Environmental Resources, approaching the state authorities on more complicated testing or if local help is unavailable. Test prices can vary greatly from no charge to several hundred dollars.

TABLE 33 ## Mineral Levels Found in Distribution Samples from Community Water Supply Study

	pH to 6.9		pH 7.0-7.4		pH 7.5-7.9		pH 8.0 or more	
	Percent Exceeding Standard	Average (milligrams per liter)	Percent Exceeding Standard	Average (milligrams per liter)	Percent Exceeding Standard	Average (milligrams per liter)	Percent Exceeding Standard	Average (milligrams per liter)
Number of Samples	425		556		550		595	
Cadmium	0.0	0.001	0.5	0.008	0.2	0.001	0.0	0.000
Chromium	0.0	0.000	0.7	0.002	0.0	0.001	0.0	0.003
Copper	5.4	0.295	1.1	0.119	0.2	0.067	0.5	0.050
Iron	10.8	0.184	11.7	0.331	7.5	0.116	3.9	0.081
Lead	1.6	0.013	2.3	0.016	0.5	0.012	0.3	0.009
Manganese	9.9	0.026	11.7	0.033	6.8	0.019	4.9	0.012
Silver	0.0	0.000	0.0	0.000	0.0	0.000	0.0	0.001
Zinc	0.7	0.225	0.5	0.321	0.0	0.180	0.0	0.056

SOURCE: Reprinted from "Problem of Trace Metals in Water Supplies: An Overview," by Leland J. McCabe, *Proceedings of the 16th Water Quality Conference*, University of Illinois, February 12-13, 1974.

You can also have your water tested by the Soil and Health Society, a nonprofit organization which is concerned with environmental issues. For a moderate fee, they will test your water for the following: arsenic, barium, cadmium, chromium, cobalt, copper, iron, lead, manganese, mercury, potassium, selenium, silver and zinc. In addition, they'll test for calcium and magnesium, as well as pH. For a sample bottle and instructions, write to the Soil and Health Society, 33 East Minor Street, Emmaus, PA 18049. Incidentally, to emphasize the importance of taking charge of your own water supply, the Soil and Health Society informed us that over 50 percent of the household water it has tested has exceeded recommended health limits for some trace minerals. (See table 34 for Limits for Minerals in Drinking Water.)

17. Beat the chlorine out of your water. Put a small amount of water in your kitchen blender and whirl it up for about 15 minutes. Or let it stand in the refrigerator overnight. Because chlorine is a gas, it's volatile, and it will escape into the air.

18. Clean chlorine from your water with vitamin C. Add a pinch of vitamin C powder or a piece of vitamin C tablet to a glass of chlorinated water immediately before drinking. Taste and odor will disap-

TABLE 34 ## Limits for Minerals in Drinking Water

Mineral	Recommended Limit (milligrams per liter)
Arsenic	0.05
Barium	1
Beryllium	no regulated limit
Cadmium	0.01[a]
Chromium	0.05
Cobalt	no regulated limit
Copper	1[a]
Lead	0.05
Manganese	0.05[a]
Mercury	0.002
Molybdenum	no regulated limit
Selenium	0.01
Silver	0.05
Tin	no regulated limit
Vanadium	no regulated limit

SOURCE: Reprinted from *Water Fit to Drink,* by Carol Keough (Rodale Press, 1980).
NOTE: Most values are based on EPA standard for drinking water quality listed in the National Interim Primary Drinking Water Regulations.
[a] From USPHS Drinking Water Standards (1962). The EPA National Interim Primary Drinking Water Regulations supercedes the USPHS Drinking Water Standards, but does not regulate the limit of this mineral in drinking water.

pear. That method works because vitamin C is an acid (ascorbic acid), while chlorine is a base. The acid combines with the base to form a compound called a salt. Therefore the chlorine is made innocuous.

19. Distill your water. If your water is very polluted with both organics (like chloroform) and metals (like cadmium), you might consider using a water distiller. Although distillation removes the good minerals with the bad, it may be the best alternative to a badly contaminated supply.

Until recently most distillers were not very effective in removing the organic contaminants, but there is a new type on the market which effectively removes close to 100 percent of chloroform present. The process is called fractional distillation—which means vaporizing and removing organic compounds before distilling the water. Cost runs in the vicinity of $400.

The major drawback of distillation is that it removes *all* minerals, including beneficial ones like calcium and magnesium. But food and supplements can easily replace them.

Protecting Home and Hearth

20. You may want to test your paint. In 1975, the Consumer Product Safety Commission set a standard requiring that only paint with less than 0.06 percent lead by weight be sold for household use. The standard went into effect in 1978 and applies to toys and outdoor furniture, too—any painted item that could be considered for household use. Any paint purchased or any home painted since then should be okay.

If the paint was applied before 1977 (or masks an undercoating from previous years), you may still be in the clear. If the paint is intact, not flaking, chipping or chalking, you would probably do best to leave it, says John Gallagher, of the Centers for Disease Control in Atlanta, Georgia. Taking it off could generate more problems by releasing lead into the air.

Still, accessible surfaces like railings, stair banisters and window-sills, intact or not, are popular teething tools for young mouths. Parents of young children may be concerned, even if the paint hasn't yet begun to peel. If you have any doubts or are concerned about the paint on your walls and woodwork, have it tested. Many local and some state health departments, particularly in larger cities, use a special instrument which, when pressed against paint, can determine the lead content. If you are concerned about older but intact paint in your home or apartment, call for an inspection.

Should the paint be chipping or peeling, take a sample to your nearest health department for analysis. They should be able to tell you if you have a potential problem. One small chip of paint could contain as much as 100 milligrams of lead—enough to trigger a medical emergency. Daily ingestion of smaller amounts over a period of days or weeks is equally serious.

The simplest and cheapest way to eradicate the problem is to cover walls with wallboard, paneling, wallpaper, or adhesive-backed paper. Should you decide to remove the old paint instead, be careful. As you fervently scrape and sand those pitted walls down to their original surface, lead particles become airborne and settle in a menacing film of dust on floors, stairs and furniture, temporarily *increasing* lead hazards.

Old putty and broken linoleum contain lead, too. Children creeping along in the rubble are more than likely to swallow a lot of dust and scrapings.

Adults are vulnerable, too. Don't forget to wash your hands before reaching for a cold beverage. Don't set down your half-eaten sandwich where it can become bespeckled with the same insidious particles. And close the door to the room you're tackling, to prevent lead-laden dust from dispersing throughout the rest of the house. Use a tarp or other floor covering, to prevent lead from being ground into carpeting or cracks between floorboards.

Farm the kids out to a neighbor or relative during major paint scraping projects. And kids or no kids, clean up as you go, to avoid powdery buildup of lead-laced residue.

21. Keep floors, woodwork and furniture dust-free. Speaking of cleaning up, good housekeeping habits can further cut down on everyday exposure to lead, particularly if you live on a busy street or near an industrialized area. Rugs, carpets and draperies trap fugitive lead blown in through windows and trekked in on shoes and clothing. Vacuum thoroughly and often. Wet-mop tile or wood floors and sponge off furniture when possible.

"Less dust means less lead," says Dr. Herbert Needleman, the Boston psychiatrist whose name is prominent in the lead field.

When asked how significant a source of lead house dust actually is, and whether housecleaning makes much of a difference, another scientist told us, "Any time you reduce lead exposure, you're better off." Eldon Savage, Ph.D., professor of environmental health at Colorado State University and head chairperson of the Committee on Environmental Toxicology for the National Environmental Health Association, added, "That's not to say that poor housekeeping by Mom or Dad will in itself account for lead poisoning in a child. But it's one more source of lead which can be controlled."

22. Plant your garden away from the street. Keep in mind that until cars running on leaded gasoline are phased out completely, auto exhaust will continue to emit lead. It might be a good idea to plan your garden accordingly. Fourteen gardens in and around the Boston area showed that the closer a garden is to heavy traffic, the higher the lead content in vegetables grown. The research was conducted by James R. Preer, Ph.D., then with the department of nutrition and food sciences, Massachusetts Institute of Technology, and Walter G. Rosen, Ph.D., department of biology, University of Massachusetts. "Lead contamination of vegetables by auto emissions is generally confined to a region within 75 to 100 feet of major highways. Many urban gardens are located well within this distance of streets, although traffic volume is often lower [than near highways]." Cadmium, too, may accumulate. Gardeners should take into consideration the wind direction and volume of traffic when planning a garden, say the researchers (*Eleventh Annual Conference on Trace Substances in Environmental Health,* June 6-9, 1977).

It might also be a good idea to test the soil itself for lead. In addition to auto exhaust, paint from old frame houses and previous landfill use can contribute lead to soil, reported Dr. Preer in later work. Leafy vegetables are the biggest accumulators, and children and pregnant women are at highest risk (*Environmental Pollution,* April-June, 1980). Contact your county extension agency of the U.S. Department of Agriculture. Even if lead content is on the high side, a new layer of topsoil can solve the problem.

23. Don't let the kids eat dirt. "This is a good opportunity to do away with the myth that a little dirt never hurt a kid," said Dr. Needleman, of Boston Children's Hospital. Dirt contains lead and is *not* harmless.

24. Bundle, don't burn, gift wrap. The same goes for color-printed magazines and newspaper ads. Colored paper often contains a variety of toxic metals, including lead and chromium. Burning colored paper in the fireplace can fill a room with potentially dangerous particles. Be careful, too, that children don't eat the paper. Put gift wrap, funnies and magazines in trash bags, seal and leave them for the sanitation department to dispose of properly.

26

Hard and Soft Water: The Inside Story

A lot more than water comes out of your water tap. Presence or absence of certain minerals depends on whether your water is soft or hard. Because that's a difference that can affect your health, water is worth a closer look.

Hard water contains large amounts of dissolved minerals, especially calcium and magnesium, which it picks up while trickling through underground deposits of dolomitic limestone. Technically, water is defined as hard if it contains more than 75 milligrams of mineral particles in a liter. But water hardness is often measured in "grains" or grains of minerals per gallon. Water is considered *slightly hard* if it contains 1 to 3 grains per gallon; *moderately hard* if it contains 3 to 6 grains per gallon; *hard* if it contains 6 to 12 grains per gallon; *very hard* if it contains 12 to 30 grains per gallon; and *extremely hard* if it contains 30 or more grains per gallon.

In other words, a boiled-down gallon of moderately hard water would leave behind a mineral deposit equal to the size of an aspirin tablet (five grains). That doesn't sound like much. But if you ever moved from an area where you enjoyed soft water to one where the water supply is hard, you know what a difference these dolomitic minerals can make (see map).

Hardness of Groundwater

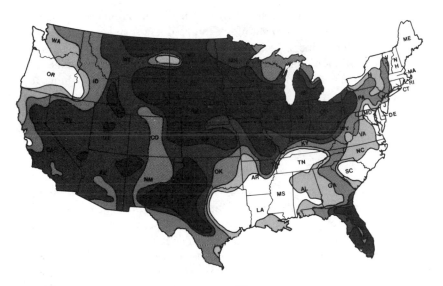

Hardness as calcium carbonate in parts per million

☐ Under 60   ■ 180-240

▨ 60-120   ■ Over 240

▨ 120-180

SOURCE: Reproduced with permission from *Water Atlas of the United States*, (Syosset, N.Y.: Geraghty and Miller, Inc.).

The bathtub develops a ring that wears longer than many wedding rings. There's no satisfying layer of soap suds in the washer. Hair doesn't squeak after shampooing. Clothes made from synthetic fabric look dingy. The bottom half of a double boiler appears to have terminal psoriasis, the chalky innards of a kettle flake into your tea, and jars processed in a canner emerge looking scabrous and unhealthy.

If yours is a hard water area, you may have been visited by a representative from the local water conditioning company. Representatives offer to test hardness with a scientific-looking kit, probably for free. Accompanying the free test is a free talk on the evils of hard water. As hard water evaporates, the story goes, it leaves behind a gritty mineral residue on the interior of the hot water heater, water pipes, radiators, and even on the inside of your bathroom cup. Conditioning companies suggest that it's cheaper to install a home water softener than to replace the household plumbing.

Soft water truly is an attractive commodity. It eliminates soap curd and detergent deposit from clothing. You need less soap for laundry and cleaning. White mineral scales no longer deposit on glasses, dishes and utensils. Soft water rinses away grime faster, and leaves no residue. It allows for luxurious bubble baths and leaves hair clean and shiny. It provides a longer life for household appliances that use water, and it protects expensive plumbing and heating equipment.

Hard Water and Heart Health

The trouble is, although soft water seems to be a plumbing panacea, it promises few benefits for personal health. Just by definition, soft water lacks calcium and magnesium—two minerals that are essential to bodily functions and optimum health. Of course, water is not our sole source of these minerals; we get much of our daily allowance in the food we eat. Yet over the past 20 years there has been considerable evidence from studies in several countries that people who drink soft water suffer more heart attacks and strokes than people who live in hard water areas. What remains in question is the magnitude of the effect: just how much difference is there?

One of the most recent studies is the British Regional Heart Study, conducted in the midst of the heat over hard vs. soft water as a protective factor, comparing water hardness and cardiovascular deaths in 253 towns. The authors of the report estimate a 10 to 15 percent excess of cardiovascular deaths in areas with very soft water compared to areas of medium hardness. Beyond medium hardness (more than 170 milligrams per liter), there was no added benefit.

The researchers are quick to concede that there is no explanation for this relationship, and don't know how long we have to drink hard water to be protected, or drink soft water to develop a risk. And we're reminded that smoking, high blood pressure, high blood cholesterol and lack of exercise have a more pronounced effect on heart disease than simple water softness (*British Medical Journal,* May 24, 1980).

Still, given the intricacies of heart health, it's hard to ignore studies that indicate the very minerals capable of clogging water pipes can prevent deaths due to clogged arteries. Or to think that something that sounds as innocuous as *soft* water might harbor some hidden health hazard. Strange as it may seem, both may be true.

For example, there's more than one reason to believe that the magnesium found in abundance in hard water supplies may somehow toughen the heart against sudden disturbances in heartbeat.

First of all, heart muscles of persons living in hard water areas (where cardiovascular death rates are low) tend to contain more magnesium than those of persons living in soft water locales. In heart muscle samples collected at autopsy from 83 cases of accidental death and analyzed for mineral content, Terence W. Anderson, M.D., Ph.D., of the University of Toronto's department of preventive medicine and biostatistics, reported that magnesium content varied significantly between hard and soft water areas. In fact, magnesium concentrations were 7 percent lower in the heart muscles of subjects who lived in the soft water areas of Ontario (*Canadian Medical Association Journal*, August 9, 1975).

What's more, heart muscles of heart attack victims contained, on the average, 22 percent less magnesium than the muscles of healthy persons who died accidentally—a finding that echoes the results of an even more recent Israeli study (*New England Journal of Medicine*, April 14, 1977).

Magnesium has been shown over and over again to play an important role in the prevention of heart arrhythmia (irregular beats) and fibrillation (rapid beats), as it is involved in reactions that are essential to the contraction of heart muscle (*American Heart Journal*, June, 1977).

But magnesium's role in heart disease doesn't stop there. A group of physicians at Georgetown University Medical Division and the District of Columbia General Hospital in Washington, D.C., report that this important mineral has a decided effect on lowering blood pressure—another serious risk factor in heart disease (*Angiology*, October, 1977).

Another theory says that spasms occurring within heart arteries may set the stage for dangerous blood clots and future heart attacks. And magnesium deficiency may be behind those spasms. "Arteries can actually go into a contracture when magnesium gets very, very low—or in other words, a spasm," says Burton M. Altura, Ph.D., professor of physiology, State University of New York, Downstate Medical Center, who's researched magnesium for over 15 years.

Furthermore, a magnesium deficiency can predispose a person to a calcium deficiency. And a calcium deficiency may also be a problem in heart disease—which is why hard water, with its ample supply of calcium, may provide double protection against heart disease. In fact, a separate English study that analyzed water from homes in 61 areas of England and Wales found calcium—not magnesium—to be the number one common denominator in the hard water-low cardiovascular death rate association (*British Journal of Preventive and Social Medicine*, September, 1977).

Soft water also lacks other minerals—silicon, selenium and

chromium—all of which have demonstrated roles of their own in prevention of one phase or another of heart disease. Obviously then, soft water's relative deficiency of essential minerals makes it a poor investment toward better health. If that were its only shortcoming, however, the solution would be simple. To make up for the minerals missing in your water supply, you could make an extra effort to concentrate on high-fiber foods as well as foods crammed with calcium (like cottage cheese, yogurt and skim milk) and magnesium (such as whole grains, spinach, beans and nuts). Or supplement your diet with mineral tablets. In fact, if you pick up a bottle of dolomite, you'll be tapping the same source of calcium and magnesium that hard water supplies do.

Soft Water Adds Unwanted Minerals

Unfortunately, though, that's only the beginning of soft water's sorry story. For one thing, naturally soft water tends to be more acidic than hard water, and acidic water is better able to corrode pipes, leaching hazardous metals such as cadmium, lead and copper into home water supplies. (More on this in chapter 25, Canceling Out Lead and Other Harmful Substances.) But in view of the correlation between soft water and increased rate of stroke and heart attack deaths, it's interesting to note that cadmium is linked to high blood pressure, a major risk factor in cardiovascular disease. A St. Louis study showed that patients with high blood pressure had 50 times as much cadmium in their urine as people with normal blood pressure (*Internal Medicine and Diagnosis News*, vol. 5, no. 17, 1972). And in Kansas City, Kansas—where the cadmium content of drinking water is three times that of Kansas City, Missouri—there is a higher incidence of high blood pressure and many more deaths due to cardiovascular disease (*Medical World News*, October 11, 1974).

On the other hand, the calcium in hard water has been shown to limit the internal absorption of lead and cadmium.

"Softened" water (that is, hard water made soft through the removal of calcium and magnesium) is no more acidic than it was before the process. But it has another drawback—salt.

Water softeners, such as the type installed in home plumbing systems, work by a method called "ion exchange." It's a complicated procedure. But what they do, quite simply, is swap electrically charged particles of salt (sodium and chlorine ions) for the water's calcium and magnesium. Water is directed into a tank filled with sodium-charged plastic beads. When a magnesium or calcium ion contacts a bead, they are drawn together like magnets. A sodium particle is released into the water and the calcium or magnesium particle takes its place on the bead.

The amount of salt that eventually ends up in your water supply depends, of course, on the amount of calcium and magnesium it had to begin with. The more grains of hardness in the water, the more salt in the softened water.

TABLE 35 ## Salt Added When Water Is Softened

Initial Water Hardness (grams per gallon)	Sodium Added by Softening (milligrams per quart)
1	7.5
5	37.5
10	75
20	150
40	300

SOURCE: Reprinted from *Water Conditioning,* by James L. Gattis (Fayetteville, Ark.: Cooperative Extension Service, 1973).

Generally speaking, Americans consume about 5 to 15 times the amount of salt the body needs to function. And because salt is linked with high blood pressure and fluid retention, the added burden placed on the body by drinking salty softened water may cause health problems. In fact, two University of Massachusetts researchers have found that sodium in drinking water appears to increase blood pressure rates in persons as young as high school age (University of Massachusetts News Release, June 27, 1978). Beyond that, softened water also creates an added burden on the ground that eventually receives it.

For these reasons, water softeners should not be installed without careful consideration. Perhaps the most important question you need to ask is, "How hard is my water?"

You can test your own water for hardness. One of the most popular test kits among both water conditioning dealers and individuals is the kit for hardness measurement. It provides you with a quick, accurate method of checking the extent to which your water is softened. Tests are relatively easy to perform, utilizing a simplified version of the titration process done in larger laboratories. First add the hardness indicator to the sample, then add the titrating solution, one drop at a time. When the solution turns color, stop adding drops of the titrating solution. The number of drops you have used to bring about the color change is equal to the hardness in grains per gallon.

The largest manufacturer of water hardness test kits is Hach Chemical Company, P.O. Box 389, Loveland, CO 80537.

The British Regional Heart Study concluded that 170 milligrams per liter (about nine grains per gallon) was about medium hardness. Softer water increased risk of heart disease, while harder water added no extra benefit. If, after testing, you find that your water is only moderately hard, pass up the softening system. If, on the other hand, you discover that your water hardness is as you suspected—the source of all your plumbing bills— consider having a water softener hooked up to your hot water system only. After all, hot water pipes are most vulnerable to the scaling residue of minerals left in the wake of water evaporation. Besides, laundry, bathing, dishwashing, cleaning and home heating can benefit from the removal of the minerals that cause hardness, while at the same time, the family can enjoy drinking and cooking without added sodium.

You don't need softened water (and the resultant maintenance and expense) for watering lawns and gardens, or for flushing the toilet—and these are the only other cold water outlets in your home. In the kitchen sink or clothes washer, a mixture of softened hot water and hard cold water will give you satisfactory results.

27

Alcohol, Drugs and Food Ingredients That Meddle with Health-Building Minerals

Back in the days when a two-room cave with a view was deemed the height of luxurious living, people didn't use alcohol, caffeine, aspirin and antacids. In the course of civilizing ourselves, though, we've concocted all manner of stimulants, relaxers and relievers. Aside from other effects on the body, many everyday drugs turn minerals topsy-turvy.

The Ins and Outs of Alcohol

We don't know anyone who doesn't have to make frequent trips to the bathroom after heavy drinking. That happens because alcohol slows down the production of the hormone that helps keep the urge to urinate down to just a few times a day. So you have to go more often after drinking a lot of wine, beer or whiskey than you do after drinking a lot of plain water. And with every trip to the rest room, some minerals are lost. Most notably, heavy drinkers flush considerable amounts of zinc, copper, calcium, magnesium and potassium out of their systems.

Unlike food, which is digested in the stomach, alcohol charges straight to the liver to be split first into a toxic substance called acetaldehyde and then into the less odious acetic acid. Acetaldehyde is so nasty that a special squad of alcohol-splitting enzymes, called dehydrogenases, are deployed by the liver to break down the poison.

Zinc is a key part of alcohol dehydrogenase, making it the drinker's most critical mineral. Even armed with a tough mineral like zinc, though, alcohol enzymes need time. It takes about an hour for the liver to process a can of beer, a glass of wine, or a highball. And it takes a couple of days at least for the body to rally all of its forces for the next attack—more if the encounter has been especially bacchanalian, like a wedding celebration. The job is hard enough without an unrelenting flood of booze. Heavy drinkers use up so much zinc that a deficiency among alcoholics is quite common. Because zinc-containing dehydrogenase enzymes also liberate vitamin A, a vitamin critical to eyesight, from the liver, night blindness and other vision problems are common in heavy drinkers.

Drink too much, too often, for too long, and the liver becomes diseased, or cirrhotic, under the stress of trying to deal with the abuse. Such liver problems, too, could be exacerbated by zinc losses. Zinc is needed for all tissue repair, including a damaged liver. Wound healing of all sorts—including recovery from surgery—is delayed by heavy drinking.

Too much alcohol also affects bone strength by interfering with the conversion of vitamin D into the active form that maintains calcium balance. When calcium metabolism goes awry, absorption is blocked, and bones weaken, increasing the risk of fractures, osteoporosis and osteomalacia (*Journal of Chemical Education,* vol. 56, no. 8, 1979).

Nonstop drinking puts rude demands on the digestive system, demands that force our body to ignore essential nutrients. Alcohol consumption results in changes in the small intestine—changes that allow food to be flushed from the body before minerals can be absorbed. (Minerals aren't the only nutrients stolen by alcohol. B vitamins, especially thiamine, folate and B_{12}, are either poorly absorbed, or excreted in larger amounts, so needs for them go up, too.)

Alcohol is a frequent but usually overlooked cause of magnesium deficiency in heavy drinkers, says Edmund B. Flink, M.D., Ph.D., professor of medicine at West Virginia University in Morgantown, West Virginia. Heavy drinkers often skip meals, deriving too many calories from alcohol and too few from food. To compound the problem, much of the food they do eat is devoid of magnesium. Dr. Flink cites sugar, starches and soft drinks as the prime offenders (*Modern Medicine,* November 15, 1979).

For those who drink moderately—and only on occasion—eating the right foods can help counteract alcohol's effect on minerals. Think back to the last cocktail party you attended. Did the host sidle up to you with a tray of frankfurters wrapped in biscuit dough? Was the buffet loaded with chips and dip? Or cheese spread and taco-flavored crackers? Those foods are notoriously low in minerals. The host who serves chopped liver is unknowingly replenishing some of the zinc and copper flushed out by champagne and whiskey sours. Nuts—cashews, pistachios, Brazil nuts, almonds—are rich in zinc, magnesium and potassium. Fresh fruit flanking the cheese wedges also offers plenty of potassium to replace that washed out by Napa Valley's best. Crisp stalks of broccoli festooning bowls of yogurt dip help bolster calcium against the ravages of alcohol.

One more thing we think you should know. Until about 25 years ago, it was widely spoken that a heavy drinker could avoid outright liver disease by eating a good diet. A number of studies since then have indicated that's just not true. Out-and-out heavy drinking is nutritional embezzlement—always on the taking end, never quite balancing the books. No matter how much he or she eats, the really heavy drinker is likely to develop nutritional deficiencies one way or the other.

All about Antacids

Antacids settle queasy, achy stomach distress for many people, evidently by temporarily reducing stomach acidity. The chief ingredients in most antacids are aluminum, magnesium, calcium and sodium, or combinations thereof (see table 36). For an occasional bout of indigestion, antacids are fairly harmless. Daily use in high doses, however, can present serious problems.

Aluminum hydroxide in high doses not only causes constipation, but also binds with phosphorus in the intestine. So instead of being passed on to the bloodstream to be installed in cells of bones and teeth, and in enzymes, phosphorus is carried out of the body as waste, like a cherished piece of silverware mistakenly thrown out with the trash. Immediate symptoms may be loss of appetite, listlessness, general discomfort, irritability and weakness—the latter because muscles are starved of phosphorus in the energy-transporting body compound, adenosine triphosphate, or ATP (discussed in chapter 4). Because phosphorus also affects calcium metabolism, use of antacids day in and day out for months or years can result in the weakened bones of osteomalacia (adult rickets). That's especially true when the diet is low in protein and phosphorus-containing food.

Most susceptible are people who turn to antacids regularly for stomach distress. Peptic ulcer is the single major reason. The traditional ulcer diet of milk, cream and bland foods (high in calcium, phosphorus and protein) is no longer routine treatment for ulcers. It's been replaced by a more liberal diet, punctuated by use of relatively high doses of antacids several times a day. That regimen is more attractive and convenient to ulcer patients, and seems to head off recurrent ulcer attacks just as well as the bland diet, if not better.

TABLE 36 ## Sodium and Chief Ingredients of Some Antacids

Product	Dosage Forms	Sodium	Ingredients
Alka Seltzer	Effervescent tablet	552 mg/2 tablets	Sodium bicarbonate, citric acid and potassium bicarbonate
AlternaGel	Suspension (to be taken with liquid)	2 mg/teaspoon	Aluminum hydroxide
Aludrox	Tablet Suspension	3.2 mg/2 tablets 1.1 mg/teaspoon	Aluminum and magnesium hydroxides
Amphojel	Tablet Suspension	2.8 mg/2 tablets 7 mg/teaspoon	Aluminum hydroxides
Baking soda	Powder	1,123 mg/teaspoon	Sodium bicarbonate
Basaljel	Tablet Suspension Capsule	4.1 mg/2 tablets 2.4 mg/teaspoon 5.6 mg/2 capsules	Aluminum carbonate and hydroxide
Basaljel Extra Strength	Suspension	17 mg/teaspoon	Aluminum hydroxide
Bisodol	Tablet Powder	.072 mg/2 tablets 157 mg/teaspoon	Calcium and magnesium carbonates, sodium bicarbonate, peppermint oil
Camalox	Tablet Suspension	3 mg/2 tablets 2.5 mg/teaspoon	Calcium carbonate with aluminum and magnesium hydroxides
Chooz	Gum tablet	6.3 mg/2 tablets	Calcium carbonate, magnesium trisilicate
Creamalin	Tablet	82 mg/2 tablets	Aluminum and magnesium hydroxides
Delcid	Suspension	15 mg/teaspoon	Aluminum and magnesium hydroxides
Di-Gel	Tablet Liquid	21.2 mg/2 tablets 8.3 mg/teaspoon	Aluminum and magnesium hydroxide, magnesium carbonate, simethicone

TABLE 36 (continued)

Product	Dosage Forms	Sodium	Ingredients
Eugel	Tablet Suspension	0.26 mg/2 tablets 3.9 mg/teaspoon	Aluminum hydroxide, magnesium carbonate, aminoacetic acid, calcium carbonate
Gelusil	Tablet Suspension	3.4 mg/2 tablets 0.8 mg/teaspoon	Aluminum and magnesium hydroxides, simethicone
Gelusil-II	Tablet Suspension	5.4 mg/2 tablets 1.3 mg/teaspoon	Aluminum and magnesium hydroxides, simethicone
Gelusil M	Tablet Suspension	5.6 mg/2 tablets 1.3 mg/teaspoon	Aluminum and magnesium hydroxides, simethicone
Kolantyl	Tablet Gel	30 mg/2 tablets Less than 5 mg/ teaspoon	Aluminum and magnesium hydroxides
Kudrox	Tablet Suspension	32 mg/2 tablets 15 mg/teaspoon	Aluminum and magnesium hydroxides and magnesium carbonate Aluminum and magnesium hydroxides
Maalox	Suspension	2.5 mg/teaspoon	Aluminum and magnesium hydroxides
Maalox #1	Tablet	1.7 mg/2 tablets	Aluminum and magnesium hydroxides
Maalox #2	Tablet	3.6 mg/2 tablets	Aluminum and magnesium hydroxides
Maalox Plus	Tablet Suspension	2.8 mg/2 tablets 2.5 mg/teaspoon	Aluminum and magnesium hydroxides, simethicone
Mylanta	Tablet Suspension	Trace	Aluminum and magnesium hydroxides, simethicone
Mylanta-II	Tablet Suspension	Trace	Aluminum and magnesium hydroxides, simethicone

TABLE 36 (continued)

Product	Dosage Forms	Sodium	Ingredients
Riopan	Tablet Suspension	1.3 mg/2 tablets 0.64 mg/teaspoon	Magaldrate
Riopan Plus	Tablet Suspension	1.3 mg/2 tablets 0.64 mg/teaspoon	Magaldrate, simethicone
Rolaids	Tablet	106 mg/2 tablets	Dihydroxyaluminum, sodium carbonate
Titralac	Tablet Suspension	0.6 mg/2 tablets 11 mg/teaspoon	Calcium carbonate, glycine
Tums	Tablet	5.4 mg/2 tablets	Calcium carbonate, peppermint oil
WinGel	Tablet Suspension	5 mg/2 tablets 2.5 mg/teaspoon	Aluminum and magnesium hydroxides

SOURCES: Adapted from
Handbook of Nonprescription Drugs, 6th ed., ed. L. Luan Corrigan National
Professional Society of Pharmacists (Washington, D.C.: American Pharmaceutical
Association, 1979).
AMA Drug Evaluations, 3rd ed., AMA Department of Drugs (Littleton, Mass.:
PSG Publishing, 1977).
NOTES: mg = milligram
For comparison purposes, 2 tablets and 1 teaspoon doses have been used. These
are not necessarily equivalent doses. Refer to manufacturers' labels for recom-
mended doses.

Quaffing down daily doses of liquid antacid resulted in crippling
pain and bone loss for one woman. The *Journal of the American Medical
Association* (December 5, 1980) tells of a 60-year-old lady—tired, depressed
and anxious—who was admitted to a hospital in Rochester, New York,
when she could no longer get out of her chair or walk due to pain and
weakness in her legs. X-rays showed overall bone loss, brittleness and a
fractured bone in her left leg. Blood tests showed phosphorus levels had hit
rock bottom. No other nutrients seemed to be affected.

Her symptoms and complaints, however, closely matched those
seen in healthy volunteers studied after prolonged treatment with aluminum-
containing antacids. As it turned out, the woman had been taking 360
milliliters or more of an over-the-counter aluminum-containing hydroxide
antacid for heartburnlike discomfort daily for the past six months—triple
what she'd been taking for the previous 12 years. That continued overuse
of antacid, say the doctors reporting the case, was the cause of her problem.

The woman was sent home with strict instructions to avoid *all* antacids. "Within one month after discharge, the patient noted dramatic ... improvement," say the authors, from the endocrine-metabolism unit, department of medicine, University of Rochester School of Medicine and Dentistry. She could once again get up out of her chair without help, and walk. The pain in her legs was practically gone. And two months later, she was walking freely about, with no pain whatsoever. X-rays showed that the fracture had healed and her bones were again growing strong and solid. Blood levels of phosphorus rose to normal.

Her case is not all that rare, the authors add. Many elderly people—already at risk due to poor dietary habits—suffer increased chances of bone loss, not only from use of over-the-counter remedies, but from routinely prescribed antacids. "Reports of this syndrome continue to appear, suggesting a need for increased awareness of this potential complication of antacid therapy."

Another doctor echoes concern that as broad use of antacids for ulcers and other disorders increases, so will phosphorus losses. And it may not necessarily take 12 years for damage to show up. According to Helen Shields, M.D., of the gastrointestinal section, department of medicine, University of Pennsylvania in Philadelphia, susceptible people can show serious phosphorus losses after only two weeks of high doses (360 milliliters) of aluminum hydroxide-containing antacids, even when eating generous amounts of phosphorus (*Gastroenterology,* December, 1978).

Magnesium compounds cause their own problem—diarrhea. For that reason, they're rarely used alone as an antacid but are usually combined with a calcium or aluminum compound, with dosage adjusted to reduce the effects. When magnesium compounds are used expressly for their laxative effect, they can raise magnesium levels undesirably high in people with faulty kidney function.

Calcium-containing antacids were once considered the ultimate in antacids, but they put people with high blood pressure or previous kidney disease at risk of kidney stones or partial kidney failure. They should be used with caution.

Baking soda, or sodium bicarbonate, is an old-time remedy for stomach woes that is neither safe nor natural. While baking soda may neutralize acid, it contains over 1 gram (1,000 milligrams) of sodium per teaspoon—as much as a few hefty sprinklings of salt on your food. Sodium encourages high blood pressure, which can damage the kidneys and cause a risk of heart failure, so that puts baking soda out of the question as a regular ulcer remedy and casts serious doubt on its place in the kitchen medicine cabinet even for occasional distress.

A few commercial antacids contain sodium bicarbonate as a chief ingredient. Alka Seltzer and Rolaids contain the most.

To top it off, all antacids suppress iron absorption when used in large amounts. So what that boils down to is that there is no ideal antacid. Certain ones may be less harmful for some people than others, but none should be used indiscriminately. Avoiding offending agents like alcohol, cigarettes, coffee, tea and cola drinks can cut down the need for antacids in the first place. Food, too, can buffer the effects of too much acid in the stomach, so small snacks may sometimes do just as well as antacids.

Aspirin Leaches Iron Out of Blood

Aspirin irritates the stomach lining and can cause bleeding. Every time you pop a couple of aspirin, you stand to lose about a teaspoon of blood. And along with it trickle out two milligrams of iron.

Granted, aspirin is one of the quickest and most effective ways to reduce fever. (The cause, of course, should be treated.) Used daily for the discomforts of arthritis, joint swelling and inflammation, muscle soreness, and nerve or headache pain, however, aspirin use can eventually lead to iron deficiency anemia. (By the way, the aspirin you take for the pounding headache of a hangover hits your stomach with a brutal one-two punch. When inflamed by overuse of alcohol, your sour and sensitive stomach is most vulnerable to aspirin's irritating effects.)

Buffered aspirin doesn't actually buffer the irritation; food and water do, though. If you absolutely must take aspirin, take it with a snack, meal, milk or a full glass of water. A diet of iron-rich foods, like liver, green vegetables, blackstrap molasses, raisins, nuts, soybeans, lentils and fish, also helps to make up for losses.

Diuretics Pull the Plug on Minerals

Prescription drugs, too, can deplete minerals. Diuretics, often prescribed to control high blood pressure, flush potassium, zinc and phosphorus out of the body. Doctors are aware of that, and many prescribe potassium supplements along with the drug, or urge patients to eat oranges, bananas or other high-potassium foods. Some diuretics, and thiazide diuretics in particular, also flush out magnesium. Physicians rarely take that into consideration, even though simultaneous potassium and magnesium losses can trigger irregular heartbeat, a serious if not disconcerting side effect.

"Magnesium deficiency [in diuretic therapy] is fairly common, but it often goes undiagnosed or simply ignored," writes Dr. Edmund Flink in the same report that discussed the diuretic effect of alcohol on magnesium (*Modern Medicine,* November 15, 1979).

Diuretics also flush phosphorus out of the body before it has a chance to be absorbed. David Juan, M.D., who studied low phosphate levels in 100 patients at the St. Vincent Hospital and Medical Center in Toledo, Ohio, found diuretics and heavy alcohol use to be two of the factors likely to cause phosphorus loss (*Annals of Internal Medicine,* December, 1978).

Thiazide diuretics also step up zinc excretion by as much as 50 percent. So chronic diuretic therapy may result in impaired wound healing with little suspicion of the cause.

What about Coffee?

Unfortunately, all those effects of diuretics have received scant attention in the medical setting and still less outside doctors' offices. And as far as we know, no one has studied the diuretic effect of coffee and tea on mineral levels in healthy people. But to the extent that those beverages send us off to the bathroom more frequently, it's highly probable that they, too, flush out minerals. And when minerals go down the drain, we're up the creek.

Corticosteroids Squander Minerals

Used to treat a long list of ailments, from asthma, hay fever and arthritis to some forms of cancer, corticosteroid drugs are synthetic versions of the hormones produced in our adrenal glands, which sit on top of each kidney. Prednisone and cortisone are two familiar examples.

Like other powerful drugs, corticosteroids (or steroids, for short) carry side effects that must be carefully watched. Aside from other metabolic effects, potassium levels nose-dive during corticosteroid therapy, leaving muscles weak. Cardiac arrest can occur unless losses are replaced by potassium-rich food or supplements. For people taking diuretics along with corticosteroids, sodium restriction is practically mandatory, and prescription of potassium supplements would also be helpful.

Corticosteroids burn up vitamin D and stifle calcium absorption, contributing to the development of osteoporosis and setting the stage for fractures—unless calcium intake is boosted. Calcium and magnesium are lost in the urine. As a result, wrists and feet can go into spasms.

Steroids also flush out zinc, leaving those under treatment more prone to bedsores and skin ulcers. Wound healing is delayed. Under increased stress—disease, respiratory infection, or surgery, for example— steroid therapy is often stepped up to help the patient get through the trauma. At that time, needs for potassium, calcium, magnesium and zinc are at their highest.

Aside from aspirin, antacids, diuretics and corticosteroids, there is a plethora of still other strong prescription drugs that, in the course of doing their duty, may carry similar liabilities.

EDTA, the Preservative
That Pries Iron Away from Food

Just as there are enhancers of iron absorption (vitamin C, copper and meat), there are also substances that stand in the way of the process.

One of the most commonly used preservatives in our food, EDTA (or disodium ethylenediaminetetraacetate, as it's known by food chemists) is a metal scavenger with a particular fondness for iron. EDTA chelates, or binds up the mineral so it can't enter our bloodstream.

EDTA pops up around every corner in the supermarket. Salad dressing and mayonnaise are its favorite haunts. Sandwich spreads and sauces have it. So do some canned foods. It works behind the scenes in soda, beer and liquor, although the labels don't tell you so. (Trade secrets prevail here.) Researchers at the University of Washington and Kansas University Medical Center estimate that the typical American diet contains about 50 milligrams of EDTA a day. To the extent that a person eats canned or commercially processed foods and beverages, it can go as high as 500 milligrams.

Knowing that EDTA holds iron hostage in our systems, James D. Cook, M.D., and Elaine R. Monsen, Ph.D., decided to measure its actual effect on iron absorption. They fed a diet containing 4.1 milligrams of iron to 45 men, divided into two groups. One diet contained 50 milligrams EDTA, the other contained none. Iron absorption was reduced by approximately half in the EDTA-loaded diet (*American Journal of Clinical Nutrition,* June, 1976). For people at risk of low iron from poor diet, such as the elderly, or with increased needs, such as menstruating women, the amount of EDTA encountered daily can make an important difference in how much iron is absorbed. Dieters, snow-blinded by mounds of cottage cheese, yogurt and skim milk (all low in iron), may at the same time be shrinking away from iron-rich foods, like liver and legumes, making themselves easy victims for iron robbery by EDTA.

How can you tell if food contains EDTA? It's not easy. Sometimes it's on the roll call of ingredients; sometimes it's not. Your best bet is to look for products clearly labeled as being preservative-free. Or make your own sauces and dressings. Try to use as few packaged foods as possible. Avoid—or at least pare down—soda, beer and liquor consumption. At the same time, be sure to eat iron-rich foods—soybeans, lentils, raisins, liver, green vegetables. And if you find yourself boxed in on all sides by EDTA, iron supplements help to shore up reserves.

Phosphates, Another Iron Blockade

Used as food additives in soft drinks, ice cream, candy, beer, baked goods and other foods, phosphates, like EDTA, bind with iron. What's more, both phosphates and EDTA are likely to show up in the same meal, putting iron in double jeopardy.

Again, labeling is a catch-as-catch-can affair. We can't say how much added phosphate you have to eat or drink before iron debts mount up. The research simply isn't there. Use your best judgment: eating too much pastry and junk food is clearly not in your best interests from a couple of standpoints, especially when they replace more nutritious goodies.

Tea and Red Wine, Bad Influences on Iron

Tannin, a natural component of tea and most red wine, is a well-known inhibitor of iron absorption.

Researchers in Sweden observed that the lowest absorption at various breakfast meals usually occurred when tea was added. Their main findings reaffirmed that dietary iron intake must be considered in terms of total meal composition, not just food sources of iron themselves.

There is a clear relationship between what you eat for breakfast and your body's absorption of iron. Tea has the greatest negative effect and orange juice the greatest positive effect. And this, the researchers conclude, is very important to know—especially for persons who are known to have a critical iron balance: for example, pregnant women and women with heavy menstrual losses, or schoolchildren, especially at periods of rapid growth (*American Journal of Clinical Nutrition,* December, 1979).

If you enjoy a hot beverage with breakfast or as a midday pick-me-up, try herb teas. They have no tannins and therefore do not block iron absorption.

And if you're in the habit of enjoying an occasional glass of wine with your evening meal, keep in mind that young red wines also contain tannins. In making red wines, the grapes' skins remain in the juice during fermentation, which may take several weeks. Heat and fermentation draw tannins and pigment out of the skins, which are discarded before bottling. In older red wine, the tannins eventually break down as the bottled wine ages. So the older the wine, the lower its tannin content. Rosés, however, are relatively tannin-free, for the skins are removed just a few hours after fermentation begins. White wines contain virtually no tannins—skins are removed before the juice hits the vats.

Sugar Jacks Up Sodium's Effect on Blood Pressure

A stampede of sugary food into the diet throws the complex regulatory systems of the body out of whack. One of those systems is our blood pressure. Too much sodium in itself sways people toward high blood pressure; adding sugar can augment that effect.

In research on rats, a team of food and nutrition scientists at the University of Maryland found that sucrose in the diet seemed to depress production of sucrose in the body, and that this in turn lowered the amount of sodium excreted from the body (*Journal of Nutrition,* April, 1980). Exactly how each of the steps in the chain of events leads to the next has not been determined, but the general hypothesis is, the more sugar you eat, the more sodium is retained by the body.

In an earlier study, Richard A. Ahrens, Ph.D., a University of Maryland nutritionist, discovered that sugar causes problems for people as well as for rats (*Federation Proceedings,* vol. 34, 1975, abstract no. 3914). "We found that people fed sucrose experienced significant elevations of blood pressure," Dr. Ahrens told us. "That was a five-week study. At an intake of 200 grams [about a cup] of sucrose a day, the blood pressures averaged 5 points higher. Those eating 200 grams averaged 78 points diastolic, while those who were not eating any sucrose averaged 73 points diastolic. That was a change of 5 points in five weeks.

"We were very careful to stay within the range of typical sugar consumption in this country," Dr. Ahrens added. "The highest levels we fed were 20 percent of the total calories in the diet. We observed striking changes in blood pressure as low as the 10 percent levels."

In a nutshell, that means that if you're free and easy with the sugar bowl, candy bars, soda and desserts, you may be bullying your heart and arteries into needless hardship.

Too Much Sodium Washes Out Calcium

Aside from sodium's sinister effect on blood pressure, it can also increase calcium losses. That's probably due to stepped-up parathyroid gland activity, which in turn speeds up turnover of bone minerals, spilling calcium into the urine. In other words, too much salt—in effect—steals calcium from the bones and flushes it out in the urine.

That could mean big trouble for a lot of people—namely anyone who eats little calcium to begin with or who doesn't absorb calcium very well—and *especially* those older people prone to the fracture-ridden bones of osteoporosis. Those implications surfaced out of experiments run by Ailsa Goulding of the department of medicine, University of Otago, Dunedin, New Zealand. In one experiment, the researcher fed extra salt to several rats at normal and low levels of dietary calcium intake. Extra salt increased urinary calcium losses for all. More critically, rats on the low-calcium diet ended up with smaller, lighter, mineral-poorer bones than did controls who ate the same amount of calcium but no added salt. Because salt exaggerates the bone loss of poor calcium nutrition, the researcher says, "a high salt intake may play a role in the [development] of

osteoporosis in some individuals" (*Mineral and Electrolyte Metabolism,*
vol. 4, no. 4, 1980).

Too Much Protein Drives Calcium Down and Out

It sometimes happens that too much of one perfectly wholesome
nutrient seriously interferes with the body's ability to use another. Protein
and calcium work that way. When we eat relatively large amounts of
protein, we can produce a serious washout of calcium.

Here's what happens. A certain amount of protein must be around
for calcium to be taken up by the cells lining the intestine. When we eat too
much extra protein—about two or more times what we need—calcium
absorption is speeded up. That would be fine, except that our kidneys seem
to panic at all that extra calcium floating their way and extravagantly dump
it into the urine before it can be delivered to bones and other tissues, where
it's direly needed.

Most of us need about 50 grams of protein a day—a little less for
women, a little more for men, and an extra 20 or 30 grams for pregnant
women or breastfeeding mothers. But many of us eat twice as much
protein as we actually need. Most of it comes from red meat and poultry,
the most concentrated forms of protein.

Ham and eggs at breakfast give us 50 grams all by themselves. A
chicken salad sandwich at lunch adds about 35 grams. Chuck roast or a
hamburger at dinner adds another 25 or 30. Total so far? About 110 or
115 grams. And that doesn't count protein in beans, milk, cheese, yogurt,
grains and other foods we may have eaten during the day.

Researchers compared calcium levels in people first eating recommended (low) levels of protein and then the elevated levels typical of most
Americans. Women in the study went from 43 grams a day during the first
part of the experimental period to 110 grams in the second. Men jumped
from 50 to 113 grams. Calcium, magnesium and phosphorus levels
remained the same. Far more calcium was carted away in the urine—and
less retained in the body—during the high-protein phase of the experiment
than the low-protein phase, report the scientists, nutritionists at the
University of Wisconsin (*Journal of Nutrition,* February, 1980). Their
work was prompted by earlier studies in the field which showed serious
calcium losses at still higher intakes of protein.

Coupled with the fact that calcium absorption seems to decline
with age, the conclusions are sobering. In women over the age of 50, that
loss of calcium can be extremely important, with serious ill effects on the
strength of bones, on posture and on muscle tone. Women of any age who
are following a high-protein diet are also creating a dangerous situation for

themselves. Supplemental calcium may not necessarily be able to offset the situation—the best bet would be to avoid a lot of extra protein.

The Anti-Iron Factor in Eggs

One large egg is listed in all the nutrition textbooks and U.S. Department of Agriculture food tables as containing 1.2 milligrams of iron, so eating two for breakfast ought to give you 2.4 milligrams of iron, which is a very useful amount. But the fact is (which many people do not realize), there is an anti-iron factor in eggs—a phosphoprotein in the yolks—which binds up the mineral and makes it very poorly available. That factor may even render iron in *other* foods you eat with your eggs less available.

Cow's Milk Is No Boon to Mineral Nutrition

Infants absorb minerals less efficiently from cow's milk than from mother's milk. For one, iron in human milk is more efficiently absorbed than that in cow's milk, which provides only small amounts anyway. And the availability and absorption of zinc from human milk is enhanced by the presence of a special prostaglandin hormone not found in cow's milk. The immune response to infection and disease depends on adequate zinc. Because a child's immune status is just beginning to develop during the first six months of life, it's important that zinc status be sound.

Calcium, too, is affected. Studies with infants show that feeding whole cow's milk results in lower calcium absorption. The long-chain saturated fatty acids in cow's milk form insoluble soaps with calcium in the intestine and slip out in the form of fatty, malodorous stools before calcium can be absorbed. Steatorrhea (by its textbook name) is less of a problem in breastfed infants.

* * * * * *

Putting it all together, we can see that a barrage of drugs and chemicals hitting our bodies one after the other is not totally kind to minerals. And to encourage mineral losses by letting reserves slip through poor diet is downright foolish.

PART IV

MAKING THE MOST OF MINERALS IN OUR FOOD

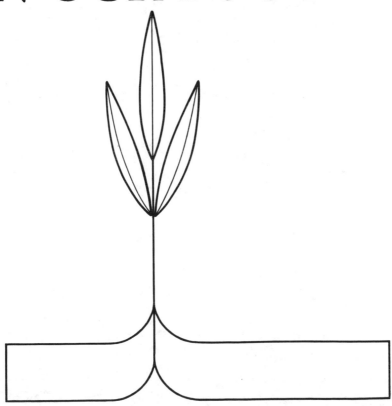

28

Vitamins and Minerals That Work Together

Some minerals are eager workers, but to perform their best they need a vitamin or two to stir them to action. And while each has its own special health-giving talents, some minerals team up with certain vitamins to tackle important jobs that would be impossible for vitamins to do alone. A few vitamin-mineral coalitions are well known; others might surprise you.

Vitamin D, the Calcium Dispatcher

Calcium, as we've seen, is undoubtedly the most important structural component of the body. Bones and teeth grow best with plenty of calcium. Membranes stay taut and tidy. Calcium also sees that muscles contract when they should and that nerve messages travel smoothly. Without vitamin D, though, calcium is caught in a deadlock. We could eat a ton of calcium and still have problems, if we didn't get enough vitamin D.

Thyroid and parathyroid hormones are substances released by our glands to regulate growth. With their help, vitamin D masterfully governs our body levels of calcium, as well as calcium's aide-de-camp, phosphorus. Vitamin D keeps circulating levels of calcium and phosphorus from dipping perilously low. First, vitamin D stimulates the intestinal absorption of calcium. Otherwise, calcium would slip right on through the body. And vitamin D stimulates the transport of phosphorus, prodding it along its way in the system.

When calcium intake slips a bit, the parathyroid hormones signal the kidneys to hold back on calcium they would otherwise unload into the urine. At the same time, the parathyroid frees vitamin D from storage—primarily in the liver. With more vitamin D around, more calcium is retained overall—a very efficient setup. If calcium intake drops *too* low, vitamin D borrows calcium from bone to keep blood and other tissues satisfied. (A lag in dietary phosphorus, although far less likely, prompts a similar release of vitamin D, but without the intercession of the parathyroid gland.)

Borrowing calcium from bone is like spending our capital for lack of income. It's all right as a short-term effort to keep nerves and muscles—like the heart—supplied. Carried on for months or years, though, it can lead to virtual calcium bankruptcy of bones—osteoporosis.

Without enough vitamin D in the first place, though, even adequate calcium can't reach the bone. In children, the result is rickets—knock knees and weak, spongy legs bowed under the simple strain of supporting the body. In adult rickets (or osteomalacia), bones don't give. They break.

Because vitamin D is essential in several phases of calcium and bone metabolism, it's the major preventive factor in rickets. By helping to maximize calcium in the diet, vitamin D may also have some role in fending off osteoporosis.

A few foods have smidgens of vitamin D—butter, cream, egg yolk and liver. But you'd have to gorge yourself on them to get any useful amounts of the vitamin. Fish—notably herring, mackerel, salmon, sardines and tuna—have far more, as do fish liver oils and vitamin D-fortified milk.

Our chief source of vitamin D, though, is sunlight. Vitamin D in sunlight is soaked up by little solar collector-like cells in the skin, passed on to the bloodstream, and carried to the liver and kidneys. (Vitamin D from food ends up there, too.) There it's zapped into its active forms. In fact, at that point vitamin D takes the form of a hormone rather than simply a vitamin. Endowed with its new entity, vitamin D is either deployed for immediate use, retained in the liver, or sent back to the skin and bones for auxiliary warehousing.

A regular spritzing of sunshine will generally supply all the vitamin D we need to keep calcium levels humming. Most of us probably get our quota of sun exposure in the course of our daily lives—at least during the summer months. People at possible risk, though, are those who:

— live in smoggy, sunless areas

— work at night and sleep during the day (actors, night auditors, some nurses or factory shift workers)

— clothe themselves from head to toe, out of custom or climatic necessity

— stay indoors, either because they are disabled or because they prefer it that way.

Some elderly people may fall into the last category. In any case, fish liver oil supplements may make up for lack of sunshine in special circumstances.

Get *too much* vitamin D, though, and the system becomes too efficient for its own good. Enormous doses over a long period of time provoke overcalcification of bone and soft tissues, among other problems. Although that's not likely, it's something to bear in mind.

Vitamin C Lends a Helping Hand to Calcium and Iron

Vitamin C, too, may aid calcium absorption. In an Egyptian study, investigators gave an oral dose of calcium phosphate to a group of rats. Some of the animals also received vitamin C; others were given pepper juice or orange juice (both rich natural sources of vitamin C). Later, the investigators measured the calcium levels in the rats' blood. "Our data showed that giving samples of ascorbic acid [vitamin C] together with calcium enhanced the rate of its intestinal absorption," the researchers reported. Pepper and orange juice also improved absorption, they added (*Zeitschrift für Ernährungswissenschaft,* vol. 15, no. 4, 1976).

As for iron, vitamin C can do more for improving iron status than adding more iron. According to studies done by James D. Cook, M.D., and Elaine R. Monsen, Ph.D., the addition of vitamin C to a meal can dramatically enhance the absorption of iron. A daily supplement of 280 milligrams of vitamin C, they report, can double iron absorption— allowing us to get twice as much out of the iron we eat, in other words. If that dose were divided and taken with each meal, they add, the rate of absorption would more than triple (*American Journal of Clinical Nutrition,* February, 1977).

Talk about squeezing the most mileage out of your nutritional fuel supply! Seventy-five to 90 milligrams at each meal from food or supplements would do it. Foods rich in vitamin C are oranges and other citrus fruits and juices; broccoli, brussels sprouts and other dark green leafy vegetables; green peppers, cabbage, pimientos, tomatoes, cantaloupes and strawberries.

B Vitamins for Iron-Rich Blood

Blood doesn't thrive on iron alone. At least two B vitamins that we know of help foster a steady stream of new blood cells from our bone marrow.

Without the B vitamin folate, the body cannot manufacture some of the molecular building blocks of DNA. DNA is the secret of cell division. Less folate means less DNA, which means a slowdown in the creation of new cells, including red blood cells—*even if iron is adequate.*

A team of University of Florida and University of Miami researchers were surprised by low folate levels when they studied blood samples from 193 elderly, low-income volunteers in the Coconut Grove section of Miami, Florida. Knowing that they would discover a high rate of nutrition-related anemia (an abnormally low concentration of red blood cells or hemoglobin) in the group, the researchers hoped to single out the cause of the anemia. The missing link wasn't iron. It was folate.

"These findings . . . point out the fallacy of the rather widespread assumption that anemia always reflects dietary iron deficiency," the Florida study noted. "It is important to reassess the true incidence of iron deficiency worldwide in view of mounting evidence of the extent of folacin deficiency" (*American Journal of Clinical Nutrition,* November, 1979).

Liver is the best source of folate (as well as other B vitamins). Conveniently, liver is also a primary source of iron, plus zinc and copper. Folate can also be found in lentils, other beans of various kinds, and most vegetables. Whole grain bread, meat and eggs are moderately good sources of folate.

Vitamin B_2, or riboflavin, also pulls iron out of the doldrums. Riboflavin seems to improve iron utilization and rejuvenation of red blood cells. A study of riboflavin-deficient school children aged 9 to 12 compared iron metabolism before and after they were given riboflavin. Hemoglobin levels rose significantly. And those children who started out with the lowest levels showed the greatest improvement.

The researchers aren't sure exactly how or to what extent riboflavin plays a part. One hunch is that, directly or indirectly, riboflavin regulates the production of red blood cells. In any case, they remark that "absorption and utilization of dietary iron depends on . . . a number of factors of which inadequate riboflavin nutrition status may play a role" (*International Journal of Vitamin and Nutrition Research,* vol. 49, no. 2, 1979).

Foods that supply us with riboflavin include almonds, asparagus, broccoli, cheese, milk, eggs, organ meats, wheat germ and whole grain products.

Vitamin E and Selenium
Rally the Immune System

Vitamin E's role in immune defense has been recognized for some time. The way research is going, it looks as if selenium is intimately related to vitamin E.

Evidently, a special enzyme, glutathione peroxidase (GSH-Px for short) is not only dependent on selenium, but thanks to selenium may also play a critical role in the immune response.

A diet low in selenium and vitamin E will result in low levels of GSH-Px activity. When GSH-Px activity is low, the health of the white blood cells suffers, lessening their natural ability to fight disease and infection. When selenium is adequate, then, GSH-Px theoretically may increase natural resistance by helping white blood cells to clear out bacteria, viruses and cancer cells. Vitamin E enhances that effect.

To varying degrees, selenium and vitamin E cancel out the harmful effects of pollution, ozone (in smog, for instance) and certain toxic metals—notably cadmium, mercury, silver and possibly lead.

Good food sources of vitamin E include vegetable oils (safflower, sesame, soybean, sunflower seed, corn and olive oils), sunflower seeds and wheat germ, and almonds and filberts.

Zinc, the Patron Mineral of Vitamin A

Since so many vitamins seem to enhance the work of minerals, it seems only natural that some minerals aid vitamins.

Zinc liberates vitamin A from storage sites in the liver and changes it into a form that improves our vision in dim light. In more than one study, people with night blindness (poor adaptation to the dark) who didn't respond to vitamin A supplements alone, did respond when zinc was added.

Several reports show that zinc also helps maintain just the right amount of vitamin A circulating in the blood (*Journal of Nutrition,* September, 1978). That's important, for vitamin A is also involved in reproduction, plus maintenance and repair of skeleton and epithelial cells (the lining of skin and organs). And, like zinc, vitamin A plays a big role in immunity. Both help boost the work of the thymus gland, a chief agent in our defense system.

Cod liver oil and fish liver oil are unusually high sources of vitamin A. Other dietary sources include animal products (liver, kidney, cheese and skim milk). Certain vegetables contain carotene, a substance the body converts into vitamin A. Go for the green and gold: dark green leafy vegetables (like collards and turnip greens), carrots, sweet potatoes, squash and yellow fruit—apricots, peaches and cantaloupes especially. The deeper green or yellow the food, the more vitamin A it contains.

Zinc Also Unleashes Folate from Food

Researchers at the University of California, Berkeley, found that when healthy volunteers were put on a diet that depleted their reserves of zinc, the absorption of that B vitamin dropped sharply. Why? The folate-containing compounds in foods, polyglutamyl folates, must be split by an enzyme before folate can be absorbed. And that enzyme, they suggest, requires zinc (*Federation Proceedings,* March 1, 1978, abstract no. 1479).

Other Partners in Health

Vitamin B_{12} depends on a couple of minerals to function. Calcium eases the absorption of B_{12} through the intestinal wall. Manganese (along with the B vitamins niacin and riboflavin) converts vitamin B_{12} into its active form. And, of course, cobalt is an integral part of the vitamin itself. Animal foods appear to be our only source of B_{12}, although there is some evidence that a few strict vegetarians may be able to manufacture it in their digestive tracts. Some fortified brewer's yeasts also contribute vitamin B_{12}.

The B vitamins thiamine and biotin contain sulfur in their molecules. Because sulfur is an integral part of protein, a diet that is adequate in protein supplies liberal amounts of sulfur.

Some research shows that manganese may help correct prolonged blood clotting time brought on by a lack of vitamin K. Vitamin K is manufactured by microorganisms in our intestines out of substances found widely in foods, especially green leafy vegetables. Vitamin K is indispensable. By ensuring that blood coagulates at a wound site, whether it be a slight scratch or a major injury, vitamin K prevents us from bleeding indefinitely.

CHAPTER

29

Super-Mineral Foods

An Eight-Step Plan for Super-Mineral Nutrition

No single food can provide all our mineral needs. Yet certain foods are such treasure troves of minerals—and often vitamins—that including them in our diet regularly goes a long way toward meeting our mineral needs.

When was the last time you ate fish? Liver? Or yogurt? How often do you eat whole wheat bread? Fresh fruit? Or dark green leafy vegetables?

Most of us probably eat some of those foods every day. For others, though, the list may look like a stretch of foreign territory. Because sales of foods like ice cream, potato chips and soda, along with fast foods and pre-prepared meal-in-a-minute foods, are at an all-time high, we can't help wondering whether people are actually eating as well as they say they are. It's been our experience that even among those of us who honestly believe we're eating quite well, some diets could use a bit of improvement. Or at least a periodic stock-taking.

As you read on, take a candid look at what you eat. Is your diet heavily populated with super-mineral foods? Perhaps the easiest way to be sure is to take a few simple steps to evaluate—or upgrade—your diet. Focus on one food category per week. Gradually, put it all together. By week eight—in less time than it takes to improve your golf swing—you can feel confident you've taken a quantum leap toward better health.

Week One: Try Liver

Because it serves as the body's processing and storage site for so many nutrients, liver—beef, calf, chicken or others—accumulates a wealth of minerals:

• Liver surpasses all other foods in iron content.

• Ounce for ounce, liver has 70 times more copper than sirloin steak.

• A 3½-ounce serving of beef liver provides five milligrams of zinc—more than a comparable serving of any other meat.

• Liver wields a bumper crop of chromium, ranking it among the finest sources of that nutrient.

Not only is liver a number one source of minerals, it's a rich reservoir of vitamin A, vitamin C and B complex vitamins as well. All those nutrients push liver into first place among super-mineral foods (see table 37).

There's more: "In addition to the known nutrients, substances are present in our diet which may be required in increased amounts during conditions of stress," says Benjamin Ershoff, Ph.D., a scientist at Loma Linda University in California. "Whole liver is a potent source of such nutrients."

When cooked properly, liver is a far cry from the tough, gray slab of stringy meat we battled with as children at the dinner table. Buy it tender, slice it thin and soak it for an hour in milk at room temperature before cooking. To mask any bitterness in the liver, you could flour it, using whole wheat or rye flour seasoned with oregano, garlic and onion. Cook liver for a minute or two on each side, in a hot frying pan with a little vegetable oil. Serving liver once a week—be it beef, calf, lamb, pork or chicken liver—boosts your mineral intake in a way no other food can.

Desiccated liver is available, too. Desiccated liver is simply dried liver. And it's a handy way to add minerals-plus to your diet when fresh liver doesn't suit your schedule or menu plan. The method of drying is unusual: the connective tissue (and in most desiccated liver products, the fat) is removed from beef liver, which is then dried in a vacuum at a temperature of about 140°F. In the process, four pounds of whole liver are shrunk down to one pound of desiccated liver—with all of the minerals and less of the bulk. A most convenient way to add this nutritional marvel to your diet.

TABLE 37   **Super-Mineral Foods**

Food	Calcium	Magnesium	Phosphorus	Potassium	Zinc	Copper	Iron	Selenium	Chromium	Manganese	Iodine	Cobalamin	Fluorine
Liver													
Yogurt													
Buttermilk													
Fish													
Blackstrap molasses													
Brewer's yeast													
Nutritional yeast													

Key

indicates minerals supplied in especially useful amounts

indicates minerals generally supplied in especially useful amounts, but actual value varies from product to product

indicates other important minerals supplied in smaller but notable amounts

indicates other important minerals generally supplied in smaller but notable amounts, but actual value varies from product to product

SOURCE: This table is based on values given in *Nutritive Value of American Foods in Common Units,* Agriculture Handbook No. 456, by Catherine F. Adams (Washington, D.C.: Agricultural Research Service, U.S. Department of Agriculture, 1975).

Week Two: Introduce Yourself to Yogurt and Buttermilk

Calcium is the body's main mineral. Reserves must be kept up without fail. While beans, nuts and greens provide useful amounts of calcium, dairy products are still responsible for most of our intake. Low-fat fermented milk foods like yogurt and buttermilk are bulwarks for fracture-prone individuals—especially women past menopause.

Yogurt is fermented by bacteria. But they're not the bacteria like the bugs that cause colds or infections. They're good bacteria, most often *Lactobacillus acidophilus* or *Lactobacillus bulgaricus.* Besides fighting various problems of the digestive tract and lowering cholesterol, there's one thing that makes yogurt a super-mineral food—calcium.

"Calcium is absorbed best when in the presence of acid in the intestine, and yogurt contains both calcium and acid," says Manfred

Kroger, Ph.D., associate professor of food science at Pennsylvania State University.

"Elderly people with brittle bones need more calcium," he told us. "Yogurt may be just the product they should be eating to strengthen their bones."

Dr. Kroger also pointed out that many elderly people have lost their ability to digest the milk sugar lactose. "When they drink milk, they get an upset stomach or gas, so they stay away from it and miss the much-needed calcium," he said. "But when milk ferments into yogurt, the bacteria reduces the amount of lactose by 25 percent. Most people who avoid milk because of lactose can safely eat yogurt."

You might want to try yogurt as a smooth topping on fruits or in blended drinks. Yogurt is also rich in protein, so for summer days, when big dinners are less appealing, try yogurt as a dressing on your salad and turn it into a complete meal. Take a look at the upcoming recipe section (chapter 31) for other serving suggestions, yogurt dishes and beverages, as well as easy directions for making homemade yogurt.

Buttermilk is also made by fermentation of milk. Like yogurt, buttermilk has the advantage over regular milk in that it, too, contains less lactose and can be easily tolerated by people who cannot digest that milk sugar. And like any milk product, buttermilk is high in calcium.

Despite its name, buttermilk contains no butter. In fact, it's practically fat-free. To make buttermilk, commercial processors add bacterial cultures, some milk solids, and often salt, to skim milk. The finished product is cultured buttermilk. Commercial buttermilk is also made by a ten-minute process in which lactic acid, stabilizers and flavorings are added to heated milk. That type of buttermilk is known as imitation, simulated, acidified or acidulated buttermilk.

Because of its slight acidity, buttermilk is an excellent ingredient in cakes, biscuits and pancakes, and helps tenderize meat. It can also be served as is, for a cool, refreshing beverage.

Lassi means "buttermilk," but it's buttermilk Indian-style—made from yogurt. According to Harish Johari, author of *Dhanwantari* (Rams Head, 1974), a book on ancient Indian principles of diet and health, *lassi* is "one of the best summer drinks."

"To make *lassi,*" writes Mr. Johari, "churn fresh, cooled yogurt with an eggbeater [or blender] until it has become well blended. . . . Now add water to make the drink the consistency of fresh milk, using honey to taste. *Lassi* is cooling, refreshing—and provides the system with a healthy measure of . . . vitamins."

Week Three: Eat More Fish

In fish we have a whole class of foods that provide us with iron, copper, potassium and selenium. Cooked fish like salmon and sardines, which have soft, edible bones, can even supply useful amounts of calcium. And unlike iodized salt, which may encourage high blood pressure, fish is an aboveboard source of iodine, necessary for healthy thyroid function. On top of all that, fish is also a good source of fluorine, cobalt and B vitamins.

What makes fish really ideal as a health-giving food, though, is what it lacks—fat. While beef cattle are overfed and raised in crowded pens to grow fat as rapidly as possible, fish are wild. Darting and dashing about after smaller fish, searching for microorganisms to eat, and plunging in quick dives to the ocean bottom to snatch mineral-rich seaweeds and grasses, a fish works hard for its meals. As a result, its flesh isn't fatty or packed with cholesterol. And most of what fat a fish does have isn't saturated like the fat of beef and pork. There is evidence that polyunsaturated fats, such as those in fish, lower cholesterol and triglycerides, blood fats that have been linked to heart disease. So fish delivers minerals to us unencumbered by unhealthy fat.

Perhaps a few of us still feel a little uneasy about eating fish, ever since the mercury scare in 1970 when the Food and Drug Administration recalled almost a million cans of tuna. Looking back, though, we can see that the mercury-in-fish scare was grossly overdone. Writing in the October, 1971, issue of the *American Journal of Clinical Nutrition,* Thomas B. Eyl, M.D., pointed out that "marine biologists are becoming increasingly convinced that the 'contaminated' fish contained perfectly normal levels of mercury, picked up from natural levels of mercury in seawater."

In other words, fish has always contained some mercury. Edwin N. Wilmsen, Ph.D., a research scientist formerly with the University of Michigan's Museum of Anthropology, checked on some preserved samples of fish from around archeological sites. He found that the "mercury concentration in prehistoric fish was of the same magnitude as is that in living fish today" (*Ecology of Food and Nutrition,* June, 1972).

Shellfish is another seafood loaded with minerals. Oysters, for example, are notoriously high in zinc. There's one big problem with shellfish, though. They're filter-feeders. That means that they pump huge quantities of water through their bodies as they feed. Some species of oysters, for instance, pump as much as nine gallons of water every hour for hours at a time. And since shellfish nestle down in coastal waters rife with pollution, they also pump toxic chemicals, heavy metals and sewage into their bodies—and accumulate and concentrate them. So, as good a food as shellfish might be, we really can't recommend it.

As for other fish, they offer such a smorgasbord of minerals, it's a good idea to eat some kind of fish at least twice a week. You may want to start by setting aside certain days of the week—say, Tuesdays and Fridays—as "fish days" until the habit becomes routine. And fish fillets cook up so quickly that they're really a convenience food—the average fillet is done in about eight minutes. Buy some fish on the way home, add a potato and vegetable, and dinner will be on the table in no time!

Week Four: Make Room for Fruit and Fruit Juices

Fruit is nature's dessert, all wrapped up in a tidy package. No fuss, no muss—and chock-full of potassium, the antisodium mineral. Fruits also tend to get high marks for vitamin C, which triples iron absorption. With high blood pressure (aggravated by sodium) and iron deficiency anemia two of the most common mineral-related disorders going, fruit can make a difference in whether you feel pooped or perky.

And to the extent that fruit juices can replace high-phosphate soft drinks, fruit gets an added endorsement. Remember to spend a few minutes of each shopping trip mulling over the fruit department. Scarf up some bananas, pineapples, apples, grapes—whatever you like.

Week Five: Switch to Whole Grain Foods

Grains are a staple in diets around the world—rice in Asia, corn in Latin America, millet in Africa, and wheat in the West. So you can see that grains aren't used only for bread and rolls. Crackers, noodles, dumplings, muffins, tortillas, crepes and cakes all spring from grain. Even the phantasmagoria of boxed cereals on the grocery shelves is basically a quartet of wheat, rice, corn and oats.

Unfortunately, refining mills away many important minerals in the embryo and husk of grains—iron, magnesium, zinc, copper, manganese and selenium, to be specific. What's left behind is the starchy mineral-poor endosperm. While it's true that minerals in whole grain foods are not quite as available as minerals in other foods, because they remain partially bound up by phytic acid in the fiber, whole grains still contribute more to mineral intake than refined white derivatives. Study after study has shown that choosing whole grain foods over refined is one factor that can make the difference between adequate and poor mineral status.

Choosing refined breads and cereals, then, can seriously undermine overall mineral intake. That's because calorie for calorie, carbohydrates make up about half our diet. And grain products, in turn, make up the lion's share of carbohydrates in the form of bread, cereal and side dishes. So it's important that the nutrient content of grain foods be tip-top.

Stock up on a couple of loaves of whole wheat bread this week. Pick up a pound or two of brown rice. Both of those are right next to the white varieties on the grocery shelves.

Week Six: Reach for Blackstrap Molasses

The dark, sticky liquid called blackstrap molasses is a very healthful food that comes from the same plants—and the same factories—that produce notoriously unhealthful white sugar. While white sugar has no minerals to speak of, molasses offers a bonanza.

A tablespoon of blackstrap molasses contains 3.2 milligrams of iron—nearly twice what you'd get from a cup of raw spinach, and more than 50 milligrams of magnesium, one-seventh the Recommended Dietary Allowance for that mineral.

That same tablespoon contains almost as much calcium—137 milligrams—as ½ cup of milk.

Blackstrap molasses has it all over fruit as a rich supply of dietary potassium. One tablespoon of that black gold has 585 milligrams of potassium, considerably more than a banana or two oranges.

The typical American diet may be woefully short on chromium, but molasses provides a sizable amount, to say nothing of valuable amounts of the B vitamins thiamine (B_1), riboflavin (B_2), niacin and pantothenic acid.

Blackstrap molasses is a kind of sheep in wolf's clothing because of its origins in sugar manufacture. When sugar cane is crushed, ground, heated and cooled, the familiar crystals of white sugar appear. Blackstrap molasses is the liquid that's left behind, usually after three extractions. Each time the process is repeated, more and more white sugar is removed, and the molasses gets thicker and darker. Blackstrap molasses—the heaviest, darkest product, has about half the sugar that was in the original cane juice. But it also has all the nutritional value that was refined out of the white sugar.

Chances are you've already tasted molasses—in baked beans, in the glaze on a baked ham or sweet potatoes, or in traditional desserts. Shoofly pie, a favorite in Pennsylvania Dutch country, is brimming with molasses.

The taste is more than sweet—it's stronger and more interesting than sugar, and it might take some getting used to. At first you might want to consider using the lighter grades of molasses, which are sweeter and less highly flavored than blackstrap (but not nearly as nourishing). Make sure, in any case, that you use *unsulfured* molasses—it's a purer product.

Substitute molasses for sugar when you bake, and you'll change a health minus into a big plus. To begin with, try a mixture of half honey, half molasses in cookies and cakes. (One cup of the mixture takes the place of two cups of sugar.) You may want to cut back on the amount of oil or milk to make up for the added liquid of the mixture.

When you make granola, experiment with molasses instead of honey. For a double bonus of good nutrition, mix a spoonful or two of molasses into plain yogurt. And for a hot drink that has lots of goodness and no caffeine, just add a teaspoon of sugar's dark, wholesome cousin to a cup of hot water. Stir, and drink up—to your health.

Week Seven: Get into Yeast

Sloshing around in the vats of a brewery, one of nature's tiniest plants ferments barley and hops into beer. The plants—brewer's yeast—

don't look like much, but those microorganisms are rich in minerals. So are other nutritional yeasts grown on molasses, grain, cheese whey or other mediums. Yeasts supply decent amounts of iron, calcium and potassium. Many yeasts are excellent sources of selenium and chromium. What's more, yeast supplies whopping amounts of several B vitamins. (Don't confuse brewer's and other nutritional yeasts with baker's yeast, though. Baker's yeast is *not* a nutritional aid.)

How do you include nutritional yeasts in your diet? Supplements are one answer. It takes about 16 tablets to equal one tablespoon of nutritional yeast, though. So as a powder, yeast is easier to work into your diet as an embellishment to food. The flavor is very mild, but varies slightly from yeast to yeast, depending on the growing medium. Brewer's yeast, as one might expect, is slightly bitter and malty, although debittered products are available. Other yeasts may be slightly tart or fruity. But in general, the flavor is mild enough to have little effect on other foods. You can add nutritional yeast to recipes for bread, pancakes, muffins and other baked goods. Or to omelets and stews, chili and tomato sauce. Mix it into hamburger patties. Stir it into vegetable juices. Sprinkle it on salads, vegetables or cottage cheese.

Week Eight: Kick the Junk Food Habit

We can make ourselves well or ill by what we put in our mouths. The choice is ours. And wise choices include mineral-rich foods. But all that attention to brown rice and yogurt can only do so much good if we're still reaching for pretzels, corn chips and gooey pastries in the junk food aisles.

How much snack food are you bringing home? Is it a steady part of your diet or a passing indulgence? More than an occasional treat means you're flirting with nutritional disaster, because any trace of nutritional value those foods might possibly have is usually diluted by salt, sugar and fat. In fact, the higher the sugar and fat content of a food, the fewer minerals it supplies, as a general rule.

We're not going to leave you with a long list of "thou shalt nots." But you can keep on your toes by stopping from time to time to ask yourself, "Why am I eating this?"

Putting It All Together

One last thing. The plan is flexible. If you want to launch your program with yogurt instead of liver, go ahead. Or plunge right into brewer's yeast. Or make whole wheat bread and pasta your first step. Whatever your approach, week eight should find your diet in pretty good shape, mineralwise.

To help you still further, recipes incorporating super-mineral foods conclude Part 4.

30

Cooking to Safeguard the Minerals in Our Food

Unlike vitamins, minerals are not destroyed by cooking. But that doesn't mean they aren't vulnerable to improper cooking. Minerals can creep out of food and dissolve into cooking water and lost juices.

By the same token, certain metal cookware can leach minerals— some good, some bad—into food. So the methods and cookware we use can make a big difference in keeping good minerals locked within food, and harmful minerals out.

Light Cooking Saves Minerals

Vegetables: Handle with Care

Of all foods, vegetables probably suffer the highest mineral losses— largely due to overcooking. There are plenty of mineral-packed vegetables.

But when we carelessly toss them into a boiling water bath, or simmer them far too long, they can emerge pale and nutritionally depleted.

Take cauliflower, for instance. Fresh, raw cauliflower has nearly twice as much magnesium as the precooked frozen kind. Yet most people are inclined to cook their cauliflower to death (in the case of frozen, they cook it again) and then make up for lost flavor by either dribbling it with butter or veiling it in a creamy cheese sauce. Unfortunately, though, nothing will make up for the minerals irretrievably lost in the cooking water.

So the next time you serve cauliflower, slice it thin and toss with bits of sweet red onion and a little minced garlic. Marinate in a vinaigrette (basically vinegar and herbs with a few drops of oil) and serve chilled. You'll welcome the change and help boost your magnesium intake. Do the same with young zucchini or tender broccoli.

Or try adding fresh peas, broccoli buds or shredded cabbage to your salads. Dandelion greens by themselves, sprinkled with vinegar and a few drops of oil, make a zesty, calcium-packed salad. Look ahead to our recipe section (chapter 31) for other suggestions, along with a vinaigrette you can make in a minute.

Never clean vegetables by soaking them. That draws out minerals, too. And cutting vegetables too far ahead destroys vitamins. Wash and cut vegetables immediately before serving, if at all possible.

The secret to keeping mineral losses to a minimum is in cooking quickly with little water. Water draws out minerals. And the longer you cook vegetables, the more minerals *and* vitamins they lose. So a vegetable that alights on your dinner plate limp, pale and lifeless-looking is likely to have little to offer nutritionally.

At the very least, cook vegetables in just enough water to keep vegetables from sticking to the pan (½ inch or so at the most) and save any residual cooking water for later use in soups, stews and sauces. Better yet, steam.

The Healthful Art of Cooking with Steam

Letting hot steam, not water, cook your vegetables is about the best way to conserve minerals. For under $5, you can buy a perforated foldout steaming basket made to hold your vegetables over boiling water in regular pots and pans. Supermarkets, hardware stores and department stores usually sell steam baskets. For a few dollars more, you can buy a steamer pot with a custom-fitted insert. Or you can quickly improvise a steamer by placing a metal colander over water in any pot with a snug-fitting lid. You can even set a regular vegetable strainer across the top of a saucepan, arrange the vegetables in that, and cover.

Steamer Basket for Cooking Vegetables

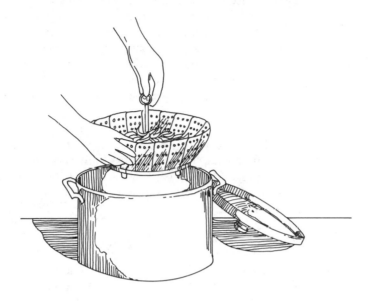

Whatever steaming method you choose, keep your apparatus handy and use it often. Whether you cook vegetables whole, halved, diced or sliced, be sure to cut them into uniform-sized pieces so they'll all be done at the same time. And pile them no more than one chunk deep, so that all cook evenly. Be sure the water is boiling vigorously before you set the steamer and vegetables in place. Cover at once and cook until the vegetables are just tender. Broccoli, string beans, greens and peas take only 3 to 5 minutes to steam. Squash, carrots, potatoes and onions take longer—up to 20 minutes or so depending on how small you cut them. For longer-cooking vegetables, check to see that the water doesn't evaporate away. Add more if needed.

Vegetables love a steam bath. They emerge bright, firm and flavorful—with most of their minerals intact. Vitamins fare well, too.

Waterless Cooking Is Nearly As Good As Steaming

The "waterless" method also makes use of steam. Cooking is done in heavy saucepans with tight-fitting lids, designed to use only the natural moisture in food and water that remains after food is rinsed. Although the waterless method is preferred over boiling, it doesn't permit quick cooking, which may cancel out the advantages of using little or no water. Nutrient loss is comparable to cooking in a small amount of water.

Stir-Frying Locks In Minerals

Stir-frying is a simple cooking method borrowed from the Chinese. The term describes exactly what we do here: a variety of vegetables are diagonally sliced into bite-sized pieces and briskly stirred in a small amount of vegetable oil over moderately high heat in an open pan called a wok. Or you can use a heavy skillet. The whole process takes three or four minutes, tops—hardly giving minerals any time to escape.

Stir-fried food is not only nutritious—it's fast and flavorful. Mixed vegetables cook up crisp and tender, with nutrients sealed in for goodness. Start with the harder, root vegetables like slivered carrots, parsnips or turnips, which take the longest to cook. Next, quickly add sliced celery, chopped onions and minced garlic. Tender foods like mushrooms, peas and leafy cabbage or other greens go in last. For a complete meal, include nuts, cooked beans, or chunks of diced chicken, fish, beef or tofu (soybean curd). Serve with cooked brown rice.

Pressure Cooking for Some Foods Only

Like steaming, pressure cooking also uses a minimum of water, but is much faster. Mineral losses are negligible. But pressure cooking involves steam under pressure and temperatures higher than boiling, which can influence vitamin losses. Some vitamin loss is made up by reduced cooking time. So the net result is comparable to cooking quickly in a little water.

The big advantage with pressure cooking is time. Potatoes, beets and beans—foods that may take discouragingly long to cook otherwise—can be pressure cooked in nothing flat. That enables us to add those wholesome foods to our menu when a busy schedule might otherwise tempt us to ferret out less nutritious convenience foods or fast food meals.

Pressure cooking isn't the best method for delicate leafy vegetables like spinach, or strong-flavored vegetables like broccoli, cauliflower or cabbage. Flavors then become too concentrated. For those foods, steaming gives better results in almost as little time.

A pressure cooker is heavy. And if not carefully attended, it can easily overcook your food. So if you have a problem lifting heavy pans or tend to be an absentminded cook, a pressure cooker is not for you.

How to Cook Flatulence-Free Beans

Beans are high in calcium, magnesium, potassium—and oligosaccharides, substances that produce gas in the lower intestine. To dodge the discomfort associated with eating beans, try the following cooking method, which breaks down gas-producing substances before they reach your sensitive insides.

Soak beans for three to four hours, allowing plenty of water for them to absorb and expand. Discard the soak water. Cook the beans in boiling water for 30 minutes, then discard that cooking water. Complete cooking in fresh water.

While it is true that soaking and boiling the beans results in mineral losses, much goodness remains. Besides, this *is* still the best way to get around the flatulence problem. And the addition of about a teaspoon of brewer's yeast for every ½ cup of dried beans after cooking will replace lost minerals and vitamins.

Table 38 is a useful guide to preparing beans and legumes.

TABLE 38 Cooking Time and Yield for Dried Beans

One Cup—Dry	Cooking Water (in cups)	Approximate Cooking Time (in hours)	Yield (in cups)
Baby lima beans	4	¾–1	2¼
Black beans	4	¾–1	2½
Black-eyed peas	4	¾–1	2½
Garbanzos (chick-peas)	4	2	3¼
Kidney beans	4	1½	2½
Lentils	4	⅓	3
Lima beans	4	¾–1	2½
Navy beans or pea beans	4	¾–1	2½
Soybeans	5	3	2¾
Split peas	4	½	2½

NOTE: Beans were soaked for four hours, then placed in a covered pot and kept constantly boiling during cooking time determinations.

Low-Salt Cooking

Cooking without salt need not be bland. The roster of herbs and spices waiting in the wings to perk up your food is long and inviting. A sprig of dill lends zip to fish. A dash of oregano adds punch to meat loaf. A grating of nutmeg jazzes up an omelet. Even if you're not sacrificing salt for health reasons, cooking with herbs and spices takes the monotony out of plain old salt-and-pepper dining.

Seasonings are best added sparingly, as they can pack quite a wallop if overdone. Don't use too many at once, or too much of any one herb or spice in one dish. Add seasonings toward the end of cooking so flavors remain fresh and pungent, yet not overpowering.

To weave flavorful flair into your favorite dishes, consult table 39 for a list of seasonings most commonly used for various foods. The list is by no means complete and absolute, but rather gives a few suggestions to help you use herbs and seasonings to replace salt.

TABLE 39 **Seasonings That Replace Salt**

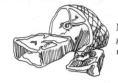

Meat (in general)—
garlic, sage, basil,
marjoram, tarragon

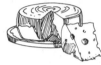

Fish –
dill, paprika, tarragon,
thyme, sage, lemon juice

Chicken –
thyme, sage, marjoram,
tarragon, rosemary,
parsely, sesame seeds

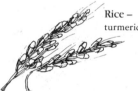

Cheese –
caraway, cayenne,
cumin

Eggs –
chives, parsley, tarragon

Rice –
turmeric, marjoram,

Beans (in general)—
mustard, savory, mint,
chili pepper

Garbanzos
(chick-peas)—
cayenne, garlic,
parsley

Lima beans—
sage, savory

Soups –
bay leaves, celery seed,
marjoram, basil,
chervil, rosemary

Green beans—
dill, lemon juice,
savory

Soybeans—
dill, garlic, thyme,
parsley

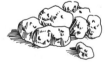

Potatoes –
parsley, chives, oregano,
rosemary, paprika,
savory, tarragon

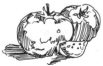

Tomatoes –
basil, bay leaves,
rosemary, oregano,
garlic, celery seed

Cauliflower –
caraway, dill, oregano,
basil, garlic, savory,
tarragon, lemon juice

Broccoli –
garlic, oregano,
dillweed

Beets –
cloves, cinnamon

Cabbage –
dill, caraway

Asparagus –
lemon juice, tarragon

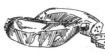

Zucchini –
garlic, basil, marjoram

Squash –
cinnamon, savory,
tarragon

Coleslaw –
caraway, dill, mustard,
turmeric

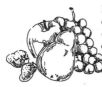

**Salads and salad
dressing –**
basil, garlic, savory,
mint, lemon juice

Vinaigrette sauce
(oil and vinegar)—
tarragon, dill, basil,
mustard, garlic

Fruit –
cinnamon, ginger,
cloves, allspice,
cardamom, lemon juice

How to Cook Brown Rice

Brown rice bears all of the minerals that milling tears away from the white fluffy kind. People who are used to instant rice, however, may be ill at ease when nudged into making the change to more nutritious but longer-cooking brown rice. No need to wince, though—cooking brown rice is quite simple. Really just a matter of patience.

Cook 1 cup of dry rice in 2½ cups of water for a yield of 3 cups of cooked rice—that's four to six small servings. Or cook 1 part rice to 2½ parts water. In other words, the dry amount will triple in volume when cooked.

Bring water (or stock) to a boil. Add grain slowly, stirring as you pour. When the water returns to boiling, lower the heat to simmer. Cover and cook until all the liquid is absorbed (25 to 30 minutes).

If at that time the grains still seem hard or tough, add a few more tablespoons of boiling water, cover again, and continue cooking. To avoid gumminess, keep stirring to a minimum.

Grains should be light and separate easily when done. Fluff with a fork before serving.

Don't Reheat Vegetables

Try serving leftover vegetables chilled, in a vinaigrette sauce. Or in a green salad. Or minced into a sandwich filling. Reheating vegetables drives out vitamins, leaving behind less than a full complement of nutrients.

Microwave Ovens: No Loss, No Gain

You may be wondering if vegetables cooked in a microwave oven come out ahead of conventionally baked vegetables. They don't. Nutritionally, there's no gain or loss over regular baking.

Meat, Poultry and Fish: Proper Cooking Means More Minerals

Cooking meat and poultry slowly will minimize shrinkage and hold in more juices, thereby conserving minerals like iron and zinc, as well as B vitamins. Braising-frying briefly to seal in moisture, followed by slow stewing, is best for poor cuts of meat or if you have a problem chewing. Nutritionally, roasting at low temperatures (about 300°F) is equally good.

Don't salt meat. Salting draws out mineral-laden juices.

Because of its high protein, low fat and rich mineral content, fish is practically a staple in healthful diets. Broiling and baking will save flavor, nutrients and calories. Cook only until the flesh flakes easily with a fork.

Choosing Safe Cookware

Naturally, you'll want cookware that's least likely to deposit harmful metals or other questionable substances in your food.

Aluminum May Be a Problem

Without a doubt, the most controversial cookware from a safety standpoint is aluminum. A strong, rustproof and lightweight metal, aluminum conducts heat well, permitting quick and even heat distribution. And it's less expensive than stainless steel or copper cookware. But aluminum does react readily with acid foods like tomato sauce and fruit, and can creep into food. Foods cooked in aluminum may also taste slightly different from those cooked in other noncorrosive cookware.

Just how much of a health threat aluminum cookware poses is not known. The American Medical Association says there is no health hazard whatsoever. "The aluminum ingested due to migration into foods from cooking utensils and cans is not enough to contribute to the total body burden or to produce toxic effects. . . . Intestinal absorption of aluminum is minimal, and any aluminum absorbed is quickly excreted by normally functioning kidneys" (*Journal of the American Medical Association,* October 3, 1977).

Allen C. Alfrey, M.D., at the Denver Veterans Administration Hospital echoed that opinion. Although his major research is on man's absorption of aluminum-containing medicines, he was able to make some interesting comments to us concerning cookware. "The amount of aluminum from cookware would be so small that I doubt it would pose any problems," he said. "Although there is a considerable variation between people in the absorption of aluminum (we don't know why), it is possible that some extremely sensitive individuals would react badly. These cases would be rare, though."

As we dug further, more misgivings arose. "It is rare, but it does happen," said Guy Pfeiffer, M.D., concerning reactions to aluminum. Dr. Pfeiffer is a specialist in environmental medicine from Matoon, Illinois. "We do not know what goes on but we do know that some people feel better when they stop using aluminum cookware. We have no scientific evidence but we do have our own practical clinical observations. Some people who are sensitive to aluminum can suffer symptoms similar to those obtained from chemicals in foods. For example, they can have indigestion, headaches, nausea, diarrhea, gas, flushing or blood pressure fluctuations."

Another doctor thinks the effects of aluminum reach much farther—to the brain and nervous system. Stephen E. Levick, M.D., of the Yale University School of Medicine, is so convinced of the case against aluminum cookware that he threw out all his aluminum pots and pans. In the wake of evidence that aluminum-contaminated kidney dialysis fluid produces a kind of mental deterioration in treated patients, he feels aluminum cookware holds more risk than is generally presumed. Dr. Levick cites a study which showed that a large group of elderly people with high aluminum levels had more nerve and behavior problems, including poor memory and eye-muscle coordination, than did elderly people with lower aluminum levels. While aluminum cookware was not specified as the source, Dr. Levick says, "Large numbers of people in our aluminum-using society may be the victims of slow aluminum poisoning from several sources. Corrosible aluminum cookware may be a nontrivial source" (*New England Journal of Medicine,* July 17, 1980).

Because the safety of aluminum cookware has not been settled one way or the other, the cautious thing to do would be to at least avoid cooking and storing the more corrosive, high-acid foods—tomatoes, fruits, and foods made of them—in aluminum.

Copper Cookware Is Fine When Lined

Copper cookware is usually lined with tin, nickel or stainless steel, so food doesn't come in direct contact with the metal. Copper itself is inert and nonpoisonous. Large amounts of copper salts, however, form when acid foods or beverages are stored in unlined copper vessels for a long period of time. There is some question as to whether cooking food in unlined copper pots would actually leach enough copper into food to cause health problems. Copper is usually lined, but for other reasons. Uncoated copper can not only discolor food, but may destroy vitamin C. Should the protective coating wear through, copper cookware can be relined.

Glass and Porcelain for Baking

Glass and porcelain enamel are the least corrosive cookware materials, with little or no possibility of affecting the safety, appearance or flavor of food. Glass is most often used as oven-to-tableware and is an ideal storage container. Porcelain enamel is a glasslike substance usually coating cast iron, aluminum or stainless steel. Enamel protects the metal underneath from rust and acids, but does chip easily. Porcelain enamel can be used in the oven or on the range.

When it comes to metal cookware itself, though, you'll want to consider resistance to wear and corrosion important factors.

Stainless Steel, Safe and Easy to Use

Stainless steel cookware is the least likely of all metal cookware to corrode into your food or to affect the flavor and appearance of foods cooked in it. It's a tough, wear-resistant alloy of nickel, chromium and iron—all harmless.

Stainless steel alone is not a very good heat conductor. So pots and pans designed for stovetop cooking often incorporate other metals, usually copper to carbon steel, to help heat spread evenly around the pan.

Three-ply stainless, for example, is usually made of two layers of steel with a layer of copper or carbon steel sandwiched between them. Some pots have an aluminum-clad bottom for better heat distribution, while the entire inside is stainless steel. Stainless steel bakeware is, as a rule, solely stainless steel.

Iron for Slow Cooking, with a Nutritional Plus

Many of those heavy black iron kettles our grandparents used are now being sold at auctions and flea markets. Ironware—old or new—is still being used today by many cooks, most of whom don't realize those rugged pots and skillets could be a source of dietary iron.

According to an editorial by Charles E. Butterworth, Jr., M.D., food cooked in an iron skillet contains significantly more iron than the same food cooked in glass (*Journal of the American Medical Association,* April 24, 1972). There are those who believe that iron cookware could contribute to our daily required intake of iron. The subject is controversial, but we do know that eating foods containing iron from cookware isn't harmful and may even be beneficial.

Some cooks like the slow cooking properties of iron for toasting foods that might burn easily, like wheat germ or sesame seeds, and for making omelets, crepes, tortillas and pancakes. Others enjoy using iron for stews, vegetable dishes and corn bread. Ironware is very heavy, however, so if you have arthritis, other cookware might be easier for you to handle.

Nonstick Cookware Needs Special Handling

Nonstick finishes like Teflon, SilverStone and Debron, to name a few, have been a great boon to people concerned about restricting their intake of fats, since cooking in nonstick cookware requires little or no added fat. The nonstick finish is achieved by applying one or more coats of a plastic called polytetrafluorethylene (or P.T.F.E.), usually to aluminum pots and pans.

The nonstick surface is basically sturdy and long-lasting—as long as it's not mistreated. And there's the rub. Nonstick coatings are soft and therefore sensitive to intense heat and scratching. Unless you're careful to use plastic or wood utensils *only* for stirring, and plastic pads for scouring, the coating will chip away into your dishwater—or food. And even with great care, the coating does wear away after a time. The Food and Drug Administration and the manufacturers of nonstick cookware claim that the plastic substances are nontoxic. Even so, what's left behind, should the plastic wear off, is the aluminum base on which the coating is applied.

CHAPTER

31

Recipes: Putting It All Together

    What we have here is not just a collection of good-tasting recipes, but dishes and beverages selected specifically with health-building minerals in mind. Until now, we've urged you to eat liver once a week for generous provisions of zinc, copper, iron, selenium and chromium. Here you can choose from seven different ways—some simple, some fancy—to prepare liver. And we've suggested using foods like yogurt and tofu (soybean curd) creatively to boost your calcium intake. So look forward to recipes that blend those with other mineral-rich foods to make the most of your diet. We've hawked fish as one of the most important sources of selenium, potassium and iodine, to name a few. Over a dozen fish recipes are included. Along the same lines, we've emphasized whole grains, beans, potatoes, fruit and vegetables for important minerals they provide. As such, our recipes incorporate all those foods in creative and tasty ways. And there's enough variety that you can shoot for high mineral intake at breakfast, lunch and dinner—plus snacktime. There are recipes to suit you whether you're on a budget, or having company.

To help you ease these recipes into your good-eating plan, we've included a list of minerals supplied by each recipe. Each mineral listed is coded to indicate the level supplied *per serving* in relation to nutritional need:

*** *Three stars.* This applies to a few very special recipes, in which just one serving yields more than a whole day's average requirement for the mineral highlighted.

** *Two stars.* One serving provides a generous portion of your daily need for that nutrient.

* *One star.* The dish is a good source of the mineral but be sure to combine several such meals—or perhaps supplement your diet in order to meet your daily needs.

Mention is also given to other minerals that are present, but in smaller amounts.

Not only should these recipes help you to prepare mineral-rich meals, you'll discover they carry no excess fat, sugar or salt—substances that, in one way or another, are partially to blame for many cases of overweight, high blood pressure, diabetes and heart disease. In fact, we'll even show you how to make your own wholesome, salt-free condiments. Moderate amounts of honey or mineral-laden molasses are the only sweetening you'll find here. And when a small amount of cooking oil is needed, we recommend you use unhydrogenated safflower, sunflower, corn, soy, sesame, wheat germ or olive oil. Hydrogenation, a chemical process, changes unsaturated fats (liquids) to saturated fats (solid). And it is the unsaturated variety that supplies essential fatty acids (linoleic and arachidonic), which are not only needed for good health but may also lower cholesterol levels. To top it off, hydrogenated or partially hydrogenated fats or oils, such as solid vegetable shortening, are also likely to be treated with antioxidant chemicals such as BHT, BHA and propyl gallate. To prevent rancidity in unhydrogenated, additive-free oils, simply refrigerate after opening and keep on hand only what you plan to use within a reasonable amount of time.

Cottonseed oil—used in a number of supermarket cooking oils—adds more saturated fat than other vegetable oils. And on a per acre basis, cotton plants are treated with more pesticides than other oil-producing crops like corn or soybeans, and so the oil carries a small, albeit unwelcome, residue of those chemicals. So we recommend you stick with the vegetable oils suggested above.

Power Breakfasts

Whether a leisurely weekend brunch or a quick nibble on the way to work, breakfast can shoulder its share of the day's minerals.

Blender Breakfast

Long on minerals and short on time,
this quick blend starts your day off right.

Serves one

1 cup milk	** Calcium
1 medium banana	** Potassium
1-2 tablespoons peanut butter	** Manganese
	* Magnesium
	* Copper
	Chromium
	Fluorine

Place ingredients in a blender and liquefy.

Toasted Granola Supreme

For a cold cereal that's far superior to any overprocessed,
highly sugared commercial brand in a box, try this homemade granola,
which can be used for a nutritious start on busy mornings.

Makes five cups

2½ cups raw wheat germ	** Magnesium
2 cups rolled oats	** Copper
1 cup coarse bran	** Manganese
1 cup rye flakes or wheat flakes	Potassium
½ cup chopped walnuts	Zinc
½ cup sunflower seeds	Iron
½ cup shredded coconut	Selenium
¼ cup sesame seeds	
½ cup liquid lecithin and/or safflower oil	
¼ cup blackstrap molasses	
¼ cup honey	

Mix all ingredients in a large bowl until the lecithin or oil, molasses and honey are evenly distributed. Then pour into a roasting pan or other large pan and toast in a preheated 350°F oven for 15 minutes, or until the granola is somewhat dry and crispy. Stir the granola occasionally while baking to produce an evenly toasted mixture.

Raisin-Spice Oatmeal

Hard-to-get selenium and chromium are just two bonuses you get with this cooked cereal. Pour on skim milk for calcium too.

Serves two

1½ cups water	** Manganese
⅔ cup rolled oats	Magnesium
3 tablespoons raisins	Zinc
½ teaspoon cinnamon	Copper
⅛ teaspoon ground cloves	Selenium
pinch of coriander	Chromium
1 teaspoon honey	
skim milk (optional)	

Bring water to a boil in a medium saucepan, and stir in oats, raisins and spices. Reduce heat and simmer, stirring, about 3 to 6 minutes, until mixture is thickened and creamy. Remove from heat, cover, and let stand for 5 minutes, if desired, for a thicker consistency.

Stir in honey before serving oatmeal plain or with skim milk.

Oats and Cheese with Fruit

A unique blend of grain and dairy foods which yields hefty amounts of key minerals.

Serves three

3 cups rolled oats	** Magnesium
2 cups apple juice	** Manganese
¼ cup almonds	* Calcium
1 cup yogurt	* Zinc
1 cup cottage cheese	* Chromium
1½ cups berries	Potassium
	Copper
	Selenium

Soak oats in apple juice 30 minutes.

Process almonds in a blender until coarsely chopped. Add yogurt and cottage cheese and process until well mixed.

Divide oats among three bowls and top each with a serving of cheese mixture. Sprinkle ½ cup berries over each portion. Serve immediately.

Quick Breakfast Cereal

Less complex than granola, this nutty-tasting blend
is easy to put together in seconds flat.

Serves one

½ cup wheat germ
1 teaspoon sesame seeds
1 banana, sliced
1 teaspoon honey or to taste
milk to taste

** Magnesium
** Zinc
** Copper
** Manganese
 * Potassium
 * Selenium
 * Chromium

Pour wheat germ into a cereal bowl. Sprinkle with sesame seeds.
Add banana.

Sweeten to taste with honey. Serve with milk.

Tofu-Mushroom Omelet

Omelets are so versatile and easy to make that this tofu-mushroom
omelet will quickly become one of your favorites for breakfast,
lunch, supper or a late-night snack. The woodsy flavor of mushrooms
and slight tang of Parmesan cheese make it special, and you'll
make it often. As with scrambled eggs (following), the tofu and yogurt
add a generous share of calcium—without the predominant
use of cholesterol-laden eggs.

Serves one

1 egg
1 tablespoon yogurt
¼ cup mashed tofu
2 teaspoons grated Parmesan cheese
½ teaspoon butter
½ teaspoon oil
1-2 mushrooms, chopped
1 teaspoon chopped scallions or chives

** Magnesium
 * Calcium
 * Manganese
 Potassium
 Zinc

Blend together the egg, yogurt, tofu and cheese with a wire whisk,
blender or electric mixer. Heat the butter and oil in a small skillet or
omelet pan. Spread the mushrooms and scallions around the pan and pour
the egg mixture over them. Cook on very low heat, covered, until
almost cooked through. With a spatula, loosen omelet around the edge
if necessary and fold over to finish cooking. The omelet is done when
lightly browned on the bottom. Serve hot.

Scrambled Egg with Tofu

Simple scrambled eggs are a good way to first try tofu.
Yogurt and tofu take the place of one egg in this recipe,
bringing the calcium total up to 141 milligrams.
That compares to 102 for regular scrambled eggs, and with less fat.

Serves one

1 egg	** Magnesium
1 tablespoon yogurt	* Manganese
¼ cup mashed tofu	Calcium
2 teaspoons grated Parmesan cheese	Potassium
½ teaspoon butter	Zinc
½ teaspoon oil	

Blend together the egg, yogurt, tofu and cheese with a wire whisk, blender or electric mixer. Melt the butter and oil in a small skillet. Add egg mixture and cook, stirring, until almost dry.

Featherlight Pancakes

For a great Sunday or holiday breakfast when the clan is on hand
and trooping in two by two, have a pitcher of this batter ready.

Makes ten pancakes

2 eggs	** Manganese
1½ cups yogurt	* Magnesium
1 cup whole wheat flour	* Copper
¼ cup soy flour	* Selenium
2 tablespoons bran	* Chromium
3 tablespoons melted butter or oil	Calcium
1 teaspoon baking powder	Potassium
½ teaspoon baking soda	Zinc

Place all ingredients in a blender and whiz just until smooth. Lightly oil a hot griddle or skillet. Pour about ¼ cup of batter for each pancake. When the cakes get bubbly, turn them over and do the flip side for about 2 minutes. For variety, add sunflower seeds or chopped apples. Top with applesauce or your favorite topping.

Liver, Meat and Poultry Dishes

*Liver's so chock-full of minerals, you'll want to serve it once a week.
Our variations help you get into the liver habit.*

Liver Dressed for Dinner

Liver takes on a new personality with a combination of spices
and ingredients guaranteed to please and surprise.

Serves two

¾ pound calf liver	*** Copper
1 tablespoon soy or corn oil	** Zinc
½ sweet red pepper, chopped	** Iron
4-5 scallions, chopped	** Selenium
3 tablespoons raisins	** Chromium
1 teaspoon chili powder	* Potassium
1 teaspoon cinnamon	Manganese
¼ cup water	Fluorine
1 teaspoon tamari	

Rinse the liver, trim away any membranes, and cut into thin
pieces. In a skillet, place the oil and add the pepper and scallions.
Stir for 5 minutes, or until the vegetables begin to become tender. Add
the raisins and spices, stir, then add the liver, the water and tamari.

Cover and steam for just a few minutes, until the liver is
lightly cooked. It should still be slightly pink inside; do not overcook.
Serve immediately.

Mexican Liver

Taste-testers gave this liver dish an "A-plus."

Serves four

2 onions, sliced in rings	*** Copper
1 green pepper, thinly sliced	** Zinc
2 tomatoes, chopped	** Iron
1 pound beef liver	** Selenium
1 tablespoon chili powder	** Chromium
1 teaspoon cumin powder	* Potassium
½ teaspoon tamari	Manganese
	Fluorine

Place onion rings and green pepper slices in a large skillet, and
steam-stir in enough water to prevent sticking until onions begin to turn

transparent. Add tomatoes and stir over medium heat until onion and pepper are tender.

Cut liver into thin strips and place over the onion mixture, add spices, and cover. Steam liver just until tender; pink juices should remain in slices. Add tamari, stirring liver and vegetables to combine, and serve with brown rice or boiled potatoes.

Polynesian Liver

Vitamin C in the pepper and pineapple enhances the absorption of iron in liver.

Serves four

1 pound calf liver	*** Copper
1 large green pepper	** Zinc
¼ pineapple (about 1½ cups sliced)	** Iron
1 cup chicken stock	** Selenium
2 cups cooked brown rice	** Chromium
	* Potassium
	Manganese
	Fluorine

Clean and slice liver into julienne strips. Remove seeds from green pepper and slice it into julienne strips. Remove skin from pineapple and core. Slice pineapple and cut slices into matchstick-sized strips.

In a medium skillet, steam-stir green pepper in a few tablespoons of the stock until it begins to become tender. Add liver and cook over medium heat, stirring, until liver is still pink on the inside and juicy, adding more stock as needed to keep mixture from sticking. Add pineapple strips and heat through, with enough of the stock to provide a sauce. Serve over brown rice.

Chicken Livers, Mushrooms and Walnuts

A winning combination of super-mineral foods.

Serves four

2 cups sliced mushrooms	*** Copper
2 cloves garlic, minced	** Zinc
2 tablespoons sunflower oil	** Iron
1 teaspoon tamari	** Selenium
1 pound chicken livers, cut into small pieces	** Chromium
¼ cup walnuts, chopped	* Potassium
1 tablespoon minced fresh parsley	Manganese
1 teaspoon basil	
½ cup chicken stock	
2 cups cooked whole wheat pasta	

In a heavy skillet, place mushrooms and garlic with the oil and tamari and stir until water has evaporated from the mushrooms and they are tender. Set aside.

Steam-stir livers in the same pan, adding a few spoonfuls of water as necessary to prevent sticking. When livers are still pink inside, add mushrooms, walnuts and remaining ingredients to the pan and heat through. Serve immediately over whole wheat pasta.

Chicken Liver Kebabs

Skewers present an array of vegetables in addition to
tasty marinated livers.

Serves two

⅓ cup water	*** Copper
3 tablespoons lemon juice	** Zinc
1 tablespoon tamari	** Iron
1 clove garlic, crushed	** Potassium
½ teaspoon finely grated lemon rind	** Selenium
¼ teaspoon thyme	** Chromium
¼ teaspoon rosemary	Manganese
¾ pound chicken livers, halved	
1 green or sweet red pepper	
1 cup mushroom caps	
1 cup cherry tomatoes	

Combine the water, lemon juice, tamari, garlic, lemon rind and herbs. Place the chicken livers in a shallow dish and pour marinade over top. Refrigerate several hours or overnight, basting occasionally with the marinade.

To prepare, halve the pepper and remove the seeds. Cut pepper into large pieces, about the size of the mushrooms. Lightly steam the pepper and mushrooms until they are only slightly tender.

On long metal skewers, arrange the tomatoes, pepper, mushrooms and liver alternately. Spoon a little of the marinade over each, then place under a hot broiler. Turn to cook both sides, and remove from broiler just when livers are still slightly pink inside. Serve immediately.

Super Chili

No one will guess that this flavorful chili is made with liver,
the super-mineral food.

Serves eight

2 cups dried kidney beans	** Potassium
1 pound lean ground beef	** Zinc
½ pound calf liver	** Copper
1 large yellow onion, quartered	** Iron
1 green or sweet red pepper, chopped	** Chromium
3 cloves garlic, crushed	* Magnesium
3-4 tablespoons chili powder	* Selenium
2 teaspoons cumin powder	Manganese
2 teaspoons oregano	Fluorine
⅔ cup tomato paste	
1½ cups bean stock	
1 cup fresh or frozen corn	
4 teaspoons tamari	
1 tablespoon blackstrap molasses	

Soak beans overnight. Next day, bring to a boil in fresh water and simmer until tender, about 1½ hours. Drain, and reserve stock.

To make chili, begin browning beef in a large, hot, lightly oiled skillet. Place the liver with ¼ of the onion in a blender and process on low to medium speed until smooth. Stir into the browning meat. When meat is cooked through, chop and add remainder of the onion, the pepper, garlic, chili, cumin and oregano. Cook together until the onion becomes transparent.

Stir in tomato paste, cooked kidney beans, bean stock, corn, tamari and molasses. Simmer chili until onions and peppers are tender. Serve hot.

Note: For hotter chili, stir in cayenne pepper or dried hot red pepper flakes to taste. Freeze leftovers for another meal.

Paté Meatloaf

A perfect way to supplement your meatloaf with liver.

Serves eight

1 pound lean ground beef	** Zinc
½ pound beef liver	** Copper
1 carrot, shredded	** Iron
½ green pepper, minced	** Chromium
1 tablespoon shredded onions	* Selenium
1 tablespoon minced fresh parsley	* Manganese
1 egg	Magnesium
1 cup soft whole wheat bread crumbs	Fluorine
1 cup rolled oats	
2 teaspoons tamari	
½ teaspoon thyme	
½ teaspoon marjoram	
¼ teaspoon oregano	
¼ teaspoon basil	

Place ground beef in a large mixing bowl. In a blender, puree liver and add to beef. Stir in remaining ingredients. Place mixture in an 8½ × 4½-inch loaf pan. Cover tightly with aluminum foil. Bake in a preheated 350°F oven for 1 hour and 10 minutes and remove foil for last 15 minutes, allowing to brown.

Note: Leftover meatloaf can be sliced, wrapped and frozen for future use.

Tofu Meatloaf

Meatloaf is so simple and basic that you probably depend on it as a staple menu item. Replacing part of a meatloaf with calcium-rich tofu restores the calcium that nature originally provided in the bones the butcher removed. Our *Tofu Meatloaf* has 59 milligrams of calcium per serving, compared to just 10 for standard meatloaf.

Serves three

⅔ cup (6 ounces) tofu	** Zinc
½ pound lean ground beef	** Copper
1 egg	* Magnesium
2 tablespoons finely minced onions	* Potassium
2 tablespoons wheat germ	* Iron
⅓ cup tomato juice	* Chromium
1 tablespoon chopped fresh parsley	* Manganese
⅛ teaspoon ground cloves	Calcium
Basic Tomato Sauce (optional)	Fluorine

Break tofu in pieces and drain thoroughly in a fine strainer. Press out as much moisture as possible. Crumble the tofu.

In a large bowl, combine all ingredients. Mix with a fork until well blended.

Press into half (one end) of a very lightly greased 8½ × 4½-inch loaf pan. Bake in a preheated 350°F oven for about 35 minutes, or until the loaf begins to shrink away from the sides of the pan and is slightly brown on top.

If desired, serve with *Basic Tomato Sauce* (see page 300).

Tired of ho-hum baked chicken and roast turkey? Read on.

Apple-Chicken Bake

Here's a quick and easy way to add potassium, chromium and iron plus to your diet. Enjoy it often!

Serves two

1 chicken breast	** Potassium
3 tart apples	** Chromium
½ cup yogurt	* Zinc
1 orange	* Iron
	Calcium
	Copper
	Fluorine

Remove skin from chicken breast, and split the breast in half. Wash, remove core and cube apples, but do not peel. Place apples in the bottom of a lightly oiled casserole dish, pour yogurt over them and stir lightly to combine. Place chicken breast halves over apple-yogurt mixture. Cut unpeeled orange into thin slices, and place these over the chicken breast to keep chicken from drying out. Bake in a preheated 350°F oven for 1¼ hours. Remove orange slices before serving.

Chicken-Fruit Salad

Here's a great way to make a gorgeous meal out of leftover chicken and serve yourself a generous helping of potassium, zinc, copper, iron and other important minerals.

Serves four

⅓ cup mayonnaise	** Potassium
½ teaspoon powdered mustard	* Zinc
juice of 2 lemons	* Copper
2 cups cooked, cubed chicken	* Iron
½ cup sliced mushrooms	* Manganese
2 bananas, sliced	Magnesium
4 pineapple slices, cubed	Fluorine
salad greens	

In a small bowl, combine the mayonnaise, mustard and lemon juice. Combine the chicken, mushrooms, bananas and pineapple in a large bowl and stir in dressing. Serve on crisp salad greens and garnish with flaked coconut, sliced almonds or sunflower seeds. A delicious high-potassium meal for a hot summer day. Nice to serve for a company buffet or on the patio.

Pumpkin-Stuffed Chicken

A new twist on turkey and pumpkin pie for the holidays—
packed with zinc, potassium and other good nutrients.

Serves six

1 chicken (about 5 pounds), cleaned	** Zinc
3 cups cooked and mashed pumpkin	** Potassium
1 cup diced apples (unpeeled)	* Copper
1 cup chopped celery	* Iron
¾ cup raisins	* Chromium
½ cup pumpkin seeds	* Fluorine
½ cup sunflower seeds	
½ cup chopped walnuts	
¼ cup whole grain cornmeal	
1 teaspoon celery seed	

Combine all filling ingredients in a large bowl and lightly stuff
into chicken cavity. Place chicken in a baking pan and cover. Bake
in a preheated 350°F oven for 2½ hours, or until chicken is tender
and nicely browned.

Turkey and Sprouts

There's more to leftover turkey than soup and sandwiches.
A bed of rice and sprinkling of bean sprouts multiplies the mineral gain.

Serves four

2 cups turkey stock	** Potassium
⅓ cup whole wheat flour	** Zinc
½ cup chopped carrots	** Manganese
½ cup chopped onions	* Iron
½ cup chopped green peppers	* Copper
½ cup chopped celery	* Chromium
2 cups diced, cooked turkey	Magnesium
½-1 teaspoon curry (optional)	Selenium
1 cup bean sprouts	
2 cups cooked brown rice	

In a large saucepan, heat stock to boiling point. Transfer 1¼ cups
of the stock to a 2-cup glass measuring cup. Stir flour into remaining
stock. Gradually add reserved hot stock, stirring constantly, until thickened.

Add all vegetables, except sprouts, and simmer for 20 minutes or
until vegetables are tender but not overcooked. Add turkey and curry
(if desired) and cook a few minutes longer. Add sprouts last.

Serve on a bed of brown rice.

Apple-Lamb Curry

Fruit, lamb and rice are a welcome change of pace,
and an appealing way to bring together a whole roster
of important minerals. Kelp adds useful iodine.

Serves four

1 pound boneless stew lamb

½ cup finely chopped onions

2 teaspoons curry or to taste

1 teaspoon tamari

½ teaspoon kelp powder

1 teaspoon honey

1 cup water

2 cups diced apples (about 2 medium),
    preferably tart

¼ cup raisins

2 tablespoons arrowroot (optional)

¼ cup water (optional)

2 cups cooked brown rice

** Potassium
** Zinc
** Manganese
** Iodine
Magnesium
Copper
Selenium
Chromium
Fluorine

Trim excess fat from meat and cut into 1-inch cubes. Brown in a heavy saucepan. Drain off any fat. Add onions, seasonings, honey and 1 cup water. Cover and simmer for 1 hour or until meat is tender. Add apples and raisins and cook 15 minutes longer. If not thick enough, mix arrowroot with ¼ cup water and stir into lamb mixture. Cook, stirring constantly until thickened. Serve over hot brown rice.

========================= Fish =========================

Fish is one of our most reliable sources of selenium,
a scarce item in many diets. Feel free to use your favorite fish
unless one is particularly specified.

Saucy Fish Fillets

No one will ever accuse you of serving bland fish if you give them this dish.

Serves three

1 pound fish fillets (cod, haddock or flounder)	** Selenium
¼ cup water	** Fluorine
2 tablespoons tomato paste	(if cod
2 tablespoons finely chopped onions	is used)
1 tablespoon cider vinegar	* Potassium
1 tablespoon honey	* Iron
	Zinc
	Copper
	Chromium
	Iodine

Place the fish fillets in a single layer in the bottom of a shallow ovenproof dish, 8 × 8 inches. Combine the remaining ingredients in a small saucepan, and bring to a boil over medium heat. Pour the sauce over the fish in the casserole and bake in a preheated 350°F oven for about 25 minutes, or just until the fish is opaque and cooked through.

Peachy Fish Almondine

When peaches are in season, enjoy this great combo.

Serves four

⅓ cup sliced or chopped almonds	** Potassium
3 tablespoons butter	** Selenium
1 pound fish fillets	* Iron
3 peaches, sliced	Zinc
	Copper
	Chromium
	Iodine

Saute the almonds briefly in the butter. Remove the almonds when they are golden. Add the fish to the hot butter. Saute for 6 to 8 minutes, depending on the thickness of fillets. Cover and allow them to heat through (3 to 5 minutes) and remove to a serving platter. Top with the toasted almonds and sliced peaches.

Fish and Tofu Kebabs

You don't need beef or a barbecue pit to enjoy a delicious kebab.
This is a fun meal the children will love,
and every bite is highly nutritious.

Serves four

¼ cup lemon juice

2 tablespoons oil

1 teaspoon tamari

1 clove garlic, crushed

¼ teaspoon dill powder (crushed seeds)

2 tablespoons chopped fresh parsley

1 pound fish fillets (flounder, haddock,
  perch, pollack or cod)

8 ounces tofu

½ pound medium whole mushrooms
  (about 3 cups)

2 onions, cut into wedges or quarters
  (depending on size)

1 green pepper, cut into 1-inch pieces

1 medium zucchini, cut into 1-inch chunks

** Potassium
** Fluorine
   (if cod
   is used)
 * Fluorine
   (others)
 * Zinc
 * Copper
   Magnesium
   Selenium
   Chromium
   Manganese
   Iodine

In a large bowl, combine lemon juice, oil, tamari, garlic, dill and parsley. Cut the fish and tofu into 1½-inch cubes and marinate in the lemon juice mixture for about 1 hour. Drain and place the fish and tofu on 4 skewers, alternating with mushrooms, onions, peppers and zucchini. Brush the kebabs with marinade, set on a broiler pan, and broil 3 or 4 inches from the heat for 5 minutes. Then brush again with marinade and broil 10 minutes longer.

Fish Stuffed with Vegetables

A mineral rich dish, perked up with vegetables. Great for a crowd!

Serves six to eight

1 4- to 5-pound fish (red snapper, striped bass or salmon), cleaned and ready for stuffing
3 tablespoons butter or oil
1 clove garlic, minced
1½ cups shredded carrots
⅓ cup chopped onions
¼ cup chopped celery
¼ cup chopped green peppers
2 tablespoons chopped sweet red peppers
2 tablespoons chopped fresh chives
2 tablespoons chopped fresh parsley
½ teaspoon dill
¼ teaspoon thyme
¼ teaspoon paprika
⅛ teaspoon rosemary
⅛ teaspoon black pepper
2 tablespoons butter, melted
parsley butter or lemon butter (optional)

** Selenium
** Fluorine (if salmon is used)
* Potassium
* Chromium
Magnesium (if salmon is used)
Copper
Iodine

Wash fish and pat dry with paper towels. Place in an oiled, shallow roasting pan.

Melt 3 tablespoons butter or heat oil in a skillet. Saute garlic and vegetables until tender. Remove pan from heat and add seasonings. Mix together well. Spoon stuffing into fish and close cavity with wooden toothpicks, or wooden toothpicks laced with string. Brush fish with 2 tablespoons of melted butter. Bake in a preheated 375°F oven until fork-tender, about 45 to 50 minutes. Baste often. Serve with parsley butter or lemon butter if desired.

Baked Haddock

Serves four

1 pound haddock fillets	** Selenium
½ cup finely chopped onions	* Potassium
½ cup shredded zucchini	* Iron
¼ cup finely chopped celery	* Chromium
1 teaspoon corn oil	Zinc
1 cup soft whole wheat bread crumbs	Copper
1 tablespoon minced fresh flat-leaf parsley	Iodine
¼ teaspoon tarragon	
⅛ teaspoon rosemary	
1–2 large tomatoes, thinly sliced	
lemon juice (optional)	

Place haddock fillets in a shallow baking pan. Combine onions, zucchini and celery in a skillet with the oil and saute until slightly tender, adding a few drops of water, if necessary, to prevent scorching. Stir in bread crumbs and herbs.

Spread bread crumb mixture over the fish in the baking pan. Place thin slices of tomato to cover the bread crumb mixture. Bake in a preheated 375°F oven for 35 to 40 minutes. Sprinkle with lemon juice before serving, if desired.

Polynesian Haddock

An exotic way to dress up an everyday fish—
and add a wealth of minerals to your supper.

Serves four

1 pound haddock fillets	** Potassium
2 tablespoons lemon juice	** Selenium
¼ cup fish or vegetable stock	** Manganese
4 tablespoons chopped onions	** Iodine
1 tablespoon chopped fresh parsley	* Iron
1 teaspoon tamari	* Chromium
1 cup crushed pineapple	Magnesium
3 tablespoons chopped almonds	Zinc
2 cups cooked brown rice	Copper

Spread the fillets in a baking pan. Sprinkle with lemon juice. In a medium saucepan combine the stock, onions, parsley, tamari and pineapple. Cook over low heat for 5 minutes. Spoon over the fish. Top with the almonds. Bake in a preheated 350°F oven for 20 to 30 minutes or until fish flakes easily when prodded with a fork. Serve over hot brown rice.

Poached Fish in Spanish Sauce

Color and flavor abound in this easy entree.

Serves two

1 onion, finely chopped	** Potassium
⅓ cup minced fresh parsley	** Selenium
1 clove garlic, crushed	* Iron
2 tablespoons tarragon vinegar	* Chromium
½ teaspoon thyme	Zinc
3 large tomatoes, chopped	Copper
1 pound haddock fillets	Iodine

Place all ingredients in a heavy pan or electric skillet, putting the fish fillets on top. When mixture has come to a boil, simmer, covered, for 10 minutes. Carefully remove fish fillets from the top of the vegetable sauce and place on a serving platter. Keep the fish warm by covering with foil while you boil down sauce. Turn up heat under the vegetables and boil quickly to reduce mixture by half. Pour the sauce over the fish and serve.

Salmon Steaks Broiled with Herbs and Garlic

This is one of our favorites, especially high in selenium and potassium.

Serves four

4 salmon steaks about 1 inch thick	** Potassium
3 tablespoons butter, melted	** Selenium
3 tablespoons chopped fresh parsley	** Fluorine
2 tablespoons chopped shallots (or	Magnesium
3 tablespoons chopped scallions)	Copper
1½ tablespoons finely chopped garlic	Chromium
juice of 3 lemons	Iodine
few grains of cayenne pepper	

Wash salmon steaks and dry with paper towels. Place in a pan suitable for broiling where steaks will rest in marinade sauce.

To make marinade, combine butter, parsley, shallots, garlic, lemon juice and cayenne pepper, and mix lightly. Spread half over steaks.

Broil for 7 minutes. Turn, spread remaining marinade over salmon, and broil another 7 minutes.

Transfer steaks to a heated serving platter and cover with marinade and pan drippings. Garnish with lemon wedges, parsley and other greens.

Poached Salmon

Try this for a refreshing alternative to fried haddock and tartar sauce.

Serves two

¾ pound salmon fillets	** Potassium
1 teaspoon crumbled rosemary leaves	** Fluorine
¼ teaspoon white pepper	Magnesium
4 cups water	Copper
¼ cup vinegar	Selenium
1 tablespoon dried celery leaves (optional)	Chromium
	Iodine

To prepare fish, wash fillets and pat dry with paper towels. Season lightly with rosemary and white pepper.

Combine remaining ingredients and bring to a boil in large skillet. Add fillets. (Be sure that liquid just covers the fish.) When poaching liquid returns to the boiling point, reduce heat to simmer and begin timing the fish. Allow 10 minutes per inch of thickness. Do not allow the liquid to boil or bubble. Fish is done when the flesh flakes apart easily when tested with a fork.

Remove immediately to avoid overcooking.

Salmon Salad Sandwich

If you have some salmon on the pantry shelf but don't quite know what to do with it, a *Salmon Salad Sandwich* is for you. Combined with yogurt and cucumber, salmon for lunch is an inviting change from the old standby, tuna fish sandwiches.

Serves two

⅔ cup canned salmon, flaked (about 4 ounces)	** Selenium
½ medium cucumber, diced into ¼-inch cubes	** Manganese
5 tablespoons yogurt	* Calcium
1 teaspoon lemon juice	* Potassium
2 teaspoons finely minced onions	* Copper
1 teaspoon chopped chives	* Chromium
4 slices whole wheat bread	* Fluorine
crisp lettuce (optional)	Magnesium
	Iodine

Combine all ingredients except bread and lettuce in a medium bowl. Chill. Tastes great with lettuce, sandwiched between toasted slices of bread. Cut each sandwich in half.

Salmon Quiche

Enjoy the subtle flavor of salmon and get a double bonus of calcium in this low-fat quiche (pronounced "keesh").

Serves six

½ cup low-fat cottage cheese	** Calcium
½ cup ricotta cheese	** Potassium
¼ cup buttermilk	** Selenium
2 scallions, finely chopped	** Manganese
2 eggs, beaten	** Fluorine
15½ ounces salmon with bones, drained	* Copper
dash of freshly grated nutmeg	* Chromium
9-inch *No-Roll Crust*	Magnesium

Place the cheeses and buttermilk in a blender and process on low speed until combined. Transfer to a large bowl and add scallions and eggs. Flake salmon meat and crush the bones; add to the cheese mixture with a dash of nutmeg.

Pour salmon mixture into the pie crust and bake in a preheated 400°F oven for 20 minutes; then turn down heat to 350°F and bake 10 to 15 minutes longer, until quiche is puffed and golden brown. Serve hot or at room temperature.

Note: You can use 1 cup of cottage cheese or 1 cup of ricotta rather than the combination above.

No-Roll Crust

Makes one 9-inch pie crust

¾ cup whole wheat flour
2 tablespoons soy flour
2 tablespoons wheat germ
¼ cup soy oil
2 tablespoons buttermilk

Combine ingredients in a 9-inch pie plate. Toss with a fork until all the ingredients are combined, then press with fingers along bottom and sides of the plate. Fill and bake according to desired recipe.

Salmon Spaghetti

The idea of salmon spaghetti may sound way-out, but don't knock it.
We tried it and loved it! When made according to this recipe from
Joanie Huggins's book *Out of the Sugar Rut* (HAH Publications,
Colorado Springs, Colorado, 1978), it is a dish you will be happy to serve
to your favorite people.

Serves four (side dish) or two (main dish)

1½ cups sliced mushrooms	** Calcium
¼ cup sliced scallions	** Potassium
2 tablespoons butter	** Selenium
15½ ounces canned salmon with liquid or	** Manganese
1 pound cooked salmon	** Fluorine
1 cup yogurt	* Magnesium
1 teaspoon whole wheat pastry flour	* Copper
⅛ teaspoon pepper	* Chromium
½ pound whole wheat spaghetti	Iodine

Saute mushrooms and scallions in butter in a large skillet over low
heat until vegetables are just tender. Add salmon and simmer for 3
minutes. Combine yogurt, flour and pepper. Stir into mixture in skillet.
Cook, stirring, for 3 minutes longer.

Meanwhile, cook spaghetti according to package directions. Drain.
Serve with salmon sauce poured over it. Serve with grated Parmesan
cheese and a tossed salad.

Tuna-Yogurt Combo

Serve it hot as a main dish—or cold as a dip.

Makes three cups

1 small onion, chopped	** Selenium
2 tablespoons oil	Calcium
1 cup sliced mushrooms	Potassium
freshly ground pepper to taste	Zinc
2 tablespoons whole wheat flour	Copper
1 cup yogurt	Chromium
6 ounces tuna, drained	Iodine
2 tablespoons water	

Saute onion in oil briefly in a medium saucepan. Add mushrooms
and pepper and cook, covered, for about a minute. Add the flour
and continue to cook for another minute. Add ½ cup of yogurt and
mix together.

Put this mixture in a blender with the tuna and water. Whiz

until smooth. Return to saucepan, add the remaining yogurt, and heat. Serve it hot as a main dish on top of brown rice or crisp whole wheat toast. Serve cold with vegetables as a dip. If you have any left over, freeze it and enjoy it again either hot or cold.

Tuna-Nectarine Salad

An unusual combination. Try it.

Serves four

⅓ cup mayonnaise	* Selenium
1½ tablespoons lemon juice	Potassium
¼ teaspoon dry mustard	Copper
⅛ teaspoon paprika	Chromium
7 ounces tuna, flaked	Iodine
2 stalks of celery, finely chopped	
3 nectarines, chunked	

Blend the mayonnaise with the lemon juice, mustard and paprika in a large bowl. Add tuna, celery and nectarines. Toss to combine and serve on crisp greens.

Tuna-Stuffed Tomatoes

This is a beautiful dish for a very special luncheon,
a buffet table or a treat for the family.

Serves four

¼ cup mayonnaise	** Potassium
¼ cup yogurt	** Selenium
2 tablespoons pineapple juice	** Iodine
2 tablespoons finely chopped onions	* Chromium
¼ teaspoon ground ginger	* Manganese
7½ ounces tuna, drained	Zinc
1 cup pineapple chunks	Copper
½ cup chopped walnuts	
4 large tomatoes	
½ teaspoon kelp powder	
salad greens	

In a large bowl combine the mayonnaise, yogurt, pineapple juice, onions and ginger. Stir in the tuna, pineapple chunks and walnuts. Chill. Place the tomatoes stem end down. Cut each tomato almost to the stem, making 5 or 6 sections. Spread apart slightly. Sprinkle with kelp. Fill with the tuna mixture. Arrange on salad greens, and garnish with parsley or watercress, if desired.

Mackerel Salad

Mackerel is rich in a fatty acid that reduces blood platelet
stickiness leading to clots.
This mackerel salad tastes like chopped herring. Make a lot and
serve several times a week, for breakfast, lunch or dinner.

Makes about 3½ cups

1 slice rye bread	** Selenium
3 tablespoons vinegar	* Potassium
2½ cups cooked mackerel, flaked	* Fluorine
1 medium onion, cut into chunks	Copper
1 large apple, chunked	Chromium
3 hard-cooked eggs	Iodine
dash of pepper	

Soak the bread in the vinegar. Put all ingredients in the bowl of
a food processor, fitted with the chopping blade. Process with the on-
off switch until it is a little lumpy. If you don't have a processor, chop
the ingredients in a wooden bowl. Taste and adjust seasoning. If you
like it more tart, add a little more vinegar. Serve with a large mixed
vegetable salad. It keeps for several days refrigerated, and should serve
6 to 8 generously.

Meatless Main Dishes

Even if you're not serving meat tonight, you can feast on mineral-rich foods.

Soy Loaf

Soybeans earn this vegetarian loaf high marks for minerals.

Serves four

1 onion, grated	** Magnesium
½ cup mushrooms	** Zinc
2 cloves garlic, crushed	** Copper
2 stalks celery, finely chopped	* Calcium
3 tablespoons oil	* Potassium
2 cups cooked, pureed soybeans	* Selenium
¾ cup wheat germ	* Manganese
½ cup cashew bits	Iron
¼ cup non-instant milk powder	Chromium
3 eggs	Fluorine
3 tablespoons oil	
1 teaspoon fresh thyme	
1 teaspoon fresh dillweed	
1 teaspoon fresh sage	
½ cup grated cheese	

Saute onion, mushrooms, garlic and celery in oil until tender.

Combine all ingredients in a large bowl and mix thoroughly. Press the mixture into an oiled 8½ × 4½-inch loaf pan.

Bake in a preheated 350°F oven for 40 minutes.

Tofu Lasagna

Just about everyone loves lasagna. Tofu easily replaces
the ricotta cheese called for in standard recipes,
but the remaining ingredients probably don't vary much
from other recipes you've tried. The whole family will enjoy
the steaming squares of noodles melted together by mozzarella,
oozing with just enough rich tomato sauce to keep it moist,
and topped with more Parmesan to give the dish extra bite.

Serves five

½ pound whole wheat lasagna noodles	** Calcium
(about 8 noodles)	** Manganese
1 cup mashed tofu	* Magnesium
½ cup grated Parmesan cheese	* Copper
1 egg	* Chromium
½ clove garlic, finely minced	Potassium
1 cup shredded mozzarella cheese	Zinc
1 cup thinly sliced mushrooms	Selenium
2 tablespoons finely chopped fresh parsley	
2½ cups *Basic Tomato Sauce* (see page 300)	

In a large pot, bring 4 quarts of water to a boil. Add a tablespoon
or 2 of oil to prevent the noodles from sticking together as they cook.
Add the lasagna noodles and continue cooking at a rolling boil for about
8 minutes, or until they are tender and begin to break apart. Stir
occasionally with a long wooden fork or spoon. Drain the noodles and
douse with cold water. Set aside.

While the noodles are cooking, mix the tofu, ¼ cup of the Parmesan
cheese, egg, and garlic. Beat till smooth and fluffy. Have the mozzarella,
mushrooms and parsley ready for assembly.

Spoon ¼ cup of the tomato sauce around the bottom of a very
lightly greased loaf pan or 1½-quart baking pan. Arrange a layer of
2 noodles on top of the sauce. Spread the tofu-Parmesan mixture over
the noodles. Arrange 2 noodles over the top of the cheese mixture.
Spread the mushrooms and parsley over the noodles and add tomato
sauce. Arrange 2 noodles and add mozzarella and sauce. Arrange the
last of the noodles and pour remaining sauce over them. Sprinkle with
the remaining Parmesan cheese. Bake in a preheated 350°F oven for 45
to 50 minutes. Allow to stand 5 to 10 minutes before serving.

Eggplant-Tofu Parmesan

The blend of lots of crumbly tofu, tender vegetables, pungent parsley and a faint hint of garlic makes *Eggplant-Tofu Parmesan* a wonderful one-dish casserole to serve with whole wheat bread and a big green salad. You'll find this version far less oily than its authentic Italian counterpart. For traditional eggplant Parmesan, the eggplant slices are first breaded and sauteed or fried. Not only is that process tedious and time-consuming, the end result is heavy with fat because of eggplant's phenomenal capacity for sponging up oil. Baking the eggplant not only eliminates all that oil but saves you a lot of work. That makes it especially appealing to folks who love ethnic dishes but can't always find the time to make them.

Serves four

1 small eggplant, sliced into ½-inch-thick slices (about 11 slices)	* Magnesium
1¼ cups tofu, mashed	* Calcium
¾ cup grated Parmesan cheese	* Copper
1 tablespoon parsley	* Chromium
½ clove garlic, finely minced	* Manganese
1 egg	Potassium
2 cups *Basic Tomato Sauce* (see page 300)	Zinc
1 small onion, very thinly sliced (about ⅔ cup)	Fluorine
½ cup diced green peppers	
⅓ cup thinly sliced mushrooms	
½ cup dry whole wheat bread crumbs	

Arrange the eggplant slices on a broiler tray or cookie sheet and bake in a preheated 375°F oven until tender—about 8 minutes on each side, turning with a fork when half done. They should be tender.

Mix tofu with ½ cup of the Parmesan cheese, along with the parsley, garlic and egg.

To assemble, first spoon a few tablespoons of the tomato sauce into the bottom of a 1½-quart loaf pan or rectangular baking pan. Arrange slices of eggplant over the sauce. Cover the layer of eggplant with half of the tofu-cheese mixture, half the amounts of each vegetable, and half the bread crumbs. Top with a thin layer of tomato sauce.

Repeat with a layer of eggplant, the rest of the cheese mixture, remaining onions, peppers, mushrooms and bread crumbs, any remaining eggplant, and tomato sauce. Sprinkle with remaining Parmesan cheese. Return to oven and bake for 45 to 50 minutes. Allow to stand for 5 to 10 minutes before serving.

Tamale Bean Pie

A potpourri of beans and spices.

Serves four to six
Crust:

2½ cups cold water	* Magnesium
1½ cups whole grain cornmeal	* Potassium
2 teaspoons chili powder	* Copper
½ teaspoon cumin powder	* Manganese
1 teaspoon tamari	Iron
	Selenium
	Chromium

Combine cold water, cornmeal, chili, cumin and tamari in a heavy saucepan and stir over medium heat until the mixture thickens and comes to a boil. Lightly oil an 8 × 8-inch casserole dish, and place two-thirds of the cornmeal mixture on the bottom and halfway up the sides of the dish. Set aside the remaining cornmeal mixture.

Filling:

1 cup cooked kidney, pinto or black beans
1 cup cooked soybeans
1 stalk celery, chopped
1 green pepper, chopped
1 medium onion, chopped
2 cloves garlic, minced
½ cup corn
3 tablespoons water
2 tablespoons tomato paste
2 tablespoons chili powder
2 teaspoons cumin powder
½ teaspoon cumin seed
1 tablespoon lemon juice
    dash of cayenne pepper
    alfalfa sprouts (garnish)

Process the beans together in a blender on low speed or with a food mill until thoroughly mashed. In a large skillet, steam-stir the celery, pepper and onion in a small amount of water until the onion is translucent; add the garlic toward the end of cooking. Add the beans and the remaining ingredients except sprouts and stir over medium heat for 5 to 8 minutes. Stir frequently, or the beans will stick.

Pour the bean mixture over the cornmeal layer in the casserole dish. Spread remaining cornmeal mixture over beans. Bake in a preheated 350°F oven for 30 minutes. Top each serving with fresh alfalfa sprouts.

Stir-Fried Tofu

If you want to try out that new wok you got for Christmas,
here's your chance. Use a large skillet if you are wok-less.
A large skillet will do just as well, however. Unadorned tofu
is most at home with stir-fried Chinese-style vegetables,
as the food originated in the Orient.

Serves four

2 tablespoons vegetable oil	** Magnesium
2 cups cubed tofu (about 1 pound)	** Manganese
2 cloves garlic, finely chopped	* Copper
½ teaspoon chopped fresh ginger or	* Chromium
⅓ teaspoon ground ginger	Calcium
1 large onion, thinly sliced and separated	Potassium
into rings	Zinc
½ pound mushrooms, thinly sliced	Iron
1 small zucchini, cut into 2-inch strips	Fluorine
1 cup broccoli florets	
2 tablespoons water	
1 sweet red pepper, thinly sliced	
1 cup chicken or vegetable broth, heated	
2 tablespoons cornstarch or arrowroot flour	
2 tablespoons tamari	
2 cups cooked brown rice	

Heat 1 tablespoon of the oil in a wok or large skillet. Add tofu
and stir-fry until browned, moving cubes around gently with a long
wooden fork. Remove from wok and drain tofu on paper towels.

Add the remaining tablespoon of oil, and the garlic, ginger, onion,
mushrooms, zucchini and broccoli to the wok. Sprinkle with the water.
Cook slightly. Add red pepper and ½ cup of hot stock. Cover and cook
3 to 5 minutes.

Combine cornstarch or arrowroot, tamari and remaining ½ cup
of the stock in a cup. Stir until blended. Pour sauce mixture into wok
with the vegetables and cook until thickened. Return drained tofu and
combine quickly with the other ingredients. Serve over hot, cooked rice.

Tofu Quiche

Quiche (pronounced "keesh") may sound exotic and complicated, but it's really quite simple. Quiche is an ideal main dish because it brings together so many protein- and calcium-rich foods. Unlike most quiche recipes, which go heavy on cream and eggs, our version has little fat by comparison.

Serves eight

Crust:

You may use either the following crust, a thin whole grain crust of your own, or the *No-Roll Crust* on page 257

** Calcium
** Manganese
 * Magnesium
Potassium
Zinc
Copper
Selenium
Chromium

⅓ cup butter
1⅓ cups whole wheat pastry flour
3 tablespoons ice water

Allow butter to reach room temperature.

In a medium bowl, mix butter and flour with pastry blender until it's the consistency of coarse cornmeal. Gradually add the ice water and press dough together into a ball. Roll out to a thickness of about ⅛ inch. Using a 10-inch pie dish as a guide, cut a circle out of the dough about an inch larger than the dish.

Transfer the dough to the inside of the pie dish. Press crust against the bottom and sides. Refrigerate while you prepare the filling.

Filling:

½ cup cold soy milk or dairy milk
2 tablespoons whole wheat flour
1 egg
½ cup dry-curd cottage cheese, uncreamed
½ cup yogurt
1 cup tofu
½ cup Cheddar cheese
¾ cup cooked, well-drained and finely chopped
    Swiss chard or spinach

Combine milk and flour in a blender. Blend until smooth. Add egg, cottage cheese, yogurt, tofu and Cheddar cheese. Again, blend until smooth.

Stir in cooked, chopped greens. Pour mixture into the quiche shell and bake in a preheated 350°F oven for 45 minutes, or until a knife inserted into the middle comes out clean. If the quiche is not brown, place under the broiler for a few minutes. Be careful not to let the edges of the crust burn. Allow to stand for 5 or 10 minutes before cutting, to set.

Note: Soy milk is often used as a substitute for cow's milk, especially for infants who are allergic to cow's milk. You can either buy it made up or you can quickly make your own for baking by combining ¼ cup soy powder and 1 cup water in a blender, mixing with an electric mixer, or combining in a jar with a tight-fitting lid and shaking vigorously.

Macaroni Salad with Cheese Dressing

An inviting version of standard macaroni and cheese.
Whole wheat macaroni adds trace minerals that white macaroni lacks.

Serves six

2 cups whole wheat macaroni	** Manganese
1 tablespoon oil	* Magnesium
1 pound snap beans, cut into 1-inch pieces	* Selenium
(approximately 2 cups)	Calcium
2 cups diced carrots	Copper
½ cup chopped scallions	
2 tablespoons chopped fresh parsley	
½ teaspoon dill	
½ teaspoon basil	
½ teaspoon black pepper	
1 cup cottage cheese	
1 cup ricotta cheese	
2 teaspoons prepared mustard	
2 tablespoons lemon juice	

Cook macaroni in plenty of boiling water to which the oil has been added. Drain and rinse with cold water. Cook snap beans and carrots according to preferred method. Drain if necessary.

Combine the macaroni, beans, carrots, scallions and seasonings in a large bowl. Process cottage cheese and ricotta in a blender. Add mustard and lemon juice and blend until smooth. Toss macaroni mixture with cheese dressing until ingredients are well coated. Chill and serve.

Buckwheat-Stuffed Cabbage Rolls

Buckwheat gives us magnesium, selenium and copper—welcome additions to our daily diet. Freeze half of these rolls for future use if you wish.

Makes 16 cabbage rolls

1 medium onion, finely chopped	** Magnesium
½ green pepper, finely chopped	Zinc
3 tablespoons oil	Copper
2 cups buckwheat groats	Selenium
4 cups boiling water	Chromium
pepper to taste	
½ cup chopped peanuts (raw or roasted)	
¼ cup chopped sunflower seeds	
1 head cabbage	
Basic Tomato Sauce	

Saute the onion and green pepper in oil until tender (approximately 5 minutes). Add groats and stir until coated with oil. Add the water, cover and simmer 15 minutes or until groats are tender and the water has been absorbed. Season and add peanuts and sunflower seeds.

While groats are cooking, core the cabbage and steam until leaves are pliable. Separate the leaves and place 2 heaping tablespoons of the groat mixture on each leaf. Roll up, tucking in the sides.

Place cabbage rolls in an oiled baking pan. Pour warm water over rolls to reach three-quarters of the way up the sides of the dish. Cover and bake in a preheated 350°F oven for 1½ hours or until cabbage is tender. Serve with *Basic Tomato Sauce* (see recipe under Condiments later in this chapter).

Squash Casserole

A hearty, very tasty main dish, sauced with yogurt, cheese and chives.

Serves four

3 cups winter squash, sliced into ¼-inch pieces	** Iodine
½ cup chopped onions	* Potassium
½ cup shredded carrots	* Chromium
½ cup chopped celery	Calcium
2 tablespoons butter	Copper
¾ cup soft whole wheat bread crumbs	Selenium
½ teaspoon basil	
½ teaspoon thyme	
½ teaspoon kelp powder	
¼ teaspoon white pepper	
1 cup yogurt	
2 tablespoons oil	
⅓ cup grated mild cheese	
1 egg, beaten	
2 tablespoons chopped chives or scallions	
¼ cup toasted sesame seeds	

Steam the squash until just tender.

Saute the onions, carrots and celery in the butter until tender. Place in a large bowl and add bread crumbs along with the basil, thyme, kelp and pepper, making a stuffing.

Put a layer of squash in the bottom of a greased 2-quart casserole dish. Place the stuffing on top, then the rest of the squash.

To make the sauce, stir the yogurt, oil and grated cheese together. Place over low heat until the cheese melts. Remove from heat. Stir a little of the hot sauce into the beaten egg, then add egg mixture to the sauce slowly to prevent curdling. Add the chives.

Pour the yogurt sauce over the squash and sprinkle with toasted sesame seeds. Bake in a preheated 350°F oven for 30 minutes.

Soups

Most soups are served as a preface to a meal.
Others are so rich they comprise a meal in themselves.

Our Favorite Borscht

Served hot or cold, this hearty soup is best made in quantity.
Freeze half for later.

Serves eight to ten

2 pounds soup meat and bone	** Zinc
3 tomatoes, chopped	* Iron
3 sprigs parsley	* Chromium
1 sprig dillweed	Calcium
2 bay leaves	Potassium
1½ quarts water	Copper
1 small cabbage, finely shredded	Manganese
2 onions, coarsely diced	Fluorine
1 cup diced carrots	
5 beets, washed and diced	
3 medium potatoes, diced	
yogurt	

Put the meat, soup bone, tomatoes, parsley, dillweed and bay leaves in a large, deep pot. Cover with water. Cover and cook over low temperature for 2 hours, or until the meat is very tender.

Remove the soup bone and the parsley, dillweed and bay leaves. Skim the fat off; or cover the stock, put it in the refrigerator to let the fat harden, then remove fat. Add the cabbage, onions, carrots, beets and potatoes to the stock and meat. Let simmer for 30 to 45 minutes and serve.

Pass the yogurt in a separate dish and stir a heaping spoonful into each dish of soup.

Chicken Gumbo

In addition to minerals mentioned, small amounts of calcium leach into the acidic broth from chicken bones.

Serves eight

1 stewing chicken (4 pounds or more)	Potassium
2 quarts water	Zinc
1 onion, chopped	Copper
4-5 green shallots	Iron
2 cloves garlic, finely chopped	Chromium
2 cups peeled, chopped tomatoes	Fluorine
1 cup chopped okra	
½ cup chopped celery leaves	
4 bay leaves	
sprig of thyme	
2 tablespoons chopped parsley	
¼ teaspoon curry	

Place the chicken and water in a heavy pot along with onion, shallots, garlic and tomatoes, and simmer for 2½ hours. Strain broth into a large bowl. Remove any meat from the bones, and return chicken and stock to the pot.

Add the okra, celery leaves, bay leaves and thyme. Simmer for 45 minutes, then add parsley and curry.

Simmer a few minutes more; then serve.

Watercress Soup

An easy, yummy way to add extra calcium to your diet.

Serves six

1 large bunch watercress	** Calcium
1 large potato	* Potassium
2 tablespoons flour	Magnesium
5 cups milk	Fluorine
3 tablespoons minced onions	
1 teaspoon chopped fresh basil	

Wash watercress and pat dry. Saving 6 sprigs for garnish, finely chop the remaining cress and set aside.

Cook potato, mash, and set aside.

Make a paste of the flour and ¼ cup of the milk in a large saucepan. Slowly stir in remaining milk, onions and basil. Cook, stirring constantly, until mixture comes to a boil. It should thicken slightly.

Stir in potato and watercress and simmer 3 minutes, not longer. Serve immediately. Garnish each serving with a sprig of watercress.

Chili Bean and Rice Soup

Beans and brown rice both contain excellent body-building nutrients.
Beans are a little short of the amino acid methionine, a deficiency
that is made up by the brown rice. Together they provide a complete
protein equivalent to what you get in meat. Many beans are rich in iron,
potassium, magnesium and manganese.

Makes eight cups

1 pound pink, red or pinto beans	* Magnesium
6–8 cups boiling water	* Potassium
2 cloves garlic, crushed	* Manganese
1 onion, diced	Copper
1 bay leaf	Iron
¼ teaspoon thyme	Chromium
¼ teaspoon marjoram	
2 cups stewed tomatoes	
1½ cups beef, chicken or vegetable broth	
½ cup brown rice	
1 teaspoon chili powder	
¼ teaspoon cayenne	

Wash the beans and soak them for 1 hour. Drain and empty
them into a large pot. Add boiling water, garlic, onion, bay leaf, thyme
and marjoram. Cover and simmer for 1½ hours. Don't let the beans boil
dry. Add hot water as needed. Now add the tomatoes, broth, rice and
seasonings. Continue to cook for another hour. When the beans are
tender, mash half of the beans (about 3 cups) with some liquid and return
to soup. Package in serving-size containers for convenience.

Salmon Bisque

Rich in calcium and selenium, this bisque also has flavor.

Serves four

1 onion, chopped	** Calcium
2 tablespoons sunflower oil	** Potassium
2 tablespoons whole wheat flour	** Selenium
1 cup whole milk	** Fluorine
15½ ounces canned salmon, drained	Magnesium
1 cup chicken stock or vegetable stock	Copper
½ teaspoon thyme	Chromium
	Iodine

Saute onion in oil until tender in a large skillet. Stir in whole
wheat flour and cook over medium heat for 2 to 3 minutes. Add milk

slowly, stirring after each addition, to prevent lumping. Simmer over medium heat until sauce begins to thicken.

Flake 1½ cups of salmon meat and set aside. Place remaining salmon with bones in a blender with the stock. Process on medium speed until smooth.

Stir flaked salmon, blended salmon and thyme into skillet with sauce, and heat through. Serve hot.

Fish Chowder

With a salad and a good whole grain bread, this chowder is a most satisfying meal.

Serves six

1 pound fish fillets	** Selenium
2 cups cubed potatoes, well scrubbed but not peeled	* Potassium
	* Chromium
2 cups boiling water	Calcium
⅛ teaspoon pepper	Magnesium
½ cup chopped onions	Zinc
2 tablespoons butter	Copper
2 cups milk	Iron
3 tablespoons whole wheat flour	Iodine
basil and/or thyme to taste	

Cut fillets into 2-inch pieces. Cook potatoes in 2 cups water for 5 minutes. Add fish and pepper. Simmer, covered, 10 to 12 minutes. Cook onions in butter till golden. Add onions and butter to fish mixture. Add the milk gradually to the flour in a bowl, and then add to chowder. Cook and stir until thickened. Add herbs to taste.

Pinto-Vegetable Soup

Here again, beans take credit for the nutrition rating.

Serves four

1 cup pinto beans	* Potassium
3 cups water	Magnesium
2 cups tomato puree	Copper
1 parsnip, chopped	Manganese
1 onion, chopped	
1 carrot, chopped	
1 bay leaf	

Soak beans for several hours.

Cook beans for 1 hour. Add remaining ingredients and cook 30 minutes more. Serve piping hot.

Cashew-Carrot Soup

Nuts and rice turn a traditional soup into a unique blend
of flavors and textures.

Serves four

2 medium onions, sliced	* Potassium
4 tablespoons oil	* Copper
2 cups coarsely shredded cabbage, turnip	* Chromium
greens or Swiss chard	Calcium
2 cups shredded carrots	Magnesium
1 cup chopped apples	Zinc
5 cups beef stock	
2 tablespoons tomato paste	
1/3 cup brown rice	
1/2 cup coarsely chopped cashew nuts	
1/2 cup raisins	
1-1 1/2 cups yogurt	

Using a Dutch oven or heavy-bottom pot, saute onions in oil,
then stir in greens and saute a few minutes; add the carrots and cook
a minute or so longer. Stir in apples, beef stock and tomato paste. Bring
mixture to a boil and add rice. Simmer, covered, for 35 to 40 minutes
or until carrots are tender and rice is cooked.

Add cashew nuts and raisins and cook until raisins are "plumped."
Serve each bowl of soup topped with a generous dollop of yogurt.

Tomato-Pumpkin Soup

Smooth and creamy, rich in flavor and nutrients,
a soup that warms the bones and cheers the heart.

Serves four

1/2 cup sliced onions	** Potassium
2 tablespoons butter	* Chromium
1 cup cooked pumpkin	Calcium
1 cup vegetable broth	
2 cups chopped tomatoes, drained	
1/8 teaspoon white pepper	
1 cup milk	
1/2 cup yogurt	
2 tablespoons toasted sesame seeds	

Saute onions in butter in a medium saucepan until tender but not
brown. Stir in pumpkin, broth, tomatoes and pepper. Bring to a boil,
cover and simmer for about 15 minutes. Pour mixture into a blender

and whiz until smooth. Return to saucepan and heat. Stir in the milk as soon as it is heated through. Add a dollop of yogurt to each bowl and garnish with sesame seeds.

Oven Split Pea Soup

A good dish to make when you are using the oven for other baking chores. If you will not be using the oven for the full 1½ to 2 hours, the soup can be finished in a pot on top of the stove.

Serves four

1 cup dried split peas	** Iodine
2 onions, chopped	* Copper
2 stalks celery, chopped	Magnesium
1 bay leaf	Potassium
1 teaspoon basil	Zinc
1 teaspoon thyme	Iron
½ teaspoon kelp powder	Manganese
¼ teaspoon celery seed	
⅛ teaspoon dried hot red pepper flakes	
1 carrot, sliced	
½ cup minced fresh parsley	
1 clove garlic, minced	
2 large tomatoes, chopped	
4 cups water	

Soak split peas for 2 to 4 hours.

Place ingredients in order given in a 2-quart casserole dish. Cover and bake in a preheated 350°F oven 1½ to 2 hours, stirring once, after 1 hour, during baking. Remove from oven; place 2 cups of soup in a blender and process on medium speed until smooth. Stir into the rest of the soup. Serve hot.

⎯ Potatoes, Rice and Other Side Dishes ⎯

*More than just an afterthought, these staples can be dressed up
to maximize the mineral supply of a meal.*

Baked, Stuffed Potatoes with Tofu

These yummy stuffed potatoes fill the kitchen with a rich, cheesy aroma
as they bake. And they're light enough to serve with any meal,
and make good companions for *Tofu Meatloaf.*
Rather than heat up the oven for only one or two potatoes,
you can boil them in their jackets for about 45 or 50 minutes
in a saucepan of water on top of the stove. If you do have
baked potatoes on hand, restuff and bake the leftovers for a fresh,
steaming side dish. Made ahead of time, stuffed potatoes can help
a busy cook serve a fancy side dish with no last-minute fuss,
while adding calcium and other extra minerals to the meal.

Serves two

1 tablespoon finely chopped onions	** Magnesium
1 teaspoon finely chopped fresh parsley	* Calcium
1 large potato, baked or boiled in its jacket	* Potassium
¼ cup mashed tofu	* Zinc
¼ cup grated strong Cheddar cheese	* Chromium
2 tablespoons yogurt	* Manganese
grated Parmesan cheese (about 2 teaspoons)	Fluorine

Steam the onions and parsley until the onions are transparent
and soft. Drain off any residual water.

Cut the cooked potato in half lengthwise. Scoop out the insides
from each half. In a blender or bowl, combine scooped potato insides
with onions, parsley, tofu, Cheddar cheese and yogurt. Blend or mix
with electric mixer until smooth.

Fill the potato shells with the cheese mixture. Sprinkle each shell
with a teaspoon or so of Parmesan cheese. Place on a lightly greased
baking sheet or in a Pyrex baking pan. Bake in a preheated 350°F
oven until lightly browned on top, about 35 minutes. Serve steaming hot.

Potato-Carrot Pancakes

Try these hearty pancakes for a Sunday breakfast that's different.

Serves four

2 cups peeled, cubed (uncooked) potatoes
1 cup sliced carrots
1 small onion, finely minced
2 eggs, slightly beaten
¼ cup whole wheat flour
½ teaspoon double-acting baking powder
½ teaspoon onion powder
    dash of pepper
    butter
    yogurt

* Potassium
* Chromium
  Magnesium
  Fluorine

In a 2-quart saucepan over medium heat, in 1 inch of boiling water, heat potatoes to boiling; reduce heat to low; cover and cook 5 minutes. Add carrots and onion and continue cooking 15 minutes more; drain.

With a potato masher, mash potatoes, carrots and onion until potatoes are smooth (carrots will still be lumpy). Add remaining ingredients except butter and yogurt, and mix well. Let stand 5 minutes.

In a 10-inch skillet over medium heat, melt about 1 teaspoon butter (or more as needed); add potato mixture by rounded tablespoonfuls. Using back of tablespoon, press each mound into a 2½-inch pancake. Fry pancake until golden on underside, about 2 minutes; turn and brown other side. Remove pancakes to platter; keep warm.

Repeat with remaining potato mixture. Serve with yogurt.

Sesame Baked Potatoes

You'll love the nutty-flavored crusts of these potato gems.

Serves two

2 Idaho or other baking potatoes
2 teaspoons sesame tahini
    wheat germ

** Potassium
 * Chromium
   Magnesium
   Zinc
   Copper
   Selenium
   Manganese
   Fluorine

Wash, dry, but do not peel potatoes. Prick them with a fork or knife. Coat with tahini and roll in wheat germ. Wrap each potato tightly in foil and bake in a preheated 350°F oven for 1 hour.

Sweet Potato Soufflé

A yummy way to "dress up" sweet potatoes.

Serves four

2 cups cooked, mashed sweet potatoes (about 3 whole potatoes)	* Magnesium * Potassium
2 egg yolks	* Chromium
½ cup pecans	Copper
1 cup milk, scalded	Manganese
2-4 tablespoons honey, to taste	
3 tablespoons butter	
½ cup raisins	
½ teaspoon nutmeg	
2 egg whites, stiffly beaten	

Mix together all ingredients in a large bowl, folding in beaten egg whites last.

Pour into an oiled 1½- or 2-quart casserole and bake in a preheated 350°F oven for 1 hour or until set as custard.

Sweet Potato-Apple Casserole

One of our all-time favorites, a great accompaniment
for a chicken dinner. Also makes a nice dessert.

Serves four

4 medium sweet potatoes	* Magnesium
½ cup water	* Potassium
3 apples	* Manganese
1 cup apple juice	Fluorine
2 tablespoons arrowroot starch	
3 tablespoons water	
2 tablespoons honey	
2 tablespoons wheat germ	

Steam sweet potatoes in a pot with a tight-fitting lid, using ½ cup water, for 15 to 20 minutes, until tender. Peel, slice lengthwise, ½ inch thick, and layer them in a casserole.

Wash and core apples, slicing them ½ inch thick. Lay apple slices on top of sweet potatoes.

Heat apple juice to the boiling point. Combine arrowroot and 3 tablespoons water and add to juice, cooking until sauce is clear and thickened. Add honey.

Spoon sauce over apples, then top with wheat germ.

Bake in a preheated 350°F oven for 30 to 40 minutes or until apples are tender.

Super Pilaf

Apricots, nuts and raisins combine with barley to make a sensational pilaf that can also be used as a stuffing for poultry or fish.

Makes four cups

2 tablespoons oil
1 medium onion, finely chopped
1 cup sliced fresh mushrooms
1 cup barley
4 cups boiling water or stock
½ cup chopped dried apricots
⅓ cup chopped almonds
⅓ cup raisins
¼ teaspoon white pepper
1 teaspoon cinnamon

* Copper
Potassium
Iron
Selenium
Chromium
Manganese

In a large heavy skillet or Dutch oven, heat the oil and saute onions and mushrooms slowly until mushrooms are soft and onions are transparent. Remove to a covered dish.

In the same pan, saute the barley briefly. Do not allow it to brown or burn. Three minutes should do it.

Add the boiling water or stock to the barley, then add the mushroom-onion mixture and the remaining ingredients. Do not stir.

Cover the pan and simmer at low heat until all water is absorbed (about 1 hour).

Stir mixture carefully, place a tea towel over the pot (to absorb excess moisture) and replace the lid. Allow to stand for 15 minutes before serving. Will serve 4 to 6 as a pilaf.

Bulgur Pilaf

This colorful assemblage of high-class nutrients makes a great dish
to set before your family or on a buffet table.

Serves four

2 medium carrots, chopped	* Zinc
1-2 stalks celery, chopped	* Copper
1 small onion, diced	* Chromium
1 medium green pepper, chopped	Magnesium
2½ cups sliced mushrooms	Potassium
½ cup chopped cashews and peanuts	Selenium
3 tablespoons butter	Manganese

2-2½ cups clear chicken broth, vegetable stock
     or water
1 tablespoon sesame seeds
1 tablespoon bran
1 tablespoon wheat germ
  garlic powder
  pepper
  chili powder
  thyme
  parsley
1 cup bulgur wheat

Chop all vegetables and nuts into small but not *fine* pieces. Saute
first 6 ingredients in the butter for about 2 minutes. Add broth, other
ingredients and seasonings to taste. Stir in bulgur. Simmer 15 minutes.
Serve with cottage cheese and sliced apples.

Vegetables and Salads

*While vegetables primarily provide the vitamins we need,
many also offer fair amounts of potassium and chromium,
among other minerals.*

Stir-Fried Vegetables

A vegetable stir-fry is almost a hot salad with all the vitamins,
minerals and juices sealed in. Serve over brown rice, or with
a baked potato and yogurt.

Serves four

2 medium onions, sliced	* Chromium
3 cloves garlic, crushed	Calcium
½ teaspoon rosemary leaves, crushed	Potassium
1 tablespoon sesame seeds	
1-2 teaspoons sesame or peanut oil	
2 large carrots, sliced diagonally	
2 stalks broccoli, sliced	
¼ head cauliflower, sliced	
1 handful mushrooms, sliced thickly	
1 handful spinach leaves	
1 green pepper, diced	

Stir-fry the onions, garlic, rosemary and sesame seeds in oil until
the onions start to brown.

Stir in the hard vegetables (carrots, broccoli, cauliflower). Put the
cover on the pan and cook until the vegetables are about half done,
about 3 minutes. Add a little water to keep everything from sticking.

Add the mushrooms, stir and cook about 2 minutes.

Add the spinach leaves and green pepper; as soon as these are
just warm and slightly wilted, serve the stir-fry.

Beets in Yogurt Sauce

A good source of chromium. Enjoy!

Serves three or four

6 medium beets
⅔ cup yogurt
2 teaspoons finely chopped fresh parsley
1 teaspoon finely chopped chives

* Chromium
Calcium
Potassium
Manganese

Scrub beets and cut off all but an inch or 2 of tops and roots. Cook until tender, about 25 minutes.

Peel and slice beets, and mix with yogurt and herbs. Heat briefly to warm sauce, or refrigerate and serve chilled.

Brussels Sprouts with Raisin-Almond Sauce

A new way to present this often-neglected vegetable.

Serves four

1 pound brussels sprouts (about 2 cups)
1 tablespoon butter
1 tablespoon whole wheat flour
1½ cups chicken stock
½ cup raisins
2 tablespoons slivered almonds

* Chromium
* Potassium

Steam brussels sprouts until tender.

Meanwhile, to prepare sauce, melt butter in a medium skillet or saucepan. Add flour and blend into a *roux*. When well blended, add stock slowly, stirring until smooth. Add raisins and allow sauce to simmer for about 8 minutes.

When ready to serve, pour sauce over sprouts and top with almonds.

Stuffed Mushrooms

The mushroom cap can be used as the container for many delectable fillings. Sesame seeds add delicious crunch to this one.

Serves four

12 large mushrooms, stems removed and set aside
1 tablespoon oil or softened butter
½ cup wheat germ
2 tablespoons minced fresh parsley
1 tablespoon minced onions
freshly ground pepper to taste
touch of ginger
3 tablespoons sesame seeds

* Copper
* Chromium
  Potassium
  Selenium

Finely chop mushroom stems and place in a medium bowl. Add the remaining ingredients except the sesame seeds and mix well. Fill the mushroom caps with the mixture and sprinkle with sesame seeds. Broil until the caps are tender (about 6 minutes).

Raw Marinated Mushrooms

Use these as a garnish on salads.

Makes five cups

5 cups mushrooms (1 pound)
6 tablespoons sunflower oil
3 tablespoons lemon juice
1 tablespoon tomato paste
1 clove garlic, sliced
1 teaspoon thyme, crushed

* Copper
  Potassium
  Chromium

Brush dirt from mushrooms. (A fingernail brush kept in the kitchen for such chores is handy.) Cut off stems, saving these for another use. Leave small mushroom caps whole; cut medium mushrooms in half, large mushrooms in quarters.

Combine oil, lemon juice, tomato paste, garlic and thyme in a large bowl. Toss with mushrooms until they are well coated. Chill 1 to 2 hours before serving.

Israeli Carrot Salad

A nice buffet dish.

Serves six

⅝ cup orange juice
4½ medium carrots, shredded
1⅛ cups chopped cabbage
⅓ cup raisins
2¼ tablespoons sesame seeds
1½ oranges, sectioned

* Chromium
Potassium

Combine orange juice, carrots, cabbage, raisins and seeds in a medium bowl. Toss. Garnish with orange sections.

Cool Summer Salad

Calcium and chromium, rolled into one.

Serves four

1 cucumber, diced
2 scallions, finely chopped
3 radishes, thinly sliced
½ cup cottage cheese
¼ cup yogurt
1 tablespoon chopped fresh chives
pepper to taste

* Chromium
Calcium

Combine vegetables in a small bowl.
Mix cottage cheese, yogurt and seasonings in a separate bowl. Pour over vegetables and toss well. Serve on a bed of lettuce, accompanied by fresh tomato wedges.

Fruits and Fruit Salads

*The great thing about fruit is that its vitamin C content
enhances iron absorption.*

Ambrosia Fruit Salad

Combining several good sources of potassium is one sure way
of hitting the jackpot for that important mineral.

Serves six

20 ounces crushed pineapple
2 oranges or tangerines
1 pound seedless grapes
1 cup sliced strawberries
2 peaches, sliced
½ cup unsweetened coconut flakes
½ cup walnuts, coarsely chopped
2 cups yogurt
    several whole strawberries

** Potassium
   Calcium
   Magnesium
   Chromium

Drain the pineapple and place in a large bowl, reserving the juice for another purpose. Peel and section the oranges or tangerines. Reserve a few sections for garnish. Add the rest of the fruit, the coconut and walnuts. Add the yogurt and mix gently to blend the ingredients. Garnish with the orange slices and a few whole strawberries. Make this heavenly salad ahead of time and let the flavors meld in the refrigerator for a few hours before serving.

Avocado-Grapefruit Salad

This dish can be described in one word—"fantastic!"
Scores high in minerals, too.

Serves four

1 grapefruit, peeled and sectioned	* Potassium
¼ pound spinach, washed and chopped	* Chromium
¼ pound mushrooms, cleaned and sliced	* Manganese
½ avocado, sliced	Magnesium
2 tablespoons honey	Copper
2 tablespoons vinegar	Fluorine
1 tablespoon oil	
1 teaspoon grated onions	
⅛ teaspoon paprika	

Cut the grapefruit segments in half and toss with spinach, mushrooms and avocado in a large glass bowl. In a separate small bowl or jar, combine remaining ingredients for the dressing and pour over the salad. This is delightful to look at as well as to eat.

Pineapple, Grape and Almond Salad

A sweet and crunchy salad that's easy to make.

Serves two

¾ cup chopped pineapple	* Manganese
¾ cup halved, seeded red grapes	Magnesium
2 tablespoons slivered, blanched,	Potassium
toasted almonds	Iron
2 tablespoons yogurt	Chromium
spinach leaves	Fluorine

Combine the pineapple, grapes and almonds in a medium bowl and toss with the yogurt. Divide between 2 plates on beds of spinach leaves. Serve chilled.

Grape-Cucumber Salad

Another taste bud teaser for you to try.

Serves four

1 medium cucumber, peeled	* Chromium
½ cup seedless grapes, halved	* Manganese
1 teaspoon tarragon vinegar	Magnesium
½ cup yogurt	Fluorine
2 teaspoons minced fresh mint	
1 clove garlic, minced	
spinach leaves	
mint sprigs (garnish)	

Cube cucumber and combine with grapes in a medium bowl. Toss with remaining ingredients. Serve on a bed of spinach with a sprig of mint as garnish.

Orange-Date Salad

Fruits plus wheat germ add up to good chromium.

Serves two

2 oranges	* Chromium
1 apple	Potassium
2 dates	
2 tablespoons yogurt	
1 tablespoon wheat germ	
dash of cinnamon	

Peel and cube oranges. Cube apple. Chop dates fine. Toss fruit together in a medium bowl with yogurt. Place in 2 serving bowls, and sprinkle with wheat germ and a dash of cinnamon.

Breads and Muffins

Whole wheat and other whole grains add precious selenium—absent in white, refined baked goods.

Oatmeal-Molasses Bread

The extra dollop of molasses makes this bread an outstanding source of potassium, while adding a fair amount of iron, too.

Makes two loaves

2 packages dry yeast	** Potassium
½ cup warm water	** Manganese
1½ cups boiling water	* Magnesium
1 cup rolled oats	* Copper
½ cup butter	* Selenium
1 cup blackstrap molasses	* Chromium
2 eggs, beaten	Zinc
6 cups whole wheat flour, sifted	Iron

Soften yeast in warm water and set aside. In a large bowl, combine the boiling water, oats, butter and molasses. Cool to lukewarm. Add the softened yeast mixture and blend well.

Blend in eggs, add flour 1 cup at a time and mix thoroughly after each addition. This is softer than kneaded dough. Place in a well-greased bowl, turning to coat the top, cover and place in refrigerator for at least 2 hours.

On a floured board, divide dough into 2 loaves and place in 2 well-greased, 9 × 5-inch loaf pans. Cover with a towel or plastic wrap and let rise in a warm place until doubled in size—about 2 hours.

Bake in a preheated 350°F oven for 1 hour or until loaves test done. Turn out onto wire rack to cool.

Honey-Orange Rye Bread

The flavor of rye delicately accented with orange and anise
makes a lovely, fragrant loaf.

Makes two loaves

2 tablespoons dry yeast	** Manganese
2½ cups warm water (105°–115°F)	* Magnesium
2 tablespoons butter	* Copper
¼ cup honey	* Selenium
⅔ cup nonfat dry milk	* Chromium
2 tablespoons freshly grated orange rind	Calcium
2 teaspoons anise seeds	Zinc
2½ cups rye flour	
3½-4 cups whole wheat flour	

Soften dry yeast in warm water in a large bowl. Add the butter,
honey, dry milk, orange rind, anise seeds and rye flour. Blend on low
speed in an electric mixer until thoroughly mixed. Change to bread hooks
and add whole wheat flour 1 cup at a time, beating at low speed until
blended; then increase to moderately high and beat for 5 minutes more.
(Of course, you can also mix with a wooden spoon and then knead
by hand for 8 to 10 minutes on a lightly floured surface.)

Shape into a ball and place in a greased bowl, turn once to coat
top, and cover. Place in a warm spot to rise until doubled in bulk
(about 45 minutes to 1 hour).

Punch down, turn out onto a lightly floured surface, knead for
1 to 2 minutes and then divide the dough in half.

Form 2 balls and place on a greased cookie sheet, leaving room
between the loaves for expansion in the oven.

Cover lightly with a towel or plastic, place in a warm spot, and let
rise again until light.

Bake in a preheated 400°F oven for 10 minutes; then lower
heat to 350°F and bake for 20 to 25 minutes more or until bread
tests done and the bottoms sound hollow when tapped.

Pineapple-Orange Bread

If you like fruit-nut breads, you'll love this loaf.

Makes one loaf

2 cups whole wheat flour, sifted	* Magnesium
1½ teaspoons baking powder	* Copper
½ teaspoon baking soda	* Chromium
1 cup crushed pineapple, well drained	Potassium
½ cup chopped walnuts	Zinc
2 teaspoons freshly grated orange peel	Selenium
1 egg, beaten	Manganese
½ cup honey	
¾ cup freshly squeezed orange juice	
2 tablespoons oil	

In a mixing bowl, sift dry ingredients together. Stir in the pineapple, nuts and orange peel. In another bowl, combine the egg, honey, orange juice and oil; then add to the dry ingredients, stirring only until moistened.

In a greased 9 × 5-inch pan, bake in a preheated 350°F oven for 50 minutes or until bread tests done. Remove from pan and cool on wire rack. This bread tastes better if you let it sit at least overnight.

Applesauce Muffins

Moist and flavorful, they're great for lunchboxes,
afternoon snacks or on the tea table.

Makes 12 muffins

1¾ cups whole wheat pastry flour	* Magnesium
2 teaspoons baking powder	* Selenium
¾ teaspoon cinnamon	* Chromium
¼ teaspoon ginger	Zinc
1 egg, beaten	Copper
¾ cup applesauce	Manganese
½ cup milk	
⅓ cup oil or melted butter	
¼ cup honey	

Grease muffin tins. (One teaspoon lecithin and 1 teaspoon oil combined and rubbed into your muffin tins will make them nonsticking.) Combine flour, baking powder and spices. Combine the remaining ingredients in another bowl. Add the applesauce mixture to the dry ingredients, stirring until the dry ingredients are barely moistened. Do not overmix. The batter should be lumpy. Fill muffin tins two-thirds full. Bake in a preheated 400°F oven for 20 to 25 minutes, until lightly browned. Serve hot or cold.

Wheat Germ Muffins

*If you love chewy, warm muffins,
you'll enjoy making—and eating—these.*

Makes 12 muffins

2 teaspoons dry yeast
¼ cup lukewarm water
2 cups oat flour
1½ cups wheat germ
½ cup nonfat dry milk
½ cup sesame seeds
½ cup whole wheat flour
⅓ cup oil
¼ cup honey
2 cups warm water
2 eggs, beaten

** Manganese
* Magnesium
* Zinc
* Copper
* Selenium
* Chromium

Soften yeast in lukewarm water. Set aside for 5 minutes. In a large bowl, combine oat flour, wheat germ, dry milk, sesame seeds and whole wheat flour. Combine oil, honey, water and eggs in a separate bowl; then add this mixture to the softened yeast. Add liquid ingredients to the flour mixture.

Let stand 10 minutes; then mix approximately 1 minute and fill well-greased muffin tins with batter. Let stand 10 minutes more. Bake in a preheated 400°F oven for 20 minutes; then lower heat to 350°F and bake for 5 minutes more.

———— Dressings, Dips and Snacks ————

Good ways to sneak extra minerals into your diet.

Basic Yogurt Dressing

Drizzling yogurt dressing over your salad adds extra calcium to your meal.

Makes about 1¼ cups
    1 cup yogurt   Calcium
    4 tablespoons lemon juice
¼-½ teaspoon dry mustard
    1 clove garlic, minced
½-1 teaspoon paprika

    Combine ingredients and let stand in refrigerator before serving.

Creamy Garlic Dressing

For creamy dressing with real zing, blend together this smoothie.

Makes about 1½ cups
    ¼ cup mild vinegar   Calcium
    1 teaspoon Dijon-style mustard
    ½ cup sunflower oil
    1 clove garlic
    1 cup yogurt

    Combine vinegar and mustard in a blender on low speed, and slowly add oil.
    Add garlic and yogurt. Store in a covered jar in refrigerator.

Tahini Salad Dressing

Sesame seeds make this nutty dressing another way to add some useful copper to your food.

Makes 1¼ cups
    1 cup sesame seeds   Copper
    ¼ cup water
    2 cloves garlic, minced
    1 lemon, peeled and diced
    few drops of vinegar
    2 tablespoons oil

    Grind seeds in an electric blender until fine. Add the other ingredients and blend until smooth.

Celery Dip

A unique nondairy way to add calcium and other minerals to
a salad or baked potato.

Makes 1¼ cups

1 stalk celery	Calcium
6 ounces tofu	Magnesium
1 scallion or ½ small onion	Potassium
2 tablespoons mild vinegar	Zinc
1 teaspoon Dijon-style mustard	Manganese

Place ingredients in a blender and process on slow, then medium speed, until smooth—about the consistency of mayonnaise.

Bean Dip

Beans make delectable dips, plus give useful amounts of
a variety of minerals.

Serves four to six

2 cups cooked soybeans or other beans	* Magnesium
3 cloves garlic	* Zinc
1 tablespoon olive oil	Calcium
1 teaspoon cumin powder	Potassium
	Copper
	Iron
	Manganese
	Fluorine

Place all ingredients in a blender. Blend, adding just enough water or bean juice (water the beans were cooked in) to give a smooth-spreading consistency to the dip.

Serve as a dip with raw vegetables or on crackers.

Cheesy Tuna Dip and Spread

Makes 3½ cups

2 cups cottage cheese	* Selenium
8 ounces cream cheese	* Chromium
14 ounces tuna	Calcium
3 tablespoons finely chopped walnuts	Magnesium
2 tablespoons finely chopped celery	Potassium
2 tablespoons shredded onions	Zinc
1 tablespoon lemon juice or to taste	Iodine
½ teaspoon paprika	
½ teaspoon chopped fresh parsley	
pinch of cayenne pepper	

Combine the cheeses in a large bowl. Beat until smooth. Add the tuna, and continue beating. Stir in the remaining ingredients. Chill. Serve some with raw vegetables as a dip, and some on your tray of spreads. It's delicious on thin slices of pumpernickel.

Zippy Sardine Spread

A handy, tasty way to take advantage of the important minerals
in these little fish.

Makes approximately one cup

½ cup mashed sardines	** Fluorine
1 hard-cooked egg	* Calcium
1 teaspoon lemon juice	* Potassium
1 tablespoon finely chopped onions	* Selenium
2 teaspoons mayonnaise	Iodine
½ teaspoon prepared mustard	

In a small bowl combine the sardines and the yolk of the egg. Mash together. Add the lemon juice and chopped onions. Combine mayonnaise and mustard, mix well and add. Spread the sardine mixture on a small, flat serving tray. Garnish with egg white forced through a sieve. Serve as a relish with salad greens or as a dip with vegetable sticks or whole grain crackers.

Sunflower Seed Spread

Here's a tasty way to add zinc to your life!

Makes 1½ cups

1 cup sunflower seed meal	* Zinc
(sunflower seeds can be ground	Magnesium
in electric blender)	Potassium
¼ cup peanut butter	Copper
3 tablespoons sunflower oil	Iron

Combine ingredients in a bowl and mix until smooth. Use as a sandwich spread, filling for stuffed celery or as a dip for raw vegetables.

Curried Pumpkin Seeds

A novel way to serve these tasty, zinc-rich seeds.

Makes two cups

2 tablespoons curry	* Zinc
¼ cup warm water	
1 clove garlic, finely minced	
1 cup water	
2 cups plain, hulled pumpkin seeds	
1 teaspoon butter	

In a saucepan, slowly add curry to warm water and garlic. When well blended, add 1 cup water and heat until liquid simmers. Add pumpkin seeds and simmer for 5 minutes.

Spread seeds on a cookie sheet and dot with butter. Toast in a preheated 250°F oven until crisp, about 25 minutes.

Salmon Party Ball

This one's pretty as a picture on the buffet table.
Save the liquid from the canned salmon for fish broth or potato soup.
If you can get fresh salmon, you'll have pure ambrosia on your hands.

Makes 2½ cups

2 cups drained salmon (1-pound can)	* Calcium
8 ounces cream cheese, softened	* Potassium
1 tablespoon lemon juice	* Selenium
1 tablespoon white horseradish	* Fluorine
2 teaspoons shredded onions	Magnesium
¼ teaspoon paprika	Chromium
½ cup chopped pecans	Iodine
3 tablespoons chopped fresh parsley	

In a medium bowl, thoroughly mix all ingredients except pecans and parsley. Season to taste, if desired. Roll into ball in waxed paper and chill several hours. Then roll in combined pecans and parsley.

Rechill until ready to serve. (This freezes nicely, too.) Serve with a platter of raw vegetables cut into convenient sizes for scooping into the salmon ball.

Salt-Free Condiments

Making your own salt-free condiments takes the frustration out of garnishing your food while trying to avoid sodium.

Ketchup

Makes 1½ cups

2 quarts tomatoes, quartered (5 pounds)
⅓ cup chopped onions
¼ cup chopped celery
1 teaspoon chopped garlic
⅓ cup white vinegar
1 tablespoon honey
2 teaspoons medium unsulfured molasses

Bouquet Garni: (tie in cheesecloth)
½ bay leaf
⅛ teaspoon celery seeds
1 small dried red chili pepper (about 1
    inch long)
¾ teaspoon mustard seeds

Puree the tomatoes in a blender. Set puree aside in a large stainless steel or enameled pot. Then puree the onions, celery and garlic, adding some of the tomato puree as liquid to work the blender.

Add the onions, celery and garlic mixture to tomato puree and bring to a boil. Stir in the vinegar, honey and molasses.

Add the bouquet garni and cook over medium heat, stirring frequently, for 30 minutes. Remove bouquet garni.

Continue to cook until the ketchup becomes somewhat thickened.

Pass the ketchup through a food mill and then transfer ½ cup to a blender. Blend at high speed, ½ cup at a time, until smooth. Cool, pour into jars and refrigerate.

Yellow Mustard

Makes ½ cup

    4 tablespoons dry mustard
    4 tablespoons hot water
    3 tablespoons white vinegar
    ⅛ teaspoon garlic powder
       pinch of tarragon
    ¼ teaspoon medium unsulfured molasses

In a small bowl, soak dry mustard in hot water and 1 tablespoon of the vinegar for at least 2 hours. Combine the remaining vinegar, garlic and tarragon in a separate bowl and let stand for ½ hour.

Strain the tarragon from the second vinegar mixture and add the liquid to the mustard mixture. Stir in the molasses.

Pour the mustard into the top of a double boiler, set over simmering water. Cook until thickened, about 15 minutes. (The mustard will thicken a bit more when chilled.)

Remove from the heat and pour into a jar. Let cool uncovered, and then put on a lid and store in the refrigerator.

Blender Mayonnaise

For best results, have all ingredients at room temperature.

Makes 1½ cups

    1 whole egg
    1 egg yolk, lightly beaten
    2 tablespoons lemon juice or vinegar
    ½ teaspoon dry mustard
    1⅓ cups oil
    2 teaspoons boiling water (optional)

Warm the blender bowl (container) in hot water and dry thoroughly.

Combine the egg, egg yolk, lemon juice or vinegar, and mustard in the blender bowl. Blend at medium speed for about 1 minute. Gradually add the oil, a few drops at a time, blending until ⅓ cup of oil has been incorporated into the egg mixture.

At this point the remaining oil can be added, 1 tablespoon at a time, until all the oil is used.

To insure against the mayonnaise breaking, 2 tablespoons of boiling water can be blended in at this point.

Store in a covered glass jar in the refrigerator.

Hand-Beaten Mayonnaise

For best results, have all ingredients at room temperature.

Makes 1¼ cups
   2 egg yolks, lightly beaten
   2 tablespoons lemon juice or vinegar
   ½ teaspoon dry mustard
   1⅓ cups oil
   2 teaspoons boiling water (optional)

Warm a glass or stainless steel bowl and a wire whisk in hot water. Dry thoroughly.

Place the egg yolks in the bowl with 1 tablespoon of the lemon juice or vinegar and the mustard. Beat to mix well.

Continue beating constantly as you add the oil, 1 drop at a time. Be sure the yolks are absorbing the oil; this may require you to stop adding the oil and just beat the yolks for a few seconds.

After about ⅓ cup of the oil has been incorporated into the yolks, the remaining oil can be added by the tablespoon, beating well after each addition of oil.

When the mayonnaise is thick and stiff, beat in the remaining lemon juice or vinegar to thin it out. Then continue to beat in the remaining oil.

To insure against the mayonnaise breaking, 2 teaspoons of boiling water can be blended in at this point.

Store in a covered glass jar in the refrigerator.

Herbal Seasoning

A good, peppery taste.

Makes ⅓ cup
   2 tablespoons kelp powder
   1 tablespoon dried parsley flakes
   1½ teaspoons dried celery flakes
   1 teaspoon ground, toasted sesame seeds
   ½ teaspoon marjoram
   ½ teaspoon onion powder
   ½ teaspoon paprika
   ½ teaspoon thyme
   ¼ teaspoon garlic powder
   ⅛ teaspoon cayenne pepper

Blend all ingredients in a blender for a few minutes. Use in a shaker as a seasoning.

Tomato Paste

Makes about 1½ cups
> 5 pounds tomatoes, preferably Italian plum

Quarter tomatoes and puree in a blender. Simmer over low heat in a large flat saucepan, stirring frequently, until all the liquid has cooked off.

Yield will depend upon the fleshiness of your tomatoes.

Basic Tomato Sauce

Makes two cups
>   5 ripe tomatoes, coarsely chopped
>   2 tablespoons olive oil
>   2 cloves garlic, minced
> 1¼ cups chopped onions
>   1 bay leaf
>   1 teaspoon basil
> ⅙ teaspoon celery seed
>   pinch of thyme
>   3 sprigs parsley, finely chopped
>   oregano and/or cayenne to taste

Puree tomatoes in a blender. In a large saucepan, heat olive oil and saute garlic and onions. Add pureed tomatoes, bay leaf, basil, celery seed and thyme. Cook over low heat for at least 45 minutes. (The longer the better.) Add parsley and cook for 2 or 3 minutes more. Season to taste with oregano and/or cayenne.

Drinks

Beverages are an ideal way to combine two or three
mineral-rich foods into a refreshing mineral "supplement."

Yogurt-Fruit Shake

Fresh, ripe fruits or berries in season make this a colorful,
smooth and refreshing "milk shake," especially for people who have
trouble drinking regular shakes but need the calcium.

Serves one

½ cup yogurt

½ cup cold water

½ cup strawberries, raspberries, apricots,
   pineapple or other ripe fruit

honey to taste

* Calcium
 Potassium
 Chromium

Combine all ingredients in a blender and blend until smooth.
Serve immediately or refrigerate.

Orange Yogurt Quencher

Try this frothy blend when you're in the mood for something different.
It's thinner and tangier than a milk shake, and better for you.
Because it takes just seconds to whip up, you'll find it quick and easy
for breakfast on the run. Or fill your thermos and sip on it
at break time or with your lunch. You may want to keep a batch
in the refrigerator for a late-night relaxer.

Serves one

½ cup yogurt

½ cup orange juice

honey to taste

* Calcium
* Potassium
 Chromium

Combine ingredients in a blender and blend until smooth. Serve
immediately or refrigerate.

Homemade Yogurt That's Easy to Make

Making yogurt is a job that's practically work-free because the bacteria that ferment milk do all the work for you.

Simply bring a quart of milk to the boiling point, then let it cool to room temperature. Mix in purchased yogurt starter (the bacteria, usually in powdered form) or 2 tablespoons of yogurt you have on hand. Pour the mixture into the containers of your yogurt maker and let it incubate until nice and firm.

If you don't happen to have a yogurt maker, there is another and perhaps slightly risky way of making yogurt. Place the mixture in a covered bowl, and put the bowl in an oven in which a 100-watt bulb or pilot light is burning. After about 8 hours, the yogurt will be ready. That method saves the expense of a yogurt maker, but might not always produce picture-perfect yogurt.

When the yogurt is ready, refrigerate it right away. For best taste and texture, let the yogurt cool for a day before eating. It keeps a week.

Banana-Strawberry Drink

Use a high-chromium yeast, and you'll make this a three-star beverage for that mineral.

Makes one large serving

1 cup skim milk	** Calcium
1 small or ½ large banana	** Chromium
2 strawberries	* Magnesium
1 teaspoon brewer's yeast	* Potassium
1 teaspoon medium unsulfured molasses	Copper
1 teaspoon peanut butter	Manganese
2 ice cubes	Fluorine

Place ingredients in a blender and process on medium speed until smooth. Serve immediately.

Cuke Cooler

Add some chromium to your life with this unusual lunchtime cooler.

Serves three to four

2 cucumbers, peeled and chunked	* Chromium
½ avocado	Magnesium
juice of ½ lemon or lime	Potassium

Process ingredients in a blender until well liquefied.

Pincapple-Carrot Juice

This unusual combo will perk you up on a hot summer day.

Serves two

1 cup chunked pineapple	Potassium
½ cup pineapple juice	Chromium
3 carrots, chopped	
¼ lemon, peeled	
1 cup ice cubes	

Process pineapple, juice, carrots and lemon in a blender until smooth. Add ice cubes and process until finely chopped.

Serve at once.

Desserts

*Dessert doesn't have to be an empty-calorie add-on.
Chosen wisely, dessert can tack useful amounts
of calcium and trace minerals onto a meal.*

Molasses Cake

If you like the flavor of molasses, you'll enjoy this moist treat.

Serves eight to ten

2½ cups whole wheat flour	** Potassium
1½ teaspoons baking soda	** Manganese
½ cup corn oil	* Magnesium
½ cup medium unsulfured molasses	* Selenium
½ cup hot water	Zinc
¼ cup blackstrap molasses	Copper
	Iron
	Chromium

Combine the flour and baking soda in a large bowl. Stir in the corn oil and molasses. Remove 1 cup of this mixture and set aside.

In a small bowl, combine the hot water and blackstrap molasses. Add to the flour mixture in the large bowl, and stir until thoroughly combined.

Place the batter in a lightly oiled 8-inch round cake pan. Sprinkle the remaining cup of flour mixture over top of the batter.

Bake in a preheated 375°F oven for 25 to 30 minutes, until done.

Tofu-Rice Pudding

Serves four

3 cups cooked brown rice	** Manganese
6 ounces tofu	* Magnesium
3 tablespoons maple syrup	* Potassium
½ teaspoon finely grated lemon rind	Zinc
½ teaspoon vanilla	Copper
⅛ teaspoon cardamom	Iron
½ cup raisins	Selenium
	Chromium

Place rice in a mixing bowl. In a blender, combine tofu, maple syrup, lemon rind, vanilla and spice. Blend on low speed until smooth. Pour over brown rice, add raisins and stir to combine. Chill before serving. Makes 3½ cups.

Banana-Sweet Potato Loaf

Plenty of good foods rolled into one!

Makes one loaf

2 pounds sweet potatoes
1 banana, mashed
¼ cup melted butter
½ cup nonfat dry milk
¼ teaspoon nutmeg
¼ teaspoon cinnamon
3 eggs, beaten
¼ cup honey
¼ cup medium unsulfured molasses
½ cup water
½ teaspoon vanilla
¼ cup raisins

* Magnesium
* Potassium
* Chromium
* Manganese
  Calcium

Boil or steam sweet potatoes until they are tender. Peel and puree them. You should have approximately 2¼ cups.

Combine sweet potatoes with banana, melted butter, dry milk and spices. Combine eggs, honey, molasses, water and vanilla in a separate bowl and add to sweet potato mixture. Then add raisins.

Turn into an oiled 9 × 5-inch loaf pan. Bake in a preheated 350°F oven for 50 to 60 minutes or until a knife inserted at the center comes out clean.

Carob-Banana Pudding

Opportunities to add calcium to the menu don't come to an end as dessert time approaches. Try this fluffy, naturally sweet blend for a bonus of 77 milligrams of calcium per serving.

Serves six

½ cup cold soy milk
1½ cups tofu (about 12 ounces)
3 medium bananas, frozen
4 tablespoons carob powder
1 teaspoon vanilla

** Magnesium
 * Potassium
 * Manganese
  Calcium
  Zinc
  Copper
  Fluorine

Combine milk, tofu, bananas, carob and vanilla in a blender. Blend until smooth. Pour into custard cups. Serve well chilled.

Note: Carob powder is much like baker's chocolate, but without the fat, sugar, caffeine and other undesirable compounds found in chocolate. You can find it in most health food stores.

Oatmeal-Peanut Cookies

A delicious way to sneak extra minerals to children.

Makes five dozen

¾ cup whole wheat pastry flour

¼ cup soy flour

½ teaspoon baking soda

½ cup peanut butter

⅓ cup butter, softened

⅓ cup honey

3 eggs

¼ cup water or orange juice

1 teaspoon vanilla

3 cups oatmeal (not the instant), uncooked

½ cup chopped peanuts

1 cup pitted dates, cut up

* Magnesium

* Zinc

Copper

Selenium

Chromium

Manganese

In a medium bowl, combine the flours and baking soda. In a large bowl cream the peanut butter and the butter. Beat in the honey, eggs, water or orange juice and vanilla until creamy. Stir in the flour mixture, then the oatmeal, peanuts and dates. Drop by teaspoonfuls 2 inches apart on baking sheet lined with parchment paper or greased with a mixture of ½ teaspoon each of liquid lecithin and oil.

Bake in a preheated 325°F oven for 15 to 20 minutes or until golden. These cookies will be soft. Allow to cool for 5 minutes on the cookie sheets placed on a rack. Remove to rack to complete cooling.

Baked Pears with Almonds and Yogurt

A quick dessert you can pop into the oven while dinner is being served.

Serves six

6 firm, ripe pears	Calcium
¼ cup honey	Magnesium
1 teaspoon vanilla	Potassium
½ cup slivered almonds	Copper
2 tablespoons butter	Chromium
1 cup yogurt	

Grease a 9-inch baking pan.

Core and slice pears (do not peel unless skins are tough, or you want the dessert to be especially fancy). Arrange the slices of pears in attractive rows in the prepared pan. Mix honey and vanilla and drizzle over pears; top with the almonds and dot with butter. Cover and bake in a preheated 375°F oven for 20 minutes or until pears are tender. Baste frequently during the baking, using the accumulated juice.

Serve hot or cold, topped with yogurt.

PART
V

PROTECTING YOUR HEALTH

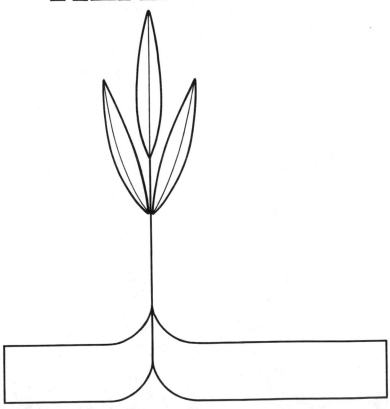

32

Osteoporosis

She notices she's a couple of inches shorter than she used to be. And her back aches. Then out of the blue, her hip breaks. Or she bumps into a chair and her thigh cracks.

She's one of the five million women a year who suffer the thin, crumbly bones of osteoporosis—the upshot of long-term embezzlement of calcium from the bones. Some one million men also share her fate.

The fracture may come as a surprise after about age 45—or after menopause in women. But the plunder begins 10, 20 or 30 years earlier. Age—plus the hormone changes that launch menopause in women—are behind much of it, especially when calcium intake is low to begin with. After all, calcium is the stuff bones are made of. Reducing diets, childbearing and breastfeeding all take their toll, too. Lack of exercise or sustained emotional stress aggravates the problem by fostering a steady trickle of calcium out of the body. Prolonged use of corticosteroids, frequently taken for arthritis, helps push calcium out of the body before it has much of a chance to nestle into bones. So does too much fat, salt, protein or phosphorus in the diet.

Osteoporosis need not team up with gray hair and wrinkles as an automatic by-product of age, though. A high-calcium diet fends off anti-bone factors. So do exercise and adequate vitamin D. Bone loss can even be *reversed* in many cases. There's no reason why we can't have the same strong bones at age 70 that we do at 25.

Not only do calcium-strong bones spare us the pain and inconvenience of a fracture, they may save our lives. One of every six people who fracture a hip due to osteoporosis withers away in a hospital bed, to die within three months. A few others last little more than a year.

And there are psychological benefits to building strong bones. Otherwise, many older people live in fear of falling. Climbing into the bathtub becomes an act of daring. The first snowflake of winter turns them into recluses, afraid to venture out onto treacherous sidewalks.

Saving Thin, Crumbly Bones

Bones are living tissue. And they go on living and growing as long as we live. Two forces are at work in bone formation—one major, one minor. The parathyroid hormone takes calcium stored in bone and distributes it to blood, nerves, muscles and other cells. The parathyroid hormone also pumps calcium into the general circulation by adjusting absorption from the intestine and excretion by the kidneys. Blood, in turn, delivers new calcium to bones. Meanwhile, the sex hormones (estrogen in women, androgen in men) influence the overall effect of the parathyroid. Together, the whole process of simultaneous stripping down and building up again is called bone remodeling.

It's also possible that excess phosphorus may goad the parathyroid into sucking too much calcium from bones or dumping dietary calcium into the urine. Excess protein—double our requirement—may also push calcium out. But generally speaking, the system works in balance to ensure that bone formation keeps pace with bone loss.

At about age 40, however, parathyroid levels take off and calcium absorption slows down considerably—in both sexes. On top of that, sex hormones in women falter toward the end of the fertile years and dwindle to nothing at menopause, with the halt of monthly periods. Or estrogen flow is cut off by surgical removal of the ovaries in hysterectomy. Either way, estrogen is no longer around to bolster bone formation in women. Bone building continues, but lags behind bone loss by about 5 percent a year. We may lose as little as two-thirds of an ounce of bone a year. Over a period of 30 years, though, that adds up to over a pound—more than a third of our total calcium. The net effect is frail, porous bones, riddled with spongelike holes (see first figure). Bones that shatter easily. Or a "dowager's hump" (kyphosis) caused by compression of the spinal bones (see second figure, on next page).

Normal (A) and Osteoporotic (B) Bones

A

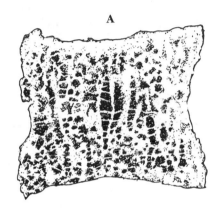

B

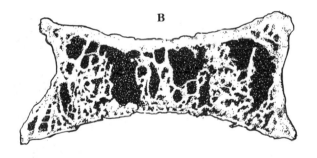

Normal bone from a 20-year-old woman (A) compared to an osteoporotic bone from a 60-year-old woman (B).
SOURCE: Adapted from *Bone Loss: Causes, Detection and Therapy* by Anthony A. Albanese (New York: Alan R. Liss, Inc., 1977).

Men are usually spared those calamities, because male sex glands continue to produce androgen throughout life, enabling them to fight off some of the effects of age on bone loss. Consequently, some doctors have turned to replacing estrogen (the female hormone) in osteoporotic women to grant them the same hormone protection enjoyed by men.

One problem, though. Cancer. Studies show that women on long-term estrogen replacement therapy are more likely to develop cancer of the ovaries, uterus or breast than those not taking estrogen. A study of 908 women who took estrogen showed that they ran a two to three times greater risk of developing ovarian cancer than women who did not take estrogen (*Lancet*, September 10, 1977). The risk of cancer of the uterus was shown in three studies to be four to eight times higher among women who used estrogen than among nonusers (*New York State Journal of Medicine*, June, 1977). In yet another study, the risk of developing breast cancer was twice as high among estrogen users (*New England Journal of Medicine*, August 19, 1976). And other studies linking estrogen with cancer add to the evidence that estrogen replacement is not such a good idea.

Loss of Height with Dowager's Hump

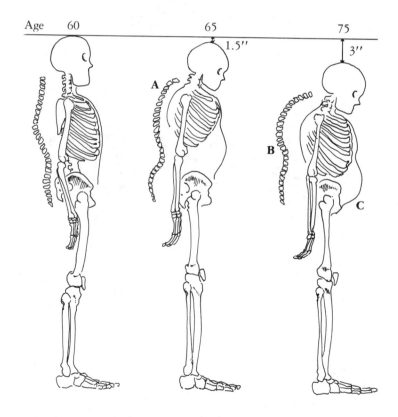

Progressive deformation of spine in osteoporosis. Result is loss of height and dowager's hump (A and B) with stomach thrust forward (C).

Calcium Builds Strong Bones

Calcium works just as well, without cancer as a side effect. Apparently, calcium tones down the destructive effects of parathyroid hormone unleashed by age and the absence of estrogen. A really protective amount seems to range between 1,000 and 1,500 milligrams of calcium a day, based on several noteworthy studies. In one such study, 61 postmenopausal women were divided into three groups. One group received no treatment; another group, 800 milligrams of calcium; and the third group, estrogen. The size of their bones was measured when the study began and again two years later. "The untreated groups continued to lose bone during the two years," write the researchers, while "the estrogen group lost none." Those in the calcium-treated group lost some bone mass, but far less than the untreated group (*British Medical Journal*, September 24, 1977).

Other studies show protective amounts of calcium clearly help bones hold their own:

• Herta Spencer, M.D., and two colleagues at the Veterans Administration Hospital in Hines, Illinois, report that an intake of 1,200 milligrams of calcium puts a halt to calcium's steady drain out of the bones (*The NIH Record*, May 7, 1974).

• A two-year study published in *Annals of Internal Medicine* (December, 1977) showed that 22 postmenopausal women who took 1,400 milligrams of calcium had *no* measurable bone loss.

Other studies show that calcium goes estrogen one better: it not only arrests bone loss, but *reverses* it! One of the studies showing that adding calcium can add new density and strength to aging bones was conducted by a team of researchers led by Anthony A. Albanese, Ph.D., at the Miriam Osborn Memorial Home in Rye, New York, and the Burke Rehabilitation Center in nearby White Plains. Twelve elderly nursing home residents (all women) were given a total of 1,200 milligrams of calcium a day, from diet and supplements, plus vitamin D (essential for good calcium utilization). Controls were given no supplemental calcium.

After three full years of boosted calcium, the women in the experimental group had denser bones. Even though they were now three years older, their bones were—for all practical purposes—actually younger! On the other hand, bone density in the women who hadn't received extra calcium decreased.

Dr. Albanese and his associates then tried extra calcium in both younger postmenopausal women and female fracture patients. After taking calcium supplements, the women had stronger bones (*New York State Journal of Medicine*, February, 1975).

In light of such evidence, justification for estrogen use pales and the case for calcium grows strong. Supplements bridge the gap. And the sooner we beef up our calcium, the better, says Jenifer Jowsey, Ph.D., professor of orthopedic research at the University of California at Davis. "Since bone loss appears to start at age 25, calcium supplementation should probably be started at this time and continued for the rest of life. That calcium supplements are effective in reducing bone [loss] has been demonstrated in persons with osteoporosis; there is every reason to think that calcium supplementation would be effective preventive therapy in normal persons," writes Dr. Jowsey (*Postgraduate Medicine*, August, 1976).

Echoing those thoughts: "Bone loss and fracture risk may be minimized or reversed by a daily intake of approximately 1 gram (1,000 milligrams) of calcium derived from the diet or through supplements" (*American Family Physician*, October, 1978).

The need for supplements is clear. You'd have to drink over five glasses of milk every day to reach levels of calcium intake that are really protective. Or eat five cups of yogurt. Or over six ounces of Swiss cheese. Or two pounds of collard greens. Or more than a pound of almonds. Not many of us could eat that as a steady diet, nor would we want to! So eating reasonable portions of those and other high-calcium foods (like broccoli, soybeans, and salmon with bones, plus nuts and cheese), then making up the difference with calcium supplements— dolomite, bone meal, or calcium compounds such as calcium carbonate, calcium lactate or calcium gluconate—is your best bet. Absorption is best when calcium is taken in small portions over the course of the day, with vitamin D from sunlight or food.

Exercise Helps Keep Bones Strong

Bone is like muscle. It will grow stronger as greater demands are placed on it. In a study at Oregon State University, the 90 participants ranged in age from 20 to 25 years old. They were divided into high-, moderate- or low-activity groups according to the amount each normally exercised. When measured, bones in the high-activity group were denser than in both the moderate and low groups. The researchers also found that calcium intake significantly influenced the bone density of participants. They concluded that increased calcium intake, combined with adequate exercise, results in stronger bones.

Vigorous physical activity for young girls was also recommended as a safeguard against early onset of osteoporosis. The exercise, they concluded, would help to build maximum bone strength and bone density in the young women. So exercise was recommended not only as a safeguard against osteoporosis but also as a treatment for it (*Nutrition Reports International*, June, 1978).

People at any age seem to benefit from exercise, so saying it's "too late" won't work as an excuse. A group of 18 menopausal women was divided in half. One group did warm-up, conditioning and circulatory exercises for one hour, three times a week. The other nine did not exercise. After one year, body calcium had *increased* in the exercise group and *decreased* in every woman who did not exercise. The researchers learned that aging and frail bones did *not* have to be accepted as a package deal. Even women past menopause could continue to *build* their bones instead of losing them if they exercised regularly (*Annals of Internal Medicine*, September, 1978).

CHAPTER

33

Heart Disease

When we talk about heart disease, we're actually talking about the heart and blood vessels—or cardiovascular system. Generally, whatever affects the arteries also affects the heart, and vice versa. Heart attack, stroke, high blood pressure and thrombosis (blood clots) are simply different expressions of the same basic disease, atherosclerosis. Atherosclerosis is marked by a buildup of fat (primarily cholesterol) in the walls of medium and large arteries, such as the heart's aorta.

Evidently, that whole business of atherosclerosis—the clogging of arteries with fatty deposits—can begin as early as early childhood. Autopsies of teenage soldiers who died in combat have sometimes shown thick fatty streaks in their heart and arteries. The reason we don't all succumb to the effects of heart disease much earlier than we do is that the process is usually much slower, albeit progressive. Also, by virtue of inherited family tendencies, some people are prone to rapidly developing heart disease, while others seem to enjoy some natural protection. In

318

between, there are a number of apparent risk factors over which we pretty much have a good deal of control. Overweight. Stress. Lack of exercise. Smoking and drinking habits. High levels of cholesterol and saturated fat in the diet. In addition, too much sodium may encourage high blood pressure, in itself a major risk factor in heart disease

Minerals and Your Healthy Heart

Although many people don't realize it, the protective role of minerals ties in with generally accepted risk factors in interesting ways. For one thing, because mineral-rich foods tend to be good in many other ways, a diet that emphasizes those foods may help steer you away from other foods that can spell disaster for your heart's health.

Overweight

A high-mineral diet won't guarantee you a slimmer waistline. But it just so happens that many foods such as fish, beans and vegetables, which are high in minerals, are also low in calories and are less likely to add on pounds than foods high in fat and sugar (which, incidentally, add very little in the way of minerals).

Saturated fat and cholesterol

Provided dairy products are chosen carefully—skim milk, low-fat yogurt and less fatty cheeses—a high-mineral diet can also reduce your intake of saturated fat and cholesterol.

Sodium

Basic, wholesome foods not only tend to be higher in healthful minerals than refined foods, they're also considerably lower in sodium.

On top of all that, five minerals stand out as playing key roles in helping guard against heart disease: calcium, magnesium, potassium, chromium and selenium. And foods high in those minerals contribute toward heart health in very specific ways.

Fiber

High-fiber diets are associated with good heart health. Complex carbohydrates—beans, potatoes, whole grains and vegetables—are not only high in fiber, but are particularly high in magnesium, potassium and selenium.

Soybeans and yogurt

Soybeans and yogurt are not only good sources of calcium, but they have a definite cholesterol-lowering effect.

Fish

Fish is not only high in hard-to-get selenium, but as an important bonus, many fish have special fatty acids which seem to protect against heart disease in populations who eat them.

All those points lead to the fact that eating a diet high in those five critical minerals constitutes one more giant step toward life-long heart health. Let's zero in for a closer look.

Calcium and Magnesium, Partners for Life

By far, the oldest association between minerals and heart health is that there appear to be fewer deaths from heart disease among people living in hard water areas. In 1960, Henry A. Schroeder, M.D., of Dartmouth Medical School in New Hampshire, determined that in areas of the United States where the water was high in certain minerals— namely calcium and magnesium—heart disease was consistently low. Towns in west Texas, for instance, have the hardest drinking water and the lowest cardiovascular mortality rate in the United States. The assumption was that hard water somehow protected against heart disease.

While controversy and many questions still swirl around the subject, what's generally agreed upon by scientists who've compiled health statistics (epidemiologists) on tens of thousands of people throughout the world, is this: people who live in areas where the underlying rocks are rich in calcium, magnesium and certain trace minerals seem to have significantly *less* chance of developing cardiovascular disease than people who live in areas where the underlying rocks are relatively impermeable and are formed of other insoluble minerals.

Regardless of whether or not that theory holds true, though, there are more specific—and probably more important—relationships between calcium, magnesium and heart disease. Water hardness is but one environmental variable. After all, only a portion of our daily mineral intake comes from drinking water. Diet contributes the most, by far.

Calcium, the Quiet Cholesterol Fighter

Whether from food or water, calcium tends to reduce cholesterol in the blood and thereby limits the extent to which it will latch onto artery walls, causing atherosclerosis. Fifteen years ago, Harold Yacowitz, Ph.D., a researcher from Fairleigh Dickinson University in Madison, New Jersey, had a hunch that there may be a connection between calcium and fat absorption. So he fed 3,370 milligrams of calcium (710 milligrams from dietary sources and 2,660 milligrams from supplements) to four men with normal cholesterol levels (less than 250 milligrams). After only four days, their blood cholesterol decreased by an average of 14 points.

Encouraged by these results, Dr. Yacowitz decided to test another group of volunteers by giving them much less calcium (a total intake of 1,600 milligrams per day) but for a longer period of time—three weeks. What he found was that the smaller amount of calcium did the job, not only of lowering cholesterol, but of decreasing other blood fats, called triglycerides, as well. And the higher the initial cholesterol and triglyceride levels, the more dramatic were the results, with cholesterol levels dropping by as much as 48 points and triglycerides by a maximum of 115. What's more, the major decrease occurred within the first week of the study and stayed at the lower levels for the remainder of the test (*British Medical Journal*, May, 1965).

Fats Carried Away

But how does calcium reduce serum cholesterol and triglycerides? "It was important to answer this question," Dr. Yacowitz told us, "since there was some concern that perhaps these lipids (fats) were being deposited in the liver, blood vessels and other tissues. Fortunately, that isn't the case. Calcium combines with fatty acids in the gut and results in the excretion of calcium soaps. Increased calcium intake resulted in increased fat excretion."

Since that time, other researchers have conducted studies which link calcium to reduction of cholesterol and other lipids.

One in particular, Anthony A. Albanese, Ph.D., of the Burke Rehabilitation Center in White Plains, New York, is noted for his studies of postmenopausal women and osteoporosis (bone loss). But while experimenting with the use of calcium to counteract that disease, he was surprised to discover that along with increasing bone density, calcium decreased the blood cholesterol "in a striking and highly statistically significant manner in the supplemented group only" (*Nutrition Reports International*, August, 1973). His study was conducted with normal, healthy elderly women, not patients with cardiovascular disease. The cholesterol-lowering effects were accomplished with only 1,025 to 1,200 milligrams of calcium per day, even less than Dr. Yacowitz had used in his second experiment.

About the same time as Dr. Albanese's study was being conducted, another experiment was getting under way at St. Vincent's Hospital in Montclair, New Jersey. This time, however, the eight men and two women tested were known to be hyperlipemic (having very high blood fats). Most had cholesterol levels between 300 and 500 milligrams at the start of the study (remember, normal is below 250) and had maintained those high levels for the previous 12 months. Yet after taking 2,000 milligrams of calcium a day for one year, their cholesterol levels decreased by an average of 25 percent. "Calcium carbonate," says Marvin L. Bierenbaum, M.D., the researcher who conducted the study, "should be considered as a potential agent for usage in long-term studies designed to produce hypolipemia [low blood lipids], since it appears to be effective and without significant side effects" (*Lipids*, vol. 7, no. 3, 1972).

The lowest serum lipid values were achieved after the first six months of supplementation and then stayed low for the remainder of the study period. "The cholesterol level would probably go right back up again if the calcium supplementation were discontinued," Dr. Bierenbaum told us. "That's because these people have a genetic tendency toward hyperlipemia. They must continue to take calcium to keep their cholesterol and other lipids lowered."

It's interesting to note that it's not just circulating cholesterol that is affected by calcium. When Dr. Yacowitz fed rabbits a high-fat and low-calcium diet, the rabbits showed pronounced aortic atherosclerosis, or fatty buildup. But two of the three rabbits fed the same high-fat diet, but with additional calcium, showed no signs of that disease. And on top of that, the cholesterol level was greatly reduced in the aortas of rabbits on the high-calcium diet.

Writes Dr. Yacowitz, "That further illustrates the beneficial effect of increased dietary calcium in reducing the severity of atherosclerosis" (*Transactions of the New York Academy of Sciences*, vol. 33, 1971).

A report published last year by U.S. Department of Agriculture (USDA) researchers also focuses on a possible calcium-cholesterol connection. Volunteers whose diets contained higher levels of calcium were found to have lower cholesterol values than other subjects. Although those findings do not prove a definite cause-and-effect relationship, "the results were consistent with other studies done in the past," Leslie M. Klevay, M.D., of the USDA's Human Nutrition Laboratory in Grand Forks, North Dakota, told us. "Dietary calcium lowered cholesterol mainly by decreasing LDL [low-density lipoprotein] cholesterol [that's the bad kind]," the scientist notes. Dr. Klevay's experiment added one more bit of information, however, not mentioned in any previous studies. While increased calcium was associated with lower cholesterol levels, the HDL (high-density lipoprotein) cholesterol (that's the good kind) remained unchanged.

"I prescribe 1 gram (1,000 milligrams) a day for my hyperlipemic patients [with high blood fats], and I take it myself," says Dr. Bierenbaum.

And he's not the only one, apparently. "Doctors *are* beginning to prescribe calcium to lower cholesterol," Dr. Albanese told us.

Magnesium, Stress and Sudden Death

Doctors generally define a heart attack as a condition that occurs when a clot blocks the flow of blood through the coronary artery to the heart. But just what prompts a clot to form at a particular time and place in the body has long been a mystery to scientists.

Now, however, several investigators report that *spasms* occurring within heart arteries may be setting the stage for dangerous blood clots and future heart attacks. If spasms should prove to be at the root of heart attacks, researchers may not have to look very far to determine what is at the bottom of spasms. In fact, research already shows us at least one reason for spasms—magnesium deficiency.

In a major report published by the National Research Council of Canada, researchers list possible causes of magnesium deficiency and a variety of illnesses that this deficiency might cause. In one study, they note the hearts of cardiac victims contained about 22 percent less magnesium than the hearts of those who died of noncardiac problems. And the magnesium shortage was most acute where the heart muscle was infarcted: dead due to ischemia, or choked-off blood circulation (*Water Hardness, Human Health and the Importance of Magnesium,* National Research Council of Canada, 1979).

Magnesium specialist Bella T. Altura, Ph.D., of the State University of New York's Downstate Medical Center in Brooklyn, also believes there is a close link between stress, magnesium deficiency and SDIHD—sudden death ischemic heart disease. Victims die of sudden heart attacks after showing no prior signs of heart disease. Dr. Altura found that stress indirectly causes the body to *excrete* magnesium, resulting in a magnesium deficiency in the heart muscle (*Medical Hypotheses,* vol. 6, no. 1, 1980).

The theory, as developed by Dr. Altura, her husband, Burton M. Altura, Ph.D., and Prasad Turlapaty, Ph.D., is this: magnesium is required for dilating or opening the blood vessels in the heart tissues, and calcium is required for constricting or closing the vessels. A delicate balance of magnesium and calcium keeps the heart beating smoothly. A shortage of magnesium means an imbalance toward constriction. A blood vessel may go into spasm and contract suddenly, cutting off circulation to a section of the heart and inducing heart failure.

Potassium Helps, Too

Potassium, we know, helps to counteract the negative effects of sodium on our blood pressure, staving off that risk for heart attack. But potassium may also be connected with the state of the heart itself under stress. A fascinating study by Carl J. Johnson, M.D., of the University of Colorado School of Medicine, and colleagues, found that there were unusually low concentrations of both magnesium *and* potassium in the heart tissues of men dying suddenly from heart attacks. Of course, it's possible that following any kind of sudden death, there could be a tendency for these minerals to leave the heart, but the studies revealed that this marked shortage of minerals in the heart does not occur in men dying a sudden death from causes other than heart attacks. What's more, they found that the four lowest potassium values were obtained for the four men who had a history of angina (pain caused by shortage of oxygen supplied to the heart, sometimes related to increased demand). And three of these four also had the lowest magnesium levels in their heart muscles. The possibility that this would occur from mere chance, they point out, is exceedingly remote (*American Journal of Clinical Nutrition*, May, 1979).

Selenium, Good Heart Insurance

Next on the roster of minerals linked to heart health is selenium. How strong is the evidence? Very strong, according to Raymond J. Shamberger, Ph.D., a researcher at the Cleveland Clinic Foundation. As Dr. Shamberger and several associates noted in a paper presented at the 12th annual University of Missouri trace element conference in 1978, rats and lambs fed selenium-deficient diets have abnormal electrocardiograms and blood pressure changes. And humans are apparently affected as well. When the researchers compared mineral intakes with heart and artery disease death rates in 25 countries, they uncovered a significant link: where selenium consumption was lowest, death rates due to coronary disease that affects the arteries leading into the heart were highest.

They found one other fascinating correlation. Coronary artery disease also tended to rise where cadmium intake was high. Cadmium is a metal pollutant that competes with selenium for binding sites— or points of activity—within the body. Cadmium is strongly suspected as a contributing cause of heart disease because it seems to raise blood pressure. Selenium may counteract that effect and protect against heart disease and stroke, which often accompany high blood pressure.

Finnish Studies Show Obvious Link

Finland has one of the highest coronary heart disease rates in the world. In central and eastern Finland, where rates run highest, people have the lowest blood selenium levels in the country. Those two factors seem to coincide geographically.

"More studies will be done, but the relationship is obvious," said Pekko Koivistoinen, Ph.D., head of the department of food chemistry and technology at the University of Helsinki, Finland. Dr. Koivistoinen told us, "On taking a closer look, we see that farming families, who subsist on food grown locally, have the lowest selenium of all, as well as the highest rates of heart disease."

Overall dietary intake of selenium is low in Finland—30 micrograms a day for men and about 20 to 25 micrograms a day for women. That compares to 50 to 200 micrograms a day judged to be essential to good health by the National Academy of Sciences in the United States and generally accepted as adequate elsewhere.

What accounts for Finland's low selenium is a combination of factors. The country has very little selenium-rich sedimentary rock, plus a humid climate, heavy rainfall and acid soil, all of which reduce selenium's availability to forage and food crops, and make Finland an ideal laboratory for further study, says Dr. Koivistoinen.

"We have low selenium to start out with. We can look at how that affects health. Added to that, we also have low chromium. Chromium is linked not only to normalization of insulin response in diabetics but to reduction of LDL [low-density lipoprotein] cholesterol [the bad kind] in the blood. Finns have high cholesterol. In that respect, those two factors together—low selenium and low chromium—could explain to a certain extent why I think we have in our country an exceptionally high rate of coronary heart disease."

Many Finns have decided to make up for low selenium on their own rather than wait for formal public health action. People are eating more fish, which is the richest source of selenium, Dr. Koivistoinen told us. And they're taking supplements.

"Stroke Belt" Low in Selenium

In our own country, a similar correlation seems to be shaping up between selenium and heart disease. Sections of the southeastern coastal plains of Georgia and the Carolinas have the highest stroke rate in the United States—so high that it's called the "Stroke Belt." Heart disease there is also very high. And it's a low-selenium area. In northwestern Georgia, by contrast, heart disease is lower and blood selenium levels are higher.

A nutrition biochemist, who's been an advocate of selenium's virtues for years, said, "I had a heart attack in 1970 and now I take selenium as insurance. Whether it's been good insurance, I don't know." He is 70 years old.

Another Kind of Heart Disease

One of the newest and most notable links in the emerging tie between selenium and heart disease was reported at the Second International Symposium on Selenium in Biology and Medicine at Texas Tech University in May, 1980. The news came from researchers from the People's Republic of China. In a study of over 45,000 Chinese—the most massive study ever done on selenium deficiency in people—supplementation with selenium wiped out a heart disorder affecting 40 out of every 1,000 children in certain areas of China.

Keshan disease is a form of cardiomyopathy—that is, heart muscle damage due to unknown causes. Symptoms include enlargement of the heart, gallop pulse, weak heartbeat, low blood pressure, fluid retention and abdominal pain. Half its victims die.

What stands out as most peculiar about Keshan disease is its distinct geographical distribution in relation to selenium in soil, food and human tissues. In areas where selenium is low, Keshan disease is common. In high-selenium areas, Keshan disease is nowhere to be found.

Low-selenium soil was noticed first. "It was as if selenium in soil acted as a physical barrier against the disease," said G. Q. Yang, Ph.D., of the Chinese Academy of Medical Sciences in Peking. Because the dividing line was so uncannily well defined, the research team felt they were on to a cure—and possibly a preventive—for Keshan disease. They tested samples of blood, hair and staple foods (wheat, corn, rice and soybeans) from affected and nonaffected areas of China. The relationship was confirmed. Low soil selenium meant low dietary and body levels of the mineral—and a high rate of Keshan disease. On the other hand, soils adequate in selenium were accompanied by adequate or high dietary and body levels, and disappearance of Keshan disease.

The answer stared them in the face. In 1973, a program of supplementation with selenium was begun for thousands of children in the affected areas, with a relatively equal number left untreated as a control group. The death rate in those treated plummeted from 50 percent to 6 percent, a spectacular show of improvement. The number of new cases per thousand dropped from 40 to 1. The program was expanded. By 1977, selenium's protective effect was so apparent that all children in the disease-prone areas studied were given selenium. Of 12,000 children so treated, none came down with Keshan disease.

There's no question that selenium was a pivotal factor in the Chinese study. "However, it's unlikely that selenium is the *only* factor in the disease," Dr. Yang pointed out to the assembly. "Other aspects of diet could be important. Protein needs to be studied. Vitamin E could be important. Both need further study." There's also some evidence that a virus could be involved to some extent, added Dr. Yang.

Even before Dr. Yang's discovery, selenium was counted among the five minerals to be studied in relation to heart disease by the World Health Organization.

Chromium Fights Diabetes and Heart Disease

It's now fairly well established that chromium improves glucose tolerance—our ability to use the carbohydrates in food—probably by enabling the body to use insulin in an efficient and effective manner. That makes it a four-star mineral for diabetics, who have abnormal carbohydrate metabolism. But it may also improve metabolism of blood fats—cholesterol and triglycerides—making it a boon to coronary-prone individuals. Diabetes and heart disease, in fact, aren't very far removed from each other. Heart attack happens to be a leading cause of death among diabetics.

The connection between the three—chromium, insulin and risk of heart disease—is summed up by Walter Mertz, M.D., chairman of the USDA Human Nutrition Research Center in Beltsville, Maryland: "The most consistent effect of marginal chromium deficiency is elevated insulin response, and the first effect of chromium supplementation is the restoration of a normal response. It appears from these data that if we improve glucose tolerance, restore normal insulin levels and at the same time lower cholesterol levels—particularly certain fractions—we may reduce the risk for cardiovascular disease."

Chromium Keeps Cholesterol under Control

The "certain fractions" of cholesterol Dr. Mertz refers to are the LDL, or low-density lipoproteins.

"Cholesterol is carried around the bloodstream in different kinds of 'packages,' " William Castelli, M.D., director of laboratories for the famed Framingham Study, told us. "In the past, we thought that all cholesterol was bad. But now, we're finding that there is one type that is really good—called HDL (high density lipoprotein). If most of the other, bad types of cholesterol are too high, they can be deposited in the lining of the arteries. But HDL is a very clever type, one which carries cholesterol away to the liver so it can be excreted. The biggest problem package is LDL.

"What we know so far," continued Dr. Castelli, "is that the higher the HDL, the better off you're going to be. And you cannot get a clear picture of the heart disease potential unless you consider the ratio of total cholesterol to HDL levels. The lower the better. Vegetarians, for example, have one of the best ratios, at 2.8. Marathon runners are 3.4, and bike riders 3 to 3.4."

What does all this have to do with chromium?

Rebecca Riales, Ph.D., a West Virginia nutritionist, believes that chromium may play a significant role in increasing HDL cholesterol levels and maybe even in decreasing LDL—the bad cholesterol.

"I didn't have a research lab with a lot of mice to be subjected to my mind's curiosity. So I took a human subject—my husband. I persuaded him to take for his persistent wife two teaspoons of brewer's yeast a day for six weeks, and to have his serum lipids measured before and after this study.

"My life has not been the same since I got his laboratory report. Contrary to expectation, the total cholesterol did not drop, but unexpectedly the HDL cholesterol took such a large jump that I thought that perhaps Mother Nature was playing a trick on me. We had it repeated, and it turned out to be a reality."

During her next trial, Dr. Riales studied eight men, all between 35 and 45, who were physicians and personal friends. After six weeks, they showed similar results.

Next, working along with another scientist, she gathered 23 men who were relatively free from known metabolic disease. She separated them into two groups—one received a daily vial of tasteless chromium chloride and the other a vial of water twice a day on an empty stomach for five days. Cholesterol, triglyceride and insulin values were measured, and glucose tolerance tests were given at the beginning of the study and again at 6 and 12 weeks.

At the time of this writing, only the data on HDL cholesterol levels had been fully analyzed. The group receiving only water maintained their HDL levels rather evenly. But the chromium-supplemented group showed a steady increase. "The effects we observed in the previous groups appear to be real," reports Dr. Riales. "A most encouraging finding."

It's Never Too Late to Start

Let's suppose, just for argument's sake, that everyone in the United States, children and older people alike, adopted a low-fat, high-mineral diet. Odds are, there'd be fewer heart attacks overall. Suppose too that everyone quit smoking. And got some regular exercise. Learned to relax. And kept their weight down. It's a good bet there'd be even *fewer* deaths from heart disease.

Sound idealistic? Maybe. Habits are tough to break. So 200 million people aren't likely to make all those changes.

But *you* can.

34

High Blood Pressure

One in every five adults has high blood pressure. That doubles his or her chances of stroke or heart attack.

Hopes for prevention are even higher, though. A combination of weight control, exercise and relaxation can help keep blood pressure comfortable. Prevailing over those factors, however, is the role of sodium. Too much sodium can jeopardize healthy blood pressure. Curbing sodium intake goes a long way toward keeping blood pressure down and avoiding ill consequences. Potassium, meanwhile, helps counteract sodium's sinister effect. There's some evidence, too, that cadmium—a major pollutant in industry, auto exhaust and cigarette smoke—also has some influence.

But the main culprit is salt.

_____How a Blood Pressure Cuff Works_____

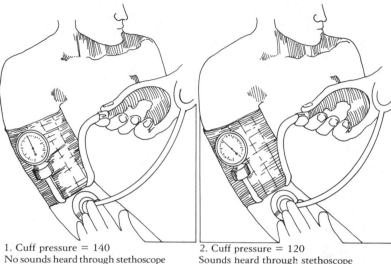

1. Cuff pressure = 140
No sounds heard through stethoscope

2. Cuff pressure = 120
Sounds heard through stethoscope

To measure blood pressure, a soft cuff is wrapped around the upper arm and inflated by a rubber bulb. Blood stops circulating momentarily and no sounds are heard through the stethoscope, pressed against the artery.

As the cuff is allowed to deflate, blood begins to flow through the artery again. Tapping sounds—the pulse—are heard through the artery. That's the point of peak artery pressure, or systolic pressure—in this case, 120, as registered on the attached meter.

Keeping Blood Pressure Free and Easy

At any one time, a total of about five quarts of blood is coursing through your blood vessels from your heart, to your kidneys, brain, other organs and back to the heart. Blood pressure—the force at which blood travels through arteries—is determined by a combination of factors: the total amount of blood, the pumping intensity of the heart, and the resistance to flow met in muscular artery walls. Resistance is determined partly by the elasticity of those walls, partly by the work load carried.

The highest pressure reached, just after the heart contracts, is the systolic pressure. The lowest pressure reached, when the heart is at rest between beats, is the diastolic (see figure). Normally, the ratio of systolic over diastolic is 140 over 90 (written 140/90) or lower. Anything greater is considered high blood pressure, or hypertension. Just how high it may be ranges from mild to moderate to severe:

Borderline or mild high blood pressure:
Systolic pressure of 140-160
Diastolic pressure of 90-95

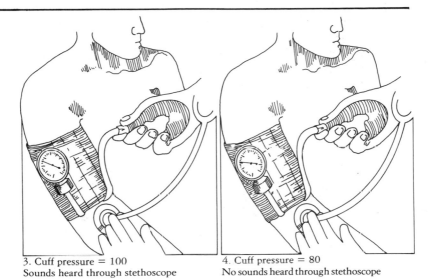

3. Cuff pressure = 100
Sounds heard through stethoscope

As the cuff continues to deflate,
tapping sounds continue.

4. Cuff pressure = 80
No sounds heard through stethoscope

A few seconds later, the tapping
sounds disappear as pressure in the
artery reaches the lowest point, or
diastolic pressure (80, in this case).

Moderate high blood pressure:
    Systolic pressure of 160-180
    Diastolic pressure of 96-114

Severe high blood pressure:
    Systolic pressure above 180
    Diastolic pressure above 115

Sodium Raises Blood Pressure

Sodium affects blood volume—and pressure—in two ways. Working with the kidneys, sodium keeps us from losing too much fluid—from dehydrating, literally. Too much sodium, however, holds back too much fluid, increasing the volume of blood to be pumped around the body. The swell in volume demands a more vigorous thrust by the heart and greater push against artery walls. Blood pressure mounts.

At the same time, sodium seems to prompt the smooth muscles around the smallest arteries to constrict, increasing resistance to flow.

Sodium may also act by accidentally stimulating angiotensin, a hormone that affects the kidneys during periods of stress and causes the heart to beat faster and the blood vessels to constrict.

That salt is a prime foe in the epidemic of high blood pressure is grounded in population studies and animal experiments. Among primitive people eating a Stone Age diet—Eskimos and villagers in the South Pacific islands, for instance—salt intake is quite low—2 to 5 grams a day. That translates into 800 to 2,000 milligrams of sodium, largely from meats, vegetables and grains. Table salt is unknown. Processed foods (which almost automatically contain salt) are unheard of. Pan over to industrialized countries such as the United States, Japan and Finland, however, and sodium intake soars—to 10 to 12 grams a day or higher, from both table salt and processed foods. And high blood pressure is rampant—affecting 35 million people in our country alone. What's more, when people move from an undeveloped country, free of high blood pressure, to our own, chances are they'll develop high blood pressure.

While the evidence is incriminating, salt is not the actual *cause* of high blood pressure. It simply encourages the condition in certain susceptible people. That's borne out by the curious fact that within nations such as ours, where salt intake and high blood pressure both run high, there are people who never develop the problem no matter how much salt they consume. Others tend to get it even when intake is moderate. Blacks, for some unknown reason, are more susceptible than others. Men under 45 are more likely to develop high blood pressure than women up to that age. (After age 45, though, women catch up.)

The difference lies in genetic disposition. That simply means some unknown factor we inherit from our parents seems to make some of us salt-sensitive and others immune to its effect on blood pressure. For salt-sensitive people who eat a lot of salt, blood pressure is likely to climb, upping their chances of stroke, heart disease, or kidney failure. Salt-immune people seem to have an inborn resistance.

The trick is in knowing if you're among the genetically prone group. But that's not always possible. If one or both of your parents has high blood pressure, you are likely to have it. But they may have had it for years and not known it. High blood pressure has no outward symptoms until it's dangerously high. For many people, high blood pressure is discovered during a routine checkup or exam for other illness.

And even if your parents seem unaffected, high blood pressure could still be in the cards for you. The American Heart Association—and many doctors—wisely recommend moderate salt intake for everyone, infants and children included. While high blood pressure may not show up until advancing years, it can start in the cradle. Cow's milk has more sodium than mother's milk, so breastfed infants are a step ahead of their bottle-fed brothers and sisters. Sodium content of commercial baby foods is now reduced compared to that of previous years. High-salt snacks for teens jeopardize adult health and should be discouraged.

If you cut down on salt, watch your weight, learn to handle stress, exercise, and don't smoke, your chances of getting high blood pressure—and its nasty consequences—are almost totally squelched. There are a few other things that also help.

Sugar and Salt, a Bad Combination

A lot of sugar in the diet may compound the threat of salt. Researchers at Louisiana State University Medical School tested three groups of monkeys for their response to high intakes of salt and sugar. The first group was fed a diet containing no added salt; the second group, a diet with 3 percent salt; and the third group, a diet consisting of 3 percent salt plus 38 percent sugar. Those amounts of salt and sugar are high, but they are "within the range of human consumption," according to the researchers.

They found that the monkeys on the salt plus sugar diet showed worse symptoms of high blood pressure than both the other groups. And they concluded their report with this cautiously worded but clear warning: ". . . the synergistic effect of dietary sodium and sucrose [sugar] on the induction of hypertension in this nonhuman primate species has a potentially important bearing on human hypertension" (*American Journal of Clinical Nutrition,* March, 1980).

Potassium Helps Flush Out Sodium

It just so happens that the diets typical of populations free of hypertension are not only low in salt but also high in potassium. And diets typical of populations beleaguered by high blood pressure—us—are relatively low in potassium. That's important, because potassium seems to exert a strong protective effect against high blood pressure. In other words, potassium may be the other side of the coin in the toss-up between getting high blood pressure or not. Sodium, you do; potassium, you don't.

A link between potassium and hypertension was made as early as 1928, when the *Canadian Medical Association Journal* carried a report saying "potassium salt regularly produced a decline in blood pressure, while sodium salt regularly produced a rise" in humans. Further research in the 1930s and 1940s also showed potassium lowering high blood pressure.

In a relatively recent study of nearly 2,000 people in three American cities, George D. Miller, Ph.D., formerly at the Johns Hopkins School of Hygiene and Public Health, found that people with low blood pressure tended to eat more potassium and less sodium (from table salt, i.e., sodium chloride) than people with high blood pressure. But the *ratio* of potassium to sodium proved to be a more accurate index of blood pressure than just sodium alone. In other words, the connection between blood pressure and sodium *and* potassium was stronger than the connection between blood pressure and sodium alone. Dr. Miller reported his results to the annual American Heart Association conference in 1978.

Subjects for Dr. Miller's study had been recruited by randomly knocking on doors and asking for urine samples. Then blood pressure readings were taken. Intakes of sodium and potassium are measured most simply by the passing of their excess into the urine, said Lewis Kuller, M.D., who worked with Dr. Miller on the study and is now chairman of the epidemiology department of the University of Pittsburgh School of Public Health. Dr. Kuller told us the results show that "the people studied who excrete more potassium in relation to sodium have lower blood pressure."

The reason *why* potassium does what it does—or seems to be doing—is "unclear at present," said Dr. Kuller. But the results are in good company, at least. "There have been other studies showing the same thing," noted Dr. Kuller.

Another contributor to the growing research in that area is Herbert Langford, M.D., of the University of Mississippi Medical School at Jackson. A few years ago Dr. Langford began making surveys with Robert Watson, D.V.M., Ph.D., of blood pressure levels among high school students in the greater Jackson area. They found that hypertension was highest among poor rural blacks. In six subsequent studies consisting of 100 students each, Drs. Langford and Watson "failed to find a significant correlation between sodium excretion and blood pressure," Dr. Langford said. The amount of potassium excretion, considered by itself, wasn't significant either.

"But what we have found, and most clearly, was that the sodium:potassium ratio correlated with blood pressure."

Dr. Langford suggested that potassium increases salt excretion, acting as a natural diuretic to assist the kidneys in flushing excess salt from the body. That's why the ratio is so critical. To some extent at least, it seems the amount of potassium may determine just how much salt we can rinse out of ourselves.

Currently Dr. Langford is giving high-potassium diets to nine patients with high blood pressure, and watching closely. "It's too soon to say much, but so far the results are encouraging," he told us.

Research with animals is terribly important for finding out things that science wouldn't dare probe for using human "guinea pigs." The principal experimenter with animals has been George R. Meneely, M.D., professor of medicine and of physiology and biophysics at the Louisiana State University School of Medicine in Shreveport.

Working on and off since 1950 on the topic, Dr. Meneely has fed super-salt diets to rats, giving them 20, 40 and 60 times what they need to survive. Alongside those rats he has a group given only what salt they need, and a group of super-salt rats which are also fed high amounts of potassium. The years of experimentation have shown that "potassium has some protective effect on blood pressure. It's not dramatic, but there's some," says Dr. Meneely. The greatest effect has been upon the rats fed 60 times the necessary amount of salt. Potassium kept their blood pressure from rising above the levels shown by rats fed only 40 times the necessary amount. What's more, the potassium-protected rats unexpectedly outlived both the unprotected rats and the control rats (those fed a supposedly "ideal" salt diet).

Doctors at London Hospital Medical College have achieved the most exciting results of all, however. They found that a high-potassium, moderate-sodium diet lowered blood pressure in hypertensive people. Two groups of people—16 with mild high blood pressure, 8 with normal blood pressure—took part in the study. Both groups were first put on a high-sodium diet for 12 weeks. Blood pressure rose slowly all across the board, but increases were highest in the high blood pressure group. Both groups were then fed a high-potassium diet with no added sodium. In the people with high blood pressure, pressure dropped to levels *below what they were at the start of the study.* (In people with normal blood pressure, levels returned to slightly above normal.) Previously, researchers were only able to do that by feeding people a very strict low-sodium diet that is hard to stick to day in and day out for months or years. So the London researchers feel that potassium offers real prospects for a practical dietary approach to long-term control of high blood pressure (*Lancet,* January 10, 1981).

Cadmium Raises Blood Pressure

The link between cadmium and high blood pressure is weaker than for sodium and potassium. But concern is growing because of cadmium's strong tendency to accumulate in the kidney, a key organ in blood pressure control. It may also affect the heart directly.

Cadmium tends to raise blood pressure in laboratory animals as it builds up in the kidneys and liver. Deficiencies of zinc, copper and iron tend to increase the adverse effects of cadmium. Conversely, doubling the required amount of zinc in animal diets can bring down the levels of cadmium in the kidneys and liver.

The same may be true for people. In a study of 50 men in Birmingham, England, both cadmium and lead levels in blood and urine were higher in those with heart disease and hypertension than in those with normal blood pressure. Whether environmental cadmium, which leaches into food, air and water, is the cause of the heart and artery disorders, or if heart disease somehow slows down excretion of the metals from those organs, is not clear, say the researchers. But their findings coincide with other work done elsewhere (*International Journal of Environmental Studies,* vol. 14, no. 4, 1980).

Selenium may help block cadmium-induced high blood pressure.

Selenium competes with cadmium for binding sites in the body. Jim Andrews, Ph.D., Curtis G. Hames, M.D., and James C. Metts, Jr., M.D., of the Community Cardiovascular Council in Savannah, Georgia, found that of 10,000 high school seniors screened in that area of the United States, 8 percent had blood pressures of 140/90 or above, considered high for their age. Cadmium was also high. And it's a low-selenium area.

"That's the time to intervene," Dr. Metts told us. "Once they leave school and get on the assembly line, we've lost them." Until they show up in their forties and fifties with heart disease, that is. Dr. Metts, an internist, has treated some of his high blood pressure patients with selenium, on an individualized basis, and has seen some encouraging results.

So if cadmium is the threat it seems to be, it may be less menacing to those whose diets are rich in zinc, copper, iron, and, particularly, selenium.

Drugs or Diet for High Blood Pressure

It may be years before we clearly understand how all those factors affect high blood pressure. In the meantime, it would seem wise to curb salt intake to remove a major agent in its development. And boost potassium as added protection. For those with established high blood pressure, the advice goes double.

Strangely enough, doctors don't always emphasize diet to their hypertensive patients. For all but the mildest cases, medication is a mainstay of treatment.

Diuretic drugs step up kidney action, flushing unwanted sodium and fluid out of the body, thereby relieving the load on the heart and arteries. Along with sodium, however, goes potassium, as well as other important minerals. Sometimes potassium supplements or potassium-rich foods are prescribed with diuretics; sometimes they're not. Rarely are other minerals taken into consideration.

In addition, extremely high salt intake can render diuretics useless, so some degree of salt moderation is appropriate even when those drugs are prescribed.

But diuretics are the least of it. There's a whole host of antihypertensive drugs on the market, each with its own set of side effects. Small doses of more than one drug are sometimes combined in order to minimize expected side effects. Unfortunately, drug interaction may sometimes produce new, unexpected effects.

The interesting thing about all these drugs, however, is that each lowers blood pressure in a way that mimics sodium restriction. Because they are powerful agents that directly manipulate the work of heart and blood vessels, they work more quickly than sodium restriction. So they're appropriate as a concerted effort to rescue a system threatened by dangerously high blood pressure of long duration. For milder cases, those drugs—and their annoying side effects—can either be avoided altogether or used in very small doses when salt is reduced. (Be sure to speak with your doctor before reducing dosage on your own.)

Studies bear that out again and again. In a two-year study of moderate salt restriction in 31 hypertensive people, diastolic blood pressure dropped by an average of 7.3 points, an effect similar to that achieved by drugs. And the patients weren't even as strict as they should have been about sodium intake. Had they followed their diet more closely, blood pressure would have probably been reduced further, say the researchers. "In persons with a diastolic blood pressure between 90 and 105 . . . salt restriction should be tried before drugs," they conclude (*Lancet*, February 4, 1978).

In Belgium, Jan Parjis, M.D., and fellow doctors told patients to avoid all food to which sodium was added in preparation and to buy low-salt bread. Sodium excretion (which reflects body sodium) over 24 hours dropped by 50 percent. Most important, systolic blood pressure dropped an average of 7.7 points and diastolic, 4.4 points (*American Heart Journal*, January, 1973).

At a cardiovascular rehabilitation center in California, 218 high blood pressure patients were treated by diet and gradual exercise for 26 days. One hundred eighty-six left drug-free and with normal blood pressure (*Chest, Heart and Stroke Journal*, vol. 3, no. 5, 1978).

In those studies, too, the results compare favorably with drug treatment. Which makes cutting back on salt as effective as taking drugs for all but the more severe cases of high blood pressure, without the troublesome side effects. When exercise is added, the results look even better.

So for controlling outright high blood pressure—with or without drugs—salt restriction does a good job. As for prevention, the argument for the low-salt regimen would seem even stronger. After all, we can't always tell ahead of time what's in store for our arteries. Yet some doctors still wag their heads, saying the case against salt hasn't been completely proved yet—although those doctors are clearly in the minority.

Probably the real reason some doctors don't take a stronger stand against salt is that low-salt diets are so unpalatable (they say) that patients don't or won't follow them. That kind of thinking is changing, too, though—largely because patients win no gold stars for taking their medication regularly, either. At least half "forget" to take their pills, or discontinue them entirely. The side effects of antihypertensive drugs can be unpleasant—and people feel perfectly well without them. So medical enthusiasm for drugs—at a high as recently as 1975—is drifting back, in favor of salt restriction for all. It's even possible that weight loss—always a key goal because it invariably helps—lowers blood pressure partly because less food eaten usually means proportionately less sodium is consumed. At the very least, salt restriction allows smaller doses of drugs to be used, when drugs are necessary.

In an editorial summarizing the turn-around in medical thought on salt and blood pressure, a leading medical journal emphasizes that the benefits of combining salt moderation with weight loss, exercise and relaxation go beyond hypertensive patients to the population at large, more than likely reducing the number of high blood pressure-related deaths for all (*Lancet,* August 30, 1980).

What *Is* a Low-Sodium Diet?

"To make it simple, begin by avoiding the known evils like pretzels, potato chips, salted peanuts, pickles, olives, and so on," said Norman M. Kaplan, M.D., head of the hypertension clinic at Parkland Memorial Hospital and professor of internal medicine at University of Texas Southwestern Medical School. "And learn to avoid the hidden sodium. Milk and milk products—ice cream and butter—have hidden sodium. So does

Hidden Sodium on Food Labels

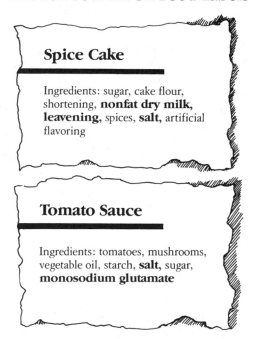

Spice Cake

Ingredients: sugar, cake flour, shortening, **nonfat dry milk, leavening,** spices, **salt,** artificial flavoring

Tomato Sauce

Ingredients: tomatoes, mushrooms, vegetable oil, starch, **salt,** sugar, **monosodium glutamate**

Watch for the words salt and sodium on food labels. Leavenings and nonfat dry milk also contribute sodium, undesirable in very low sodium diets.

processed food—anything prepared before we touch it. Unfortunately, processing usually means salt has been added." (And potassium is lost.)

"Eat more fresh foods. Fresh meats are okay. Sausages, ham and other cured meats are not. Bacon is the world's most evil food," added Dr. Kaplan. "Not only does it have too much sodium, it has fat, calories, everything.

"And, of course, don't salt food while cooking or at the table," said Dr. Kaplan. (See chapter 30, Cooking to Safeguard the Minerals in Our Food, for helpful hints on seasoning food with herbs and other flavorings.)

"By doing all those things, we can halve the amount of sodium in the typical American diet—from the present equivalent of 10 to 12 grams of salt to 5 or 6 grams. That will bring most of us to the 2,000 milligrams of sodium a day typical of diets eaten by people with little or no high blood pressure."

At first, fresh, natural unsalted food may taste "like nothing" to many people who have been reaching for the saltshaker for years. "After a few weeks, though, they get used to it," observed Dr. Kaplan, who's treated hundreds of patients with reduced salt diets.

"We're not after a rigid, low-sodium diet," said Dr. Kaplan. "People won't eat it and I don't expect them to. Halving their intake doesn't really require a massive intrusion in their diet and is often sufficient."

Foods tend to fall into three general categories as far as sodium is concerned. Many are very low in sodium, a few have moderate amounts, and many more are very high. Table 40 (on the following pages) tells you approximately how each type of food rates, sodiumwise. (See our recipe section, chapter 31, for salt-free condiments and sauces.)

The eating plan that's right for you will depend on the state of your blood pressure. If it's quite high, your doctor may limit you to 500 milligrams of sodium a day—probably from foods closest to the center ring on table 40. If your blood pressure is only mildly high, you may be advised to keep sodium to about 1,000 milligrams a day—still near the center of the target, plus small amounts of milk or milk foods, plus an extra 500 milligrams or so from regular bread and butter, or some cheese, or a little salt (¼ teaspoon only) or some other concession. (A 250-milligram diet, used more often in cases of kidney disease or toxemia of pregnancy than high blood pressure, is quite strict—low-low sodium foods only, with low-sodium milk and a check on the sodium in your drinking water.)

As for prevention, the closer we stick to foods in the center ring—with limited consumption of foods in the middle ring, and avoidance of foods outside the rings—the better our odds of sidestepping high blood pressure. On the other hand, the more foods we eat from the middle ring and outer area, the closer we come to the 10 or 12 grams of salt that gets so many of us in trouble.

TABLE 40   **Sodium-At-A-Glance**

frozen turkey
(unless unsalted)

pancake or waffle mixes

commercial spaghetti
macaroni and noodle
dishes; rice mixes

commercial breads
and baked goods,
self-rising flour,
crackers

low-sodium
breads and rolls

most commercial cereals

oatmeal, wheat germ,
farina, grits,
puffed rice or wheat,
shredded wheat and
low-sodium cereals

sauerkraut and
canned vegetables

potatoes, rice,
spaghetti, macaroni
and noodles

frozen vegetables

most fresh
vegetables;
low-sodium
frozen or
canned vegetables

commercial desserts
(read the label)

cooked beets,
beet greens, carrots,
celery, spinach
and Swiss chard

fresh fruit;
low-sodium
frozen or
canned fruit

chemically softened
community or
home drinking water

fruit desserts,
unsalted;
plain gelatin,
and low-sodium
cakes or cookies

fruit processed with
sodium and fruit dried
with sodium sulfite

carbonated beverages

Foods in the center of the
diagram are lowest in sodium
and can be eaten freely if prepared
or eaten without added salt.
Foods in the next ring have considerable
amounts of sodium and should be eaten less
frequently. Foods outside the rings are very high
in sodium and should be avoided.

cocoa mixes

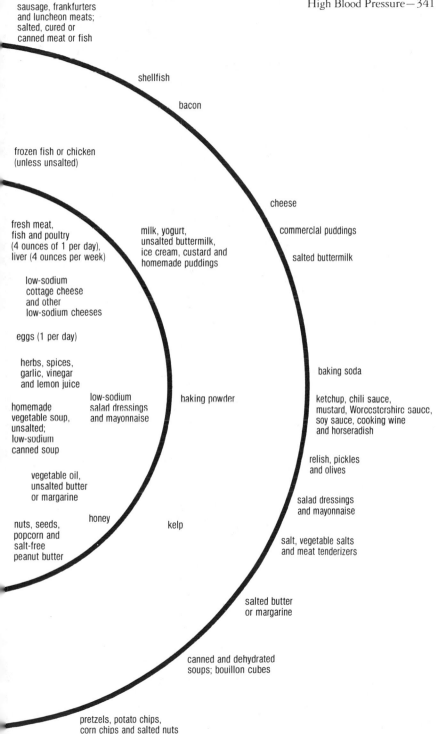

sausage, frankfurters
and luncheon meats;
salted, cured or
canned meat or fish

shellfish

bacon

frozen fish or chicken
(unless unsalted)

cheese

fresh meat,
fish and poultry
(4 ounces of 1 per day),
liver (4 ounces per week)

milk, yogurt,
unsalted buttermilk,
ice cream, custard and
homemade puddings

commercial puddings

salted buttermilk

low-sodium
cottage cheese
and other
low-sodium cheeses

eggs (1 per day)

herbs, spices,
garlic, vinegar
and lemon juice

baking soda

homemade
vegetable soup,
unsalted;
low-sodium
canned soup

low-sodium
salad dressings
and mayonnaise

baking powder

ketchup, chili sauce,
mustard, Worcestershire sauce,
soy sauce, cooking wine
and horseradish

relish, pickles
and olives

vegetable oil,
unsalted butter
or margarine

salad dressings
and mayonnaise

nuts, seeds,
popcorn and
salt-free
peanut butter

honey

kelp

salt, vegetable salts
and meat tenderizers

salted butter
or margarine

canned and dehydrated
soups; bouillon cubes

pretzels, potato chips,
corn chips and salted nuts

35

Diabetes

Who would think a little extra sugar in the blood could cause so much mischief? Yet that's precisely what happens when insulin—a hormone released by the pancreas—fails to properly regulate carbohydrate metabolism. Diabetes—the single name for certain conditions marked by elevated blood sugar—predisposes one to a host of problems. For reasons that are not entirely clear, diabetics are prone to certain complications. The disease produces changes in both the large and small blood vessels, which, directly or indirectly, may have serious consequences. Diseased large blood vessels increase diabetics' chances of atherosclerosis and heart attack. Those same changes in small blood vessels up their chances of senility, slow-healing leg ulcers, stroke, kidney failure and even blindness. The last complication, called diabetic retinopathy, involves tiny hemorrhages in the retina of the eye. Tight control of blood sugar metabolism, however, can head off those complications.

Drugs have come a long way toward reducing the long-term effects of diabetes. Diet and nutrition can go even further. Research clearly points to the fact that everyone—but diabetics especially—should avoid certain dietary errors and pay special attention to other factors (see accompanying box, Guidelines for Prevention and Dietary Control of Diabetes). Simply put, things to avoid are sugar, fat, salt, overweight and too much alcohol. Things to stress are exercise, fiber, complex carbohydrates—and the mineral, chromium.

Guidelines for Prevention and Dietary Control of Diabetes

1. Avoid overweight
2. Cut down on sugar intake
3. Cut down on fat intake
4. Reduce salt intake
5. Limit alcohol consumption
6. Eat complex carbohydrates such as beans, potatoes and whole grains, and other high-fiber foods
7. Eat plenty of chromium-rich foods such as liver, brewer's yeast, chicken and mushrooms
8. Exercise regularly

In addition, a diet high in zinc and magnesium may be helpful.

Chromium Aids Carbohydrate Metabolism

Why chromium?

"We still aren't sure of the exact function chromium has in the onset and treatment of diabetes," says Victoria J. K. Liu, Ph.D., assistant professor in the department of foods and nutrition at Purdue University. "But it definitely seems to aid insulin in body metabolism of glucose."

The young scientist became increasingly interested in the mysterious connection between chromium and diabetes during her postdoctoral training several years ago at the University of Missouri's Trace Substance Research Center and Research Reactor Facility. Two of her mentors were Richard J. Doisy, Ph.D., and Walter Mertz, M.D., both pioneers in research linking blood sugar problems to inadequate chromium intake.

Dr. Liu's focus concerns only the maturity-onset condition (or adult-onset diabetes), which first strikes its victims in their fifties and sixties. Unlike its counterpart, juvenile diabetes, in which the pancreas doesn't secrete normal insulin amounts, in maturity-onset diabetes, *too much* of that hormone is secreted. But maturity-onset diabetics cannot keep the levels of sugar in their blood down in spite of that fact.

Yeast Is a Rich Source of Chromium

It was Dr. Mertz, the godfather of chromium research, whose seminal work first suggested the association with diabetes. Dr. Mertz, the chairman of the USDA Human Nutrition Research Center in Beltsville, Maryland, determined that insufficient glucose tolerance in rats could be corrected by adding a product rich in chromium—brewer's yeast—to their diet. Later he identified the chromium compound that facilitates the body's metabolism of sugar, and called it the glucose tolerance factor.

In fact, only by hooking up with a specific combination of niacin and amino acids does chromium become more active and accessible to the body's cells. Unfortunately, not all chromium in food has that characteristic. The problem is aggravated by the fact that not all people can convert enough of the independent chromium to the active state to meet all their physiological needs. Furthermore, the body's chromium content is known to dwindle with age, increasing our midlife vulnerability to a deficiency. Such is the case in maturity-onset diabetes.

Armed with this knowledge, Dr. Liu devised her own experiment five years ago to study the effects of chromium supplementation in 27 women, aged 40 to 75. The subjects were fed a daily extract of brewer's yeast over a three-month period. Twelve of the older women were diagnosed as hyperglycemic (a high blood sugar condition which may lead to diabetes); 15 women had no apparent difficulties with sugar metabolism. After 90 days, the insulin, glucose and even cholesterol levels were significantly lower in the hyperglycemic group. In the normal group, only the cholesterol levels and total insulin levels were reduced.

Thus, Dr. Liu concluded that chromium, by easing the absorption of available energy into the bloodstream, would reduce the risk or delay the onset of diabetes. In fact, she told us, people with high insulin secretion such as the obese, those suffering from an infection, pregnant women, persons with elevated blood sugar levels and victims of mild adult diabetes may require extra amounts of chromium.

To further explore the cause of the "intimate relationship between chromium levels and sugar metabolism," Dr. Liu is currently analyzing the results of glucose tolerance tests administered to volunteers. What's more, she is one of the few scientists in the country able to study human blood samples with a neutron activation technique and other sophisticated instruments. The findings from blood samples taken every 30 minutes to an hour over a three-hour period are being recorded graphically to correlate insulin response and glucose entry within the cells.

Researchers at St. Luke's Hospital and Columbia University in New York saw similar results with chromium-rich brewer's yeast in 24 volunteers, including eight mild insulin-independent diabetics. Those people (average age 78) were divided into two groups. One group was given chromium-rich yeast daily for eight weeks, the other was not. Before and after yeast supplementation, blood glucose and insulin response to 100 grams oral glucose were measured every 30 minutes for two hours.

Chromium-rich yeast improved both glucose tolerance and insulin response in the experimental group. As an added bonus, cholesterol and serum lipids (blood fats) fell. Esther G. Offenbacher, Ph.D., and Xavier Pi-Sunyer, M.D., of the department of medicine at St. Luke's and Columbia conclude, "This supports the thesis that elderly people may have a low level of chromium, and that an effective source for chromium repletion, such as brewer's yeast, may improve carbohydrate tolerance and cholesterol levels" (*Clinical Research,* April, 1980).

Low Blood Sugar, a Related Problem

The overwhelming evidence that chromium helps the body use insulin in a much more efficient way strongly suggests that the mineral may help another type of blood sugar problem—hypoglycemia, or low blood sugar. Symptoms range from simple fatigue and inability to concentrate, to shaking, sweating and anxiety. Even though the problem is essentially the opposite of diabetes—low blood sugar—the basic problem is the same: poor control of blood sugar. Low blood sugar can arise as a problem in itself or as a prelude to diabetes.

With chromium at work in blood glucose regulation, less insulin is needed to control blood sugar. So there's less likelihood of extreme fluctuations in blood sugar in either direction, up or down.

High Sugar and Fat Mean Little Chromium

The more sugar you eat, the more sugar gets dumped into your bloodstream, the more insulin you'll make, and the more chromium must be mobilized from tissue stores to handle the whole process. Since refined sugar has very little chromium, you're going to be losing more than you're replacing.

Scientific literature supports the theory that the high-sugar American diet places a heavy demand on what otherwise would be adequate chromium consumption. When chromium is low, high sugar intake means double jeopardy (see chapter 11, Chromium).

You can perk up your body's chromium content by filling your shopping cart with foods like calf liver, cheese, wheat germ, whole wheat bread or other whole wheat products, chili pepper and mushrooms. And don't overlook one of the richest dietary sources of chromium—brewer's yeast. If used imaginatively, it may not only spice up your soups and stews but provide that extra oomph that could be lacking in your diet.

Zinc and Magnesium May Help

In addition to chromium's influence on blood sugar control, some evidence indicates that zinc and magnesium may each play a special part in the control of diabetes.

Some diabetics have been found to lose more zinc than usual in their urine. Why is not exactly clear. Presumably, some diabetics lose zinc without an obvious drop in blood levels of zinc. "Perhaps the failure of some diabetics to heal ulcers of the feet (and elsewhere) is related to zinc deficiency," says Ananda S. Prasad, M.D., Ph.D., a leading zinc researcher from Wayne State University School of Medicine in Detroit. "Healing of such ulcers in diabetes has been reported [following] zinc therapy."

In addition to those observations in people, Dr. Prasad describes rat studies which show that glucose tolerance after fasting was depressed in zinc-deficient rats, but adequate in others that were not deficient in zinc. "The reasons for poor glucose tolerance of zinc-deficient animals are not clear," says Dr. Prasad. Perhaps the rate of insulin secretion drops during zinc deficiency. Or while actual blood levels of insulin stay the same, the potency of the hormone may somehow be reduced by zinc deficiency. Either is plausible, since zinc has been found to participate in the synthesis and storage of insulin in the pancreas (*Zinc in Human Nutrition,* CRC Press, 1980).

Low levels of magnesium in the blood may be an important risk factor in the development of diabetic retinopathy, one of the major complications of diabetes. When a team of doctors in Denmark examined 71 insulin-treated diabetics who had had the disease for at least 10 years, they found "a definite lowering" of blood magnesium levels, compared with 194 nondiabetics. And those patients with the most advanced and severe retinopathy had the *lowest* magnesium levels of all (*Diabetes,* November, 1978).

The researchers hope future studies can determine if magnesium supplements will slow down such harmful changes.

36

Cancer

Most people probably expect the cure for cancer to come in a sudden flash of insight at a multimillion-dollar research lab. But that's not quite the way it's happening. Research is a continuum—each day new findings contribute to our understanding of this mysterious disease. What's more, because cancer is not one but many diseases, affecting various organs in different ways, the ultimate answer is likely to be multifaceted. As for both cure and prevention, what we're seeing—rather than a brilliant flash—is a brightening glow on the horizon.

Part of that glow is due to minerals like selenium. From basic population data to actual medical treatment, evidence is growing that this special trace mineral holds great promise for the fight against cancer.

Cells Gone Haywire

All living cells reproduce by dividing. Normal growth and repair take place in an orderly manner. If they don't, a mass of irregular tissue—a tumor—builds up. A tumor may be harmless (benign), in which case it stays put, or harmful (cancerous, malignant), and will most likely grow or spread to other tissues and organs.

Substances that stimulate cancer directly are called carcinogens. Chemicals in tobacco smoke, ultraviolet sunlight and charbroiled meat are only three. Just how much of a carcinogen it takes to produce cancer isn't easy to pin down, however. Some substances cause cancer only when combined with other substances. And certain conditions—eating too much animal fat or too little fiber, for instance—seem to make some people more vulnerable to carcinogens than others. Yet we're all exposed to some carcinogens somewhere along the line. Why do some of us get cancer, while others do not?

The answer seems to lie, for a large part, in immunology—our inborn defense system against not only cancer, but viruses and infections as well. And because all metabolic activities, including immunity, are fundamentally influenced by our diet, good nutrition is critical to our defenses. We already know that several nutritional factors—including iron, zinc, protein and calories—build basic immunity. Now it looks as if selenium may play a major role in a very specialized line of defense.

In areas of low selenium intake, there's a high cancer incidence. In Bulgaria, for example, where the daily average intake of selenium is relatively high—about 250 micrograms per person—the number of deaths due to breast cancer in women is one of the lowest of the countries studied. On the other hand, in the United States, where daily selenium intake is judged to be relatively low—about 50 to 100 micrograms per person—the number of deaths from breast cancer is among the highest (*Illinois Research,* Winter, 1980).

Taking a closer look, surveys show that people in geographical areas of high selenium have high blood selenium levels, whereas people in low selenium areas have low blood selenium. On the surface, then, it appears that selenium offers some protection against cancer.

But it doesn't stop there. Several investigators using different animals have found that selenium is capable of squelching tumors in animals, whether the growths are chemically induced, transplanted from other animals, or pop up spontaneously.

Speaking at the Second International Symposium on Selenium and Biology in May, 1980, A. Clark Griffin, Ph.D., a biochemist from one of the largest cancer research centers in the world, M.T. Anderson Hospital and Tumor Institute in Houston, Texas, said, "Several papers have reported the protective effect of selenium. There are more than a dozen reports showing major reduction of tumors in several species of animals by injection of selenium. It prevents tumors in quite a few organs—colon, liver, skin. The mammary [breast] tumor picture looks particularly exciting."

Gerhard N. Schrauzer, Ph.D., at the University of California at San Diego, added selenium to the drinking water of specially bred mice that normally develop spontaneous breast tumors. Instead of the usual cancer incidence of 80 to 100 percent, only 10 percent developed tumors. The implications for people are real: the fact that breast cancer is a familial trait makes the high-risk woman very much like a specially bred mouse in that respect. Most American diets are very low in selenium, says Dr. Schrauzer, and increasing the amount of that nutrient could significantly reduce the incidence of breast cancer as well as other forms of cancer. Yet, he explains, "Cancer is not a selenium deficiency disease. If you're not susceptible to cancer, selenium won't help. But if you are, it will. It's like an insurance policy."

Why the National Cancer Institute Takes Selenium Seriously

Aware of those significant reports, the National Cancer Institute (NCI) held a special program in September, 1980, to piece together the prevailing state of selenium/cancer research and chart the direction of future investigations. The participants were virtually a Who's Who in the area of selenium/cancer research: biochemists, epidemiologists, cancer researchers and practicing doctors. One panelist, a noted research chemist with the USDA Human Nutrition Research Center in Beltsville, Maryland, explained what he saw to be the purpose of the workshop: "People are going to their doctors and asking about selenium. The doctors don't know, so they look to NCI. And NCI looks to us."

The fact that the workshop was set up for the free exchange of information—and that the panel listened attentively to a potential therapy outside the realm of drugs, radiation and surgery—says something quite significant, not only about the future of nutrition research, but also about changes in the way traditional medicine deals with cancer—formerly in an after-the-fact manner only. If the chain of events that creates a tumor (see figure on next page) can be blocked at one or more points before the cancer works its way through the system, the chances for nipping it in the bud—and saving a life—are actually pretty good. Traditional therapies try to exorcise the cancer in three different ways. Surgery cuts out the main tumor. Radiation aims to wipe out neighboring maverick cells or to prevent recurrence of the disease. And drugs (chemotherapy) travel to remote parts of the body via the bloodstream, destroying cancer cells encountered en route. Those drugs kill cancer cells either by jamming cellular metabolism or by interfering with their reproduction.

Selenium Blockades in the Pathways to Cancer

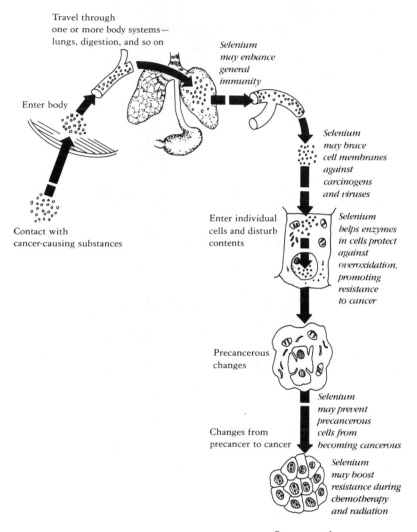

Travel through
one or more body systems—
lungs, digestion, and so on

Selenium
may enhance
general
immunity

Enter body

Selenium
may brace
cell membranes
against
carcinogens
and viruses

Contact with
cancer-causing substances

Enter individual
cells and disturb
contents

Selenium
helps enzymes
in cells protect
against
overoxidation,
promoting
resistance
to cancer

Precancerous
changes

Selenium
may prevent
precancerous
cells from
becoming cancerous

Changes from
precancer to cancer

Selenium
may boost
resistance during
chemotherapy
and radiation

Cancer spreads

Cancer-causing substances (small circles) may enter the body and find their way into various metabolic activities, possibly leading to the formation of cancer in one or more organs. Breaks in the arrows show points where selenium may cut off that chain of events.

SOURCE: Adapted with permission of the publisher from "The Laboratory Approach to the Identification of Environmental Carcinogens," by Umberto Saffiotti in *Proceedings of the Ninth Canadian Cancer Research Conference*, ed. P. G. Scholefield, University of Toronto Press, 1971.

Chemotherapy has evolved from a last-ditch effort to a primary mode of treatment and seems to do fairly well against many common cancers. But there are real problems. The drugs used aren't choosy about what kind of cells they kill—chemotherapy doesn't always spare normal, life-sustaining cells. And the side effects are unpleasant, to say the least: loss of hair, nausea and vomiting, plus immunity often lowered to a point where cancer victims can die of malnutrition or an everyday infection, not necessarily the cancer itself.

And, of course, none of those major treatments can be turned around and used to prevent cancer in the first place.

Aware of the shortcomings of current treatments, scientists realize there's got to be a better answer somewhere. And selenium seems to offer hope. At the same time, they want to be absolutely sure, through more well-controlled research, *how* it works.

Selenium Stimulates Immune System

Part of selenium's anticancer effect may lie in the way our immune system responds to disease. Both selenium and vitamin E are known to independently stimulate the formation of antibodies, special proteins that act as the body's defense agents. Antibodies charge after invading bacteria, viruses and cancer cells (collectively called antigens), rendering them harmless. Antibodies only prevail, however, when armed with selenium and vitamin E.

Vitamin E's role in immune defense has been recognized for some time, but just how selenium fits into the picture has only recently begun to grow clear. Evidently, a special enzyme, glutathione peroxidase (GSH-Px for short) is not only dependent on selenium but may also play a crucial role in the immune response made possible by the presence of selenium. It works this way. Too much oxygen is toxic to cells. Evidently, oxygen not only damages cell membranes, but sets them up for cancer. Selenium-containing GSH-Px is responsible for normal metabolism of peroxides (oxygen compounds) in cells, thus protecting tissues from overoxidation—and possibly cancer.

Julian Spallholz, Ph.D., associate professor of food and nutrition at Texas Tech University, has been studying the relationship between selenium and immunity for many years and speculates that in the normal course of controlling oxidation, selenium-containing GSH-Px may help cells resist bacteria and viruses.

As we discussed in an earlier chapter, a diet low in selenium and vitamin E will result in low levels of GSH-Px activity. When GSH-Px activity is low, the health of the white blood cells suffers, lessening their ability to fight disease. When selenium is adequate, then, GSH-Px theoretically may increase natural resistance by helping white blood cells to clear out bacteria, viruses—and cancer cells. Vitamin E enhances that effect.

Selenium Toughens Cells against Cancer

At the NCI workshop in September, 1980, the role of selenium in oxidation and cancer was probed at considerable length. Eduardo A. Porta, M.D., pathologist from the University of Hawaii School of Medicine, showed conclusively that cells supplemented with vitamin E and selenium had far healthier, better-defined membranes than tissues not supplemented. And less oxidation occurred, thus implying that the deficient cells were probably prone to cancer.

A membrane specialist from the University of California at Berkeley added that a good stiff membrane exposes more surface receptors for antibodies, providing a means to attack and kill cancer cells, as well as any other antigens.

All that fits in well with a philosophy that says prevention and successful treatment of cancer lie in the use of substances normally present in the body and required for us to stay alive. Other such anticancer substances also being studied are vitamins A and C. By changing the amounts of those substances in the human body, it is hoped that cancer will be thwarted from taking hold—or choked off in its earlier stages. Apparently, though, it takes abnormal doses to deal with abnormal cells. And that opens up a whole, virtually uncharted field for cancer research.

Cancer Patients Respond

For doctors who have to face the man or woman who's stricken with cancer, the time lag is frustrating. So perhaps the most exciting news at the NCI workshop came from a doctor who has been using selenium, along with other nutrients, to treat people whose cancer had persisted despite surgery, radiation treatment and chemotherapy. The results are encouraging. But because of the pioneering nature—and delicate implications—of his work, however, the doctor told us he'd prefer we didn't refer to him directly by name.

The doctor started by giving nutritional levels of selenium, 200 micrograms a day, then gradually increased the dosage. But he is not yet sure exactly what level of selenium is high enough to affect the cancer, yet not be toxic to the patient.

John Milner, Ph.D., a professor of food science at the University of Illinois, who has had similar success using selenium against tumors in animals, was supportive of his colleague's work. He commented, "Our main goal is to wipe out tumor cells. If we can do it by any means, why then, let's do it."

Later in 1980, at another cancer symposium, yet another scientist reported on the role of cancer prevention and treatment, first in animals, then in people. Emanuel Revicci, M.D., director of the Institute for Applied Biology in New York, shared his research with colleagues gathered at Cancer Dialogue '80. Like others, much of his early work involved certain mice prone to spontaneous tumors. About 40 percent of those mice usually die from tumors, over twice the death rate of healthy controls of the same age. After treatment with selenium (in the form of selenium sulfate), only 8 percent of the tumor-prone mice died—even fewer than the number of healthy controls. The selenium compound not only seemed to prevent cancer, but it evidently prolonged the normal lifespan in mice.

Encouraged by such work with animals, Dr. Revicci then treated some of his cancer patients with selenium, often bound to fatty acids. His approach is too complicated to discuss at length here—much has to do with the nature of the cancer and the acid-base balance of the individual—but he does seem to be on to something.

Of those patients who have responded well, Dr. Revicci tells of two notable cases. Some years ago, an 11-year-old boy had come to him. Biopsy showed he had a brain tumor. "We treated him with selenium with splendid results. Recently I came across the address of his mother and I called her. 'I'd like to see your son,' I said. She said, 'Please, don't. He's married now, with two children. He's a carpenter. He was 11 years old when he had the tumor. He has forgotten all about it. Don't remind him.' I said, 'All right.' I didn't call him."

A more recent case, says Dr. Revicci, is a woman who came in with cancer in the abdomen. Her husband was told she had two weeks to live, or perhaps a month at the most. Dr. Revicci started her on a selenium-based treatment. "In less than a month, she was out of bed. In three months, she was playing golf. She had no trace of the tumor," says Dr. Revicci.

Her husband didn't want her to know she had cancer. "The woman felt all was well and stopped the treatment. A year later, she was in the hospital again. She was again dying of cancer. I put her on the treatment again. She got better. Again off the bed. Again playing golf. And again stop the treatment," says Dr. Revicci. A year later, the same thing happened. For a third time, the cancer recurred and disappeared with treatment.

"She lived almost 12 years more—and died of pneumonia," says Dr. Revicci.

"Now, I heard at least a hundred times, 'Oh, they were spontaneous remissions.' Spontaneous remission the first time? Spontaneous remission the second time? *The third time?* Improbable."

"We are not pretending we have *the* treatment for cancer," says Dr. Revicci. "But I think we have opened a door."

How does Dr. Revicci think selenium works?

"In normal animals, selenium taken in is eliminated after two or three days. But if the animal has a tumor, almost the entire amount is fixed on the tumor and remains there a long time," he said. Dr. Revicci feels that's significant, and aims to find out more. Right now, he believes that selenium works along with fatty acids as a catabolic (or breaking down) agent on the tumor, forcing it to reduce or disappear. The results of treatment in people are not always consistent—much seems to depend on how much chemotherapy a patient has had, plus many other factors, of course.

Hunting for the Right Dose

In an earlier address, at the Selenium Symposium at Texas Tech University in May, 1980, Gerhard N. Schrauzer, Ph.D., one of the pioneers of selenium research, said, "It comes down to drugs versus nutrients. I think if we really want to consider nutritional cancer prevention in national populations, we have to include selenium either through a change of diet or supplementation—or both."

Selenium is a two-edged sword, though. In very high doses, over a period of time, selenium is toxic to animals. So there is some question as to how much selenium is too much for people. We know that there's no problem of toxicity to people at accepted nutritional levels of 50 to 200 micrograms of selenium a day. Apparently, though, you only get elevated blood levels of selenium—that is, levels high enough to boost cell resistance—at higher doses such as the anonymous doctor in the Midwest used to treat his patients.

The most widely recognized sign of selenium toxicity in animals is liver damage. Yet that doctor reported to NCI that at 2,000 micrograms a day, none of his patients showed liver damage—even after as long as a year of supplementation. So he's fairly confident that his doses didn't approach the level of toxicity for selenium in human adults—whatever that level may be.

A parallel situation exists among the vitamins. Vitamin A appears to be of prophylactic value against cancer, probably because that vitamin is required for the manufacture of the protective (epithelial) tissues lining our organs. But in very high doses, vitamin A is toxic. And the potential toxicity of high, therapeutic doses of any substance raises some questions.

The first concerns zeroing in on the right dose. "Before we go dumping selenium into people, we have to ask if we might do more harm than good," cautions William G. Hoekstra, Ph.D., a biochemist and nutrition scientist at the University of Wisconsin, who's published reams of material on selenium. In other words, Dr. Hoekstra feels it's a matter of carefully balancing toxicity against therapeutic effectiveness.

And how much should be responsibly publicized about research considered preliminary by its investigators? On one hand, some say, "Let's not be premature. It's not fair to hold out hope to cancer patients and their families until we know for sure." But on the other hand, the public feels it has a right to know about any promising treatment, especially one legitimate enough to be supported by the NCI (National Cancer Institute), a major grant-giving body and the government's principal agency for cancer research. And as with any hint of a breakthrough of this kind, there's the problem of how to handle a barrage of phone calls from families of cancer patients once you're on to what looks like an effective treatment. People can't be cured over the phone.

On top of that, the use of selenium is regulated by the Food and Drug Administration (FDA). Because selenium taken in very high doses would probably be toxic to people, investigators are cautious to the point where most are very close-mouthed about even insinuating that people should take selenium to prevent or cure cancer. They worry that if the FDA thinks people are taking too much, too freely—for any reason—the agency might yank selenium supplements off the market, setting back years of progress.

Looking even further below the surface, we should pause to consider two strong and intertwining medical attitudes. First, scientists tend to treat any conclusion gingerly unless the research is overwhelmingly convincing. That's rarely the case, though. For every known discovered, a hundred unknowns seem to arise. And paradoxically, the medical establishment appears to encourage new research while at the same time leaning toward reinforcement of prevailing attitudes. The tendency is to react to new ideas with apathy or ridicule until it's no longer possible to ignore the evidence. At this time, medical people are not overly enthusiastic about dealing with cancer through diet.

Some, of course, think it makes a lot of sense. James C. Metts, Jr., M.D., a doctor of internal medicine from Savannah, Georgia, told us, "I'll tell you one thing for sure. If I had cancer, I'd take selenium."

For you and me, one option is to wait for 5, 10 or 20 years, until the results are officially in. Not everyone can afford that kind of patience. As Dr. Schrauzer said, "Yes, I take supplements. I wish I had started 15 years ago and not believed the nutritionists."

37

Wound Healing

Most of us probably don't give much thought to a little scrape or burn. We nick ourselves shaving, burn our hand on the range or stub our toe on the stairs and just naturally expect the wound to heal. It may sting a little at first and look unsightly for a few days, but gradually the damage is repaired and the wound fades away.

Larger wounds command more notice. We slip with a kitchen knife. Or tear a tendon climbing down a ladder. Or a stray dog decides to munch on our ankle. Or our surgeon says our gallbladder must come out. At best, we get away with a small scar. At worst, our sores linger until it seems they're around to stay. And then there is also the hazard of infection. In any case, we grit our teeth and wait it out, hopeful that nature will do what it's supposed to do.

How *long* we wait may depend on zinc. A close-up look reveals that wound healing is a dynamic chain of events, highly affected by zinc.

Thousands of new cells must be manufactured to help replace damaged tissue, whether ravaged by a bruise, a scalpel or a sprain. Many vital nutrients are needed for the healing job: protein, carbohydrates, vitamins (notably A and C) and minerals. Iron deficiency, for instance, will slow down healing. A key healing nutrient, though, is zinc. Without zinc, healing is next to impossible.

Zinc for Pinker, Cleaner, Faster-Healing Wounds

Wound healing is a unique manner of growth. The way new cells are manufactured and laid down in a wound depends on DNA, a special substance in the nucleus of each and every cell of the body. DNA programs cells to duplicate themselves during any kind of growth and in so doing, takes charge of the healing process. When we gash or burn ourselves badly, a spurt of DNA activity prompts cells to divide rapidly, multiplying six times faster than normal to meet the emergency. And cells continue to multiply until well after the wound is closed, to be certain healing is complete. And zinc, among other things, is essential to the synthesis of DNA.

Rapid cell division begins within hours of the injury, and peaks in the areas just beyond the edge of the wound. A front line of old cells, meanwhile, has begun to migrate over the wound. In this phase of wound healing, old cells close in from the perimeter. The migrating cells stick to each other in sheets and continue to creep across the surface until they bump into cells advancing from the other side. The converging fronts meet head on and stop in their tracks. New cells then move in to fill in their ranks. (In burns, there's a slight difference: first, cells divide and pile up at the edge for a week or so before moving in.)

After those surface (epithelial) cells are laid down, zinc again goes to work—this time through the manufacture of another kind of tissue—collagen. Collagen is the tough, fibrous protein of connective tissues. Collagen fibers weave their way over the wound, meshing new tissue with old, as early as the second day after injury. Lucky for us: collagen keeps the wound from splitting apart during healing. Scar tissue is basically a bundle of collagen.

Zinc also liberates vitamin A from the liver. Vitamins A and C both play roles in collagen formation, too. Vitamin A also influences the rate at which epithelial cells migrate across a wound during the first hours of healing.

Zinc also stabilizes individual cell membranes, keeping them strong and resilient under stress. And zinc musters up white blood cells to fight bacteria, warding off infection—always a potential problem with damaged tissue.

The healing pattern is the same at all levels of a wound, like matching like through all layers. Skin cells link with skin, nerve with nerve, muscle with muscle, and so on. And it's the same in all organs—heart, lung, colon, spleen.

Such a tall order makes any wound a zinc sponge, sapping body stores of the mineral. When you gash your foot or have your appendix out, zinc rushes to the site of the wound. That's been measured: levels in the area of the wound go up; body levels go down. As the wound heals, the body must continue to send out reinforcements of zinc, or the battle becomes a long, drawn-out—and frustrating—affair. If body stores are low to begin with—due to poor diet or lack of appetite—healing can drag on and on. Incisions refuse to close up for lack of collagen to keep edges firmly knit, leaving an open sore. New cell growth slows, falling short of the wound center, leaving only a thin web of easily broken tissue. The slightest irritation sets healing back days. Or infection takes over.

On the other hand, healing is a breeze if zinc is in good supply. Wounds heal up tight, smooth and clean. Infections have less of a chance of making your recovery miserable. The Recommended Dietary Allowance for zinc is 15 milligrams a day. But at least double that amount is needed for optimum wound healing.

Harnessing the Healing Power of Zinc

Some wounds—like surgery—are planned. Or at least anticipated. Poor wound healing afterwards is not. The surgeon sews up his incision and exits the operating room, but that's only the beginning for you. Researchers have found that zinc levels before and after surgery are a good barometer of how well we heal.

Before and after injury

Eight patients—young, healthy people on good diets—underwent minor surgery (removal of cysts). Zinc levels (as measured by hair analysis) in all eight people were compared to the amount of time their incisions took to heal. Results showed a definite correlation between hair zinc levels and the rate of wound healing. *The higher the zinc level, the faster they healed.*

In a separate study, one patient who was given a zinc supplement (220 milligrams of zinc sulfate, three times a day) healed exceptionally fast. Walter J. Pories, M.D., and William H. Strain, Ph.D., who report both studies, call the second results "provocative." They add, "With zinc therapy, healing is definitely promoted, perhaps to the optimum rate." Their results, however, could not be duplicated by others (*Zinc Metabolism,* Charles C Thomas, 1966).

Tonsillectomy has long been one of the most common operations performed. Thousands upon thousands of children are reassured that the operation "won't hurt a bit" and that they'll be able to soothe their pain with gobs of ice cream, anyway. The ice cream may help with the soothing, but the healing requires zinc.

Fredric W. Pullen II, M.D., of the University of Miami School of Medicine, tested zinc's ability to speed healing after tonsillectomy. Dr. Pullen's study was "double blind," meaning neither the doctors nor the patients knew who was getting dummy pills, or placebos. Those who did get zinc were given a total of 477 milligrams spread out over the day.

By the end of two weeks, 21 of the 24 people getting zinc were completely healed. Only 13 of 22 people not getting zinc were completely healed that soon. Dr. Pullen, reporting his study in a book, *Clinical Applications of Zinc Metabolism* (Charles C Thomas, 1974), says, "The results are even more striking when one realizes that these tonsillectomies were performed in otherwise healthy individuals and not those with cirrhosis, or other debilitating diseases. . . . it is very apparent that zinc is a necessary ingredient within the healing mechanism."

And the sooner zinc is bolstered, the better. All but the most trivial of injuries cause some degree of distress to the body even if only for a short time. Any event that involves breakdown or rapid turnover of cells—major surgery, accidental injury or bone fracture—prompts the body to dump large amounts of zinc into the urine—perhaps two to five times the norm, depending on how severe the damage. Magnesium, potassium, phosphorus and nitrogen are also lost.

Zinc losses do not always show up on a blood test. A blood sample (if one should be taken) could very well show normal zinc when body levels are precariously low.

We spoke to one surgeon in particular who takes the role of zinc in healing quite seriously: Sheldon V. Pollack, M.D., assistant professor of medicine and chief of the chemosurgery unit at Duke University Medical Center in Durham, North Carolina. Dr. Pollack is planning a trial of zinc and vitamin C supplements in 100 skin surgery patients over the current year.

"The average skin surgery wound—a hole two or three inches big—heals by itself in four or five weeks, six at the most. With zinc and vitamin C, it's possible that such wounds may heal 25 percent sooner," speculated Dr. Pollack.

"If this helps, I'll recommend supplements to all my patients after surgery . . . and probably before surgery, too," Dr. Pollack told us.

What Dr. Pollack has in mind is about 55 milligrams of zinc a day. That amount, he says, is arbitrary. Thirty milligrams of zinc a day might be a good place to start for most people facing surgery.

Burns heal faster with zinc

Doctors have found that burn patients usually have low levels of zinc—due to the highly destructive nature of a burn. Zinc supplements definitely speed healing of charred skin. What's more, skin grafts, when needed, "take" better after zinc supplementation (*Clinical Applications of Zinc Metabolism,* Charles C Thomas, 1974).

Drs. Pories and Strain report a similar outcome of a one-year followup of 43 burn patients at Case Western Reserve University's teaching hospital. Hair samples taken showed that the zinc content of hair plummeted after a severe burn, indicating probable zinc deficiencies in all the patients. That "not only supports the hypothesis that zinc is important to healing, but also suggests that zinc therapy may offer a promising approach to the treatment of burns" (*Zinc Metabolism,* Charles C Thomas, 1966).

Bedsores vanish with zinc

Bedsores are not only ugly and painful, they can keep you in the hospital long after your illness is over. Prolonged pressure on elbows, heels or buttocks—usually in people laid up in bed for weeks or months— produces a craterlike sore, called a decubitus ulcer. The skin simply breaks down under the continual pressure and friction of skin rubbing against sheets. And because of their vulnerable locations, bedsores continue to fester, resistant to treatment. Taking pressure off the wound, applying salves and allowing air to circulate over the wound may help. Some reports also indicate that, like other skin damage, bedsores will respond to zinc supplements.

Steroid Drugs Leach Zinc

Even if zinc intake is pretty good, other factors can take their toll. Long-term usage of cortisone and other steroid drugs (corticoids, corticosteroids, gluticosteroids) is often to blame for draining zinc from the system. And that can delay wound healing. Arthur Flynn, M.D., and Orville A. Hill, Jr., M.D., along with Drs. Pories and Strain at Case Western Reserve University School of Medicine and Cleveland Metropolitan General Hospital, measured blood levels of zinc in patients receiving long-term corticosteroid therapy. Blood levels of zinc were low. And the patients healed far more slowly than similar patients given zinc supplements —660 milligrams a day of zinc sulfate (*Lancet,* April 14, 1973).

Other doctors have found the same thing. In a review of the role of zinc in wound healing, researchers from the University of Leeds in England and Edinburgh University in Scotland say, "In patients . . . receiving long-term corticoid therapy, there will be decreased serum zinc levels and poor wound healing. Zinc supplements appear to increase the rate of wound healing in these patients." They also remind us of other conditions that call for more zinc—surgery, injury, cirrhosis of the liver, and of course zinc deficiency in itself. Furthermore, they say that patients low in zinc are likely to be low in other nutrients which must also be corrected before healing can be restored (*Surgery, Gynecology & Obstetrics,* October, 1976).

Poor Diet, Poor Wound Healing

The people who need zinc the most may not be getting it. Over the past ten years, evidence has surfaced to show that hospital diets are poor in the very nutrients that will most help the ailing and injured get back on their feet. And zinc is among the conspicuously absent. What's more, it's not only hospital patients who are missing out. The rest of us may stand vulnerably low in that mineral.

Researchers led by Leslie M. Klevay, M.D., conducted a landmark study for the U.S. Department of Agriculture and the University of North Dakota—a hard look at 20 hospital diets as well as diets consumed by the general public. The startling results show that hospital diets averaged 9.4 milligrams of zinc per day—about 35 percent below the 15-milligram requirement for healthy people. And about 70 percent below the 30-milligram *minimum* needed for optimum wound healing! (Copper levels, too, were low. Copper is essential to health because it builds strong nerve fibers and stimulates iron absorption.) (*Journal of the American Medical Association,* May 4, 1979.)

Supplements Bridge the Gap

Beef liver is the number one food source of zinc. But we'd have to eat nearly a pound and a half *every day* to reach the 30 milligrams needed to insure fast and final wound healing.

That's where supplements step in. Added to a regular diet well supplied with zinc-rich foods—liver, turkey, fish, nuts, seeds and beans—zinc supplements can help prepare us for those unexpected kitchen injuries, workshop mishaps or dog bites. It sometimes takes a few weeks for us to adjust to stepped-up zinc intake—that is, to utilize it most efficiently. So routine supplementation is the best way to meet unforeseen injuries head on. And wise people would probably want to fortify themselves when facing intentional injury—be it cyst removal or hip replacement. Big wound or small, the sooner we heal, the better we feel all over.

CHAPTER

38

Leg Ulcers

Zinc for Stubborn Leg Ulcers

Leg ulcers are another stubborn "wound" that zinc helps heal faster.

Some leg ulcers are due to a breakdown of healthy skin under pressure, as is also the case with bedsores. Many result from poor circulation, or decreased supply of blood flowing through arteries or veins. That can happen as a result of deep vein thrombosis, varicose veins or diabetes. With an insufficient amount of blood reaching out to nourish the extremities, the skin deteriorates and is subject to infection.

The first and foremost goal, of course, is to get circulation well routed again—through exercise, leg elevation, elastic bandages, or all three. And you don't want to bump or bruise the wound. But the wound itself needs special attention. It must be kept moist and germ-free in order to speed healing and stave off infection.

Most leg ulcers, however, resist treatment. And they're debilitating. Knowing that zinc is a wound healer, surgeons at Jewish Hospital and Washington University School of Medicine in St. Louis, Missouri, devised an effective cream by combining zinc with two other healing aids. Silver being a known germ-killer, silver nitrate was chosen as an antimicrobial agent. Allantoin, a uric acid derivative, promotes new growth and acts as a wound scavenger, carrying away dead tissue to make way for the new. The new compound, silver-zinc-allantoinate in a 1 percent cream, was applied to 400 stubborn leg ulcers in 264 patients. In some of those patients, the surgeons had tried everything, including medical wrappings and antibiotics. Still, some ulcers had defied treatment.

After just a week of treatment with the zinc compound, bacteria were 99 percent wiped out. And of the 400 ulcers, 339 (nearly 85 percent) had completely healed, in an average of about 10 weeks (*Archives of Surgery,* June, 1977).

Oral zinc may speed healing even further, according to work done by Dr. S. Latafat Husain, a dermatologist at the Royal Infirmary in Glasgow, Scotland. When the doctor gave zinc supplements (220 milligrams, three times a day) to half of a group of 104 hospital patients with leg ulcers, zinc cut healing time by more than half. The average healing time for people who didn't get zinc supplements in Dr. Husain's study was 77 days. But those who got zinc healed in an average of only 32 days (*Clinical Applications of Zinc Metabolism,* Charles C Thomas, 1974).

39

Cold Sores and Mouth Ulcers

Those awful cold sores. You can always tell when one is coming on. It starts as a burning sensation on your lip. Then a white spot or a red blister erupts. The next thing you know, it smarts like the dickens and you're walking around for two weeks with an embarrassing red blotch right on your kisser.

Cold sores and other kinds of mouth ulcers (often called fever blisters, collectively) are painful and frustrating—but not hopeless. An extra helping of zinc, plus a few other simple precautionary measures, can help you get the jump on the jinx.

Blisters from a Virus

Cold sores are caused by a virus—*herpes simplex* type 1, one of a large family of similar herpes-type viruses. Closely related is genital herpes (*herpes simplex* type 2), which provokes similar sores and discomfort in and around the genital area in both men and women. Still another type of herpes affects the cornea of the eye and in extreme cases can affect sight. Cold sores are by far the most common form of herpes and can show up along with genital herpes in the same person. Both are contagious.

Canker sores also affect the mouth and are often hard to distinguish from cold sores. Canker sores are often lumped together in discussion of cold sores. The major difference is that the cause of canker sores is still a mystery. They do appear to respond to the same treatment, however, that works for cold sores.

Once a *herpesvirus* enters your system—usually, but not always, through direct physical contact with someone who's actively infected—it can act in one of two ways. Either it launches a full-fledged attack and then retreats to live peaceably among healthy tissues for the rest of its life, or it sneaks up on you again and again. Some people suffer the outward effects of a herpes attack—painful, ugly sores—twice a year or more. Most, however, seem to be immune, rarely—if ever—succumbing to the bug. The tendency generally runs in families. If both your parents are plagued with recurrent sores, chances are nine out of ten that you will be too. If only one parent suffers, you have about a 60 percent chance of getting them regularly. When neither parent gets mouth ulcers, your chances are about one in four.

The pattern is always the same. Cold sores begin as a small tender bump (or cluster of bumps) on the lips, tongue, roof of the mouth, gums or cheek—usually preceded by an ominous tingling or itching sensation. The bumps quickly rupture into painful ulcerations. They form a crust or a scab in about a week and take about ten days to three weeks to heal completely. (A mouth ulcer that persists for weeks, growing larger and deeper, is not your garden-variety cold or canker sore, and warrants attention. Some systemic diseases, for instance, produce mouth ulcers that mimic cold sores. Have your doctor check it out to be sure.)

After the first infection, the *herpesvirus* hides in the nerve roots in the skin. And there it remains dormant—for most people—most of the time. Under certain circumstances—some known, some unknown—the virus can become reactivated and travel up the nerve path to the skin surface to rekindle the fire of a cold sore.

Three out of four outbreaks of herpes ulcers can be traced to physical or emotional stress, although the actual biochemical changes that reawaken the virus remain obscure. A whole throng of physical irritations can incite the virus to resurface: sunburn, vigorous kissing, intercourse, dental work, shaving, smoking, and eating sharp-edged foods. (Potato chips and hard pretzels are known offenders.)

Overwork or anxiety can provoke an attack. And fever, colds and respiratory disease can also trigger the sores: hence the names cold sore and fever blister. Hormonal changes during the menstrual cycle can bring on a round of blisters. Some women report complete absence during pregnancy of otherwise regular herpes outbreaks.

Eventually, cold sores and canker sores heal by themselves. Two weeks is about the average, although it may seem like forever to anyone who's vexed with the problem. Treatment focuses on relief of symptoms, although antibiotic ointments are sometimes prescribed to forestall secondary infection by bacteria. Aspirin and anesthetic mouthwashes temporarily relieve inflammation inside the mouth and make eating less painful. Salt water rinses and application of alum and baking powder are sometimes used, but you must be careful not to swallow either one. One dentist reports that sauerkraut juice, for those who don't mind the taste, can be helpful.

Zinc to the Rescue

Studies have indicated that many cases of cold sores and canker sores may respond to zinc, possibly through some inhibition of the *herpesvirus's* reproduction or boosting of the immune system—or both. In one Australian clinic, ten people with stubborn cases of genital herpes were given 220 milligrams of zinc sulfate (equivalent to about 50 milligrams of zinc) every day, along with 50 milligrams of magnesium sulfate and 5 milligrams each of vitamins B_1 (thiamine) and B_2 (riboflavin).

In the month before treatment began, the people had collectively suffered 22 outbreaks of herpes. During the first month of supplementation, outbreaks decreased to 19. In the second month, there were only 12 attacks and in the third, 9. Not only were the actual number of repeat attacks cut by more than half, says Dr. Rodney Jones of the clinic, but those who did suffer recurrences had smaller, less painful blisters than usual. Two patients told Dr. Jones that they temporarily doubled their zinc as soon as they felt the first warning signs of local tingling and burning, thereby preventing attacks altogether.

Dr. Jones calls his report preliminary, but said it "shows an apparently beneficial effect of therapy with zinc . . . with improvement in both objective criteria and general morale." In other words, with the virus under control, everyone felt better (*Medical Journal of Australia,* April 7, 1979).

A few weeks later in that same journal, Dr. J. C. Fitzherbert wrote of an informal trial of zinc for cold sores that followed the same healing pattern. Dr. Fitzherbert enlisted cold sore sufferers from the ranks of friends, family and hospital colleagues. All began taking 100 milligrams of zinc sulfate (approximately 25 milligrams of zinc) plus vitamin C (250 milligrams), twice a day for six weeks. Effectiveness ranged from no more cold sores in some, to violent eruptions in a few. In between were people who reported tingling sensations as if a sore was about to erupt, but which did not, or tingling with only slight swelling and tiny blisters lasting only one day. Individual differences account for the variation in success, explains Dr. Fitzherbert. "The level of concentration of zinc within the cells seems to be vital. Factors which may result in reduced availability and absorption of zinc, or cause increased excretion, can adversely affect the . . . result. Alcohol, particularly, may cause excess loss, necessitating increased dosage." In other words, if you drink, take zinc.

As an aside, Dr. Fitzherbert mentions that zinc also blocks reproduction of cold viruses (*Medical Journal of Australia*, May 5, 1979).

Although their underlying cause is probably different, canker sores may also respond to zinc supplementation. In a study of 17 patients with canker sores, 12 improved after taking zinc supplements: they had either no or fewer sores, and the sores they did have were smaller, less painful and didn't last as long—similar to the results achieved in the two Australian studies on cold sores. Three patients who were completely healed stopped taking zinc and their sores returned—only to heal again when they resumed their supplements (*Southern Medical Journal*, May, 1977).

Because of what we know about zinc's ability to fight infection and clear up other skin problems, the results make sense. The latest thinking behind canker sores is that they result from an incompatibility that arises between the slippery mucosal lining of the mouth and certain white blood cells (lymphocytes), a key part of the immune system. For some unknown reason, both the mouth lining and lymphocytes may undergo simultaneous changes that set off a destructive reaction in the host. The result is the canker sore.

Topical applications of zinc may work just as well for both cold sores and canker sores. In one study, 18 people with herpes skin infections were treated with a wet dressing of 4 percent zinc sulfate in water, applied to their sores four times a day for 4 days. In all patients, pain, tingling and burning were completely gone in 24 hours. In most, crusting took place within 2 days, rather than the 7 normally anticipated. Healing was complete in an average of just under 10 days, compared to the usual average of 16.

The authors call for more extensive studies, but say that "topical zinc may prove to be a safe, easily available and inexpensive form of treatment for this condition" (*Acta Dermatovener*, vol. 60, no. 2, 1980).

Topical zinc may also do the trick for canker sores. One man reported his perhaps unscientific but nonetheless successful method:

> I have experienced the misery of mouth ulcers (canker sores) for 40 years, and have tried every remedy recommended by scores of doctors.
>
> What works for me is zinc gluconate. More than a year ago, I decided to experiment with zinc, since it is an age-old ingredient of many pharmaceutical preparations for skin problems. Zinc gluconate was a natural selection, since it is already available in a grade suitable for oral consumption. I pulverize several tablets by using a teaspoon and a tablespoon as a mortar and pestle. I then dip a moistened cotton-tipped applicator into the zinc gluconate

powder and apply it topically to the ulcer every three to four hours. Healing is usually complete in two to three days instead of the usual week or more.

Iron May Help Too

Perhaps because it plays such a big part in the body's immune system, good iron stores may be another deciding factor in whether or not you get canker sores. Two studies done by Dr. David Wray and other researchers at the Glasgow Dental Hospital and School in Scotland showed that people who suffer repeated episodes of canker sores are more likely to have deficiencies of iron, folate (a B vitamin) and vitamin B_{12}. Of the three, iron was the nutrient lacking most often.

Of 39 people with canker sores and proven nutritional deficiencies of one or all of the above, all responded well to supplements of the missing nutrients. Twenty-three had no canker sores for at least six months. That's quite a blessing for canker sufferers, some of whom had suffered on and off for up to 40 years. Eleven others had only occasional ulcers. Five were not helped, possibly due to underlying disease.

In addition to oral supplements, some canker victims rinsed with a mouthwash of zinc chloride or zinc sulfate, boosting healing by about 10 percent.

As a result of his work, Dr. Wray suggests a tendency toward canker sores in some people may be due to an unknown physical ailment that, when combined with a dietary deficiency, may cause the sores to erupt (*Journal of Oral Pathology,* December, 1978).

Preventing Future Attacks

It's not the *duration* of cold or canker sore episodes that bothers people so much as their recurrence. If you always seem to break into blisters just before a big date, it certainly can cramp your social life. If you have to speak in front of a group or sing in the front row of the choir on Easter Sunday, the last thing you want is a mouth decked out in red sores.

The studies cited earlier strongly suggest that zinc may help keep mouth ulcers at bay. Besides zinc, there are other preventive steps you can take. If the sun seems to provoke attacks, use protective lip gloss or sunscreen lotion. Or try to stay out of the sun except for short intervals. If shaving with a razor blade stirs up the sleeping germs, be sure to lather generously with shaving cream to reduce irritation. Or switch to an electric rotary shaver. Don't eat tortilla chips or other offending foods.

And, of course, don't spread your misfortune around. Misery loves company, but not when it comes to cold sores. Close physical contact with other people is the primary route for spreading herpes infection. Keep family and friends at arm's length when trouble does erupt.

40

Acne

Acne isn't the end of the world. But for those so plagued, it may seem like it runs a close third—right behind leprosy.

Zinc can take it out of the race altogether, though.

By age 17, 86.4 percent of American teenagers have acne. Many try one ointment after another to wipe out pimples and blotches on the face, neck, chest, shoulders and back. Or scrub so hard and often they make Lady Macbeth look like a slob.

Of those who run to a dermatologist (skin disease specialist) for help, many will most likely walk away with a lifetime prescription for antibiotics. In the very worst cases, acne sufferers may submit to having their skin peeled, planed or sanded.

Until recently, the only real hope for cure seemed to be that if you could hang in there long enough, you would just outgrow the scourge. Sometimes even that doesn't work, though. Acne has been known to hang on until the twenties and thirties.

True, nobody dies of acne. Perhaps that's why research has come up with little in the way of an honest-to-goodness cure. Within the past few years, though—almost by accident—doctors have found that zinc may be the answer.

What *Is* Acne?

In response to sex hormones unleashed at puberty, the many sebaceous (oil) glands in the skin secrete a fatty substance called sebum. Those glands are largest and most numerous on face, neck, chest, shoulders and back—acne's favorite haunts. Normally, sebum escapes through surface pores. In acne-prone people, however, sebum plugs the pores. If the pore remains plugged but open, the result is a blackhead—unsightly, but no hazard. If the plugged pore closes up, trapping the fatty oils, the result is a whitehead. And that's where trouble starts.

Certain bacteria *(Corynebacterium acnes)* grow in sebum. And they absolutely *thrive* in plugged pores. The infected pores can fill with pus (pimples) and the surrounding skin may become inflamed (red and blotchy).

Some acne pimples become so large that, untreated, they leave ice-pick scars or craters when they do clear up. Don't squeeze them, though. Merciless self-lancing of blemishes also leaves scars. That's where the most drastic approach—dermabrasion, or skin planing—comes in. It's a medical technique for removing scars.

Keeping skin as grease-free as possible helps to remove some of the oils that make skin ripe for acne, but most of the bacterial dirty work is rooted below the surface. There's controversy over the effects of eating chocolate and greasy foods like french fries and potato chips. Some dermatologists swear they have no effect; others swear they do. Some mysterious acne cases are sparked, not by the grease in food, but by iodine-containing additives and kelp.

Drugs for the Bug on the Mug
Or: Pills for pimples

Tetracycline and other antibiotic drugs seem to suppress acne in some people by fighting off acne-forming bacteria. Notice we said suppress, not cure. As soon as the antibiotic is stopped, acne usually returns in full bloom.

A full one-tenth of all the tetracycline produced in this country is used to fight acne. Yet the success rate is not 100 percent. It's more like 65 percent. That's not all that great. Even placebos (dummy pills with no active ingredients) work up to 56 percent of the time. Why some people respond and others do not, no one knows. And the sad fact is, antibiotics are least likely to work for those people who have the worst acne.

Even those for whom antibiotics work may not be home free. While allergic or toxic reactions and other side effects are uncommon, they do occur to some degree in one out of ten users, and there are other drawbacks. Vaginal infections (especially the *Candida albicans* or yeast variety) are more prevalent in young women who take antibiotics for months or years. And while many young people initially improve on an antibiotic, the bacteria become resistant to one drug and therapy must be switched to another and another. Growing out of the disease is about the only thing that gets one off the merry-go-round of antibiotic therapy.

Topical applications of peeling agents, such as benzoyl peroxide, are often used along with oral antibiotics to coax out blackheads and whiteheads—but not without some redness and irritation.

Zinc Triumphs over Acne

Unlike antibiotic therapy, zinc lets bacteria die a natural death by choking off their life-support system. It's not only safe, but seems to be more effective than antibiotics—about 85 percent, according to the few trials that have been done.

Zinc therapy for acne was first stumbled upon by a doctor in Sweden who was treating people for a different skin disease, a rare disorder of zinc metabolism called acrodermatitis enteropathica.

When Gerd Michaelsson, M.D., and his colleagues at Uppsala University Hospital in Sweden gave zinc to one of their patients with acrodermatitis enteropathica, they noticed a welcome and unexpected side effect. The patient's acne cleared up almost completely!

Next they decided to give zinc to groups of teenagers and young adults with acne. The results were heartening. After 12 weeks of treatment, those persons taking zinc experienced a decrease in their acne scores from 100 to approximately 15 percent. "Indeed," they conclude, "the effect of zinc therapy in some of our patients with severe inflammatory acne has been remarkable."

"Eight patients in the zinc groups spontaneously remarked that the skin on their faces was less oily than before treatment and rather dry," the Swedish doctors reported. In addition they noted, "Many patients also had acne of the back and chest, and these lesions usually healed to the same extent as those of the face."

Nine of 13 people who had previously not been helped by antibiotic treatment showed an improvement of more than 50 percent after taking zinc for four weeks.

"We do not yet know how to explain the effect of zinc treatment in acne," Dr. Michaelsson and his co-workers admit. "It is possible that there is an absolute or relative zinc deficiency in puberty. Zinc deficiency seems to be more common than previously known, and a daily intake below the recommended 15 to 20 milligrams is probably not uncommon. Some diets in hospitals, as well as in average households in the United States and Europe, have been found to contain only 4 to 7 milligrams of zinc."

Working backwards from that premise, Dr. Michaelsson feels that a zinc deficiency at puberty could disturb certain hormone-enzyme relationships. Zinc is essential to dozens of enzymes, some of which are tied in with the activity of sex hormones (androgen and estrogen) beginning with puberty. As it happens, some of those enzymes are located in the sebaceous, or oil-producing glands of the skin—the seedbed of bacterial acne. Without zinc, says Dr. Michaelsson, the enzymes are disturbed, and the visible result is acne pimples.

As a general anti-inflammatory agent, zinc may also help to suppress acne in progress by reducing the irritation, wiping out the characteristic red blotches that often accompany pimples (*Archives of Dermatology,* January, 1977).

Later that same year, a separate study, also in Sweden, showed similar results. Of 91 acne patients, 48 were given 45 milligrams of zinc (in the form of zinc sulfate) twice a day for 12 weeks. Forty-three acne patients were given identical-looking placebos. Based on before-and-after photos and the patients' own judgment, Dr. Lars Hillstrom and other dermatologists found that, compared to a placebo, zinc definitely helped acne. "After 12 weeks' treatment with zinc sulphate 75 percent of the patients were content with therapeutic results," they report (*British Journal of Dermatology,* December, 1977).

In light of the Swedish studies, and well aware of the drawbacks of long-term antibiotic treatment, a contributor from New South Wales, writing in a medical journal, recommends the following approach for successful treatment of acne:

"(1) A short course, if necessary, of tetracycline to control infection; and (2) administration of zinc sulfate (approximately 100 milligrams/day) at night (and not with cereal food [which partially binds up zinc]) which is continued intermittently during the period of high zinc demand. No tetracycline should be administered during this phase . . .

"In teenagers, 100 milligrams of zinc sulfate is approximately equivalent to their daily requirement of zinc," says Dr. J. C. Fitzherbert. Dr. Fitzherbert adds, "It seems logical to combine the zinc with vitamin C which also has a role in maturation of skin collagen" (*Medical Journal of Australia,* November 12, 1977).

No More Acne

People who've learned about zinc's victory over acne have thrown away hopeless creams and instead reach for zinc. A few of their comments, as reported to *Prevention* magazine's "Mailbag":

Lately I've felt like a different person. I had the world's worst skin, thanks to acne. I hated putting all that "garbage" on my face but I tried every kind of commercial medication. Then I read about zinc. I started taking about 50 milligrams of zinc daily, along with other vitamin supplements. You can judge the results by how happy I am now.

I am 25 years old and have had a problem with acne for ten years. I could not get rid of the pimples on my chin. That is, until I tried zinc.

I started out with 50 milligrams and am now down to 30 milligrams a day. I also take vitamins A and D, dolomite, C and I also make sure I get two tablespoons of brewer's yeast a day.

I can't believe how good my skin looks now. I used to always have at least one pimple on my chin but for the last two weeks I have not had one and I can't believe it yet. Every day I keep thinking I'll get a zit but it must be zapped by the zinc.

Recently I hit upon a letter which described zinc as a help for acne sufferers. It works wonders. I started to take it, and my skin (always loaded with blemishes) has never looked clearer. Believe it or not, I had acne into my thirties! No amount of scrubbing or lotions has ever done what zinc supplements accomplished in one short week.

I want to mention my discovery to every young adult who is still plagued with those awful zits!

A jubilant mother writes:

Our son had bad acne all across his back with the usual soreness, scarring and large pustules. Only three weeks after he started taking zinc, we began to notice improvement and now there is no trace of the acne—only an occasional pimple or two.

And finally:

I had bad acne for about 10 years. Then I read about the benefits of zinc. For three months I have been taking zinc, and I've never had better results with anything I've tried. My acne is healing up very nicely.

41

Itching

Itching has too many possible causes to name them all here. Dry skin. Irritation. Allergic reactions to food, clothing, drugs, plants or pets. Underlying disease.

If all those have been ruled out and you *still* itch, the problem may be low iron.

Iron Soothes Her Itch, Finally

One August a few years ago, a 62-year-old woman walked into a clinic in San Angelo, Texas. For the previous six months, for no apparent reason, she itched all over. It was driving her crazy.

Doctors at the clinic gave her a checkup and skin tests and found nothing wrong. She was taking estrogen regularly and aspirin from time to time. The doctors tried giving her one drug after another over the next few months, but nothing worked. Her itching didn't let up. By December of that year, the woman gave up on drugs. The doctors at first suspected the problem was psychogenic—that is, either emotional or all in her head.

Then they did more tests. Blood tests showed that iron levels were quite low. So was total iron binding capacity, another index of iron status. Bone marrow—the breeding ground for healthy red blood cells—also showed some abnormalities. Apparently, she'd been anemic all along.

The woman was immediately started on 300 milligrams of ferrous sulfate (equivalent to 60 milligrams of iron) three times a day, for a total of 180 milligrams of iron daily. (That's within the dosage range of 150 to 200 milligrams of iron that is standard treatment for such cases of out-and-out iron deficiency anemia.)

Within a few short days, the woman felt better. Estrogen and aspirin were stopped, then started again, to see whether those drugs had anything to do with the itching. They didn't. No underlying disease was responsible, either. Itching cleared up completely with iron supplements.

"Iron deficiency should be considered as one of the causes of generalized [itching]"—especially when other disease has been ruled out, says E. Michael Lewiecki, M.D., one of two doctors who report the case.

Dr. Lewiecki and his colleague, Fazlur Rahman, M.D., a hematologist (blood specialist), say that in iron-deficient people, there seems to arise some sort of defect in epithelial tissues—that is, the lining of organs such as the skin. Numbness and tingling are also common, pointing to some slight nerve dysfunction. Drs. Lewiecki and Rahman suggest that those skin and nerve changes associated with iron deficiency could very well be one cause of generalized itching, as was evidently the case with their patient (*Journal of the American Medical Association,* November 15, 1976).

A few months later, the above report caught the attention of a doctor at the University of California in San Francisco. John R. T. Reeves, M.D., reports, "I have examined serum iron levels in several patients with unexplained pruritus [itching] and have found at least two who were iron deficient; they subsequently responded to iron therapy" (*Journal of the American Medical Association,* April 4, 1977).

Dr. Reeves based his work on work by yet another doctor, Dr. C. F. H. Vickers, a British dermatologist who has probably reported more cases of itching due to low iron than any other researcher. Seeing Dr. Reeves's letter prompted Dr. Vickers, of the Liverpool Royal Infirmary and University of Liverpool in England, to bring readers up to date on his findings. As of 1974, reports Dr. Vickers, he had seen a total of 87 cases of itching directly attributed to low iron (*Journal of the American Medical Association,* July 11, 1977).

Low-Iron Itching, Not As Rare As You Might Think

On top of all that, a Finnish doctor trots out some interesting statistics. Between 1967 and 1972, over 23,000 men and almost 20,000 women in Finland were screened for hemoglobin, the oxygen-carrying molecule in blood and a good indicator of iron status. According to a questionnaire, 13.6 percent of the men—about 1 in 7—with iron deficiency anemia also had frequent itching. That's over twice as many as men with normal hemoglobin levels. Among the women with iron deficiency anemia, about 1 in 13 also itched, as compared to 1 in 20 for those with normal iron status.

Heikki Takkunen, M.D., of the Helsinki University Central Hospital, feels that iron deficiency anemia can cause changes in the skin and mucous membranes, and that itching may be one manifestation of those changes (*Journal of the American Medical Association,* April 3, 1978). His explanation is very close to that proposed by Dr. Lewiecki.

The important thing, says Dr. Reeves, is that iron doesn't necessarily have to reach rock bottom for itching to start. Many patients reported by Dr. Vickers, the British dermatologist, were not actually anemic, but nonetheless had iron levels low enough to provoke itching (*Journal of the American Medical Association,* April 4, 1977).

CHAPTER

42

Eczema

Eczema is difficult to define exactly. A general type of skin inflammation, eczema is assumed to be an allergic reaction to a whole host of potentially irritating substances—foods, dust, the sun, dry air, cold air, soap, cosmetics, jewelry, even fungus and yeasts. You name it, and somebody's skin is allergic to it.

To deal with that dilemma, many dermatologists define eczema as simply "anything that looks like eczema." Technically, it goes by the terms atopic eczema, atopic dermatitis, or eczematous dermatitis. What it looks like is red, weeping patches of tiny round bumps and blisters. And it itches like crazy. In later stages, eczema crusts over, forming scales. The affected skin then thickens, hardens and turns brown. Some forms of eczema go through all of those stages; others only some. The typical features, though, are the small, water-filled blisters. The term eczema, in fact, comes from a Greek word meaning "to boil over."

Characteristically, eczema is worse on the areas of the skin in front of the elbows and behind the knees. The skin may be rough, red, cracked, scaly and, in places, bleeding. The rest of the skin on the forearms may vary between nearly normal, and smaller, scattered spots of rough, scaly red skin. Wrists may be affected, and hands covered.

Eczema may be an upshot of nervousness, anxiety and tension. If not, it can leave you quite irritable, at best. For eczema is not a pretty picture.

Flareups tend to be acute, and repeat attacks the norm. Eczema typically begins early in childhood and recurs throughout life. Sometimes it disappears for months, or shows up just a little. Other times it's really bad. Three out of four eczema sufferers come from families with a strong history of allergies, and are quite likely to have hay fever or asthma themselves.

Yet the allergic reaction behind many eczema cases may be only the surface of the problem. The real problem may lie in a basic immunodeficiency—a failing of the body's natural defense system against irritating substances.

As far as medicine goes, treatment with corticosteroids is standard for eczema. Systemic steroids bring dramatic relief of eczema, but the drugs are too powerful to be used in all but acute flareups. For long-term therapy, steroid ointments, gels, lotions and creams are more appropriate. But they are absorbed through the skin into the bloodstream and cannot be used indiscriminately. Sometimes they work, sometimes they don't.

Research, in fact, shows up very little in terms of prevention of eczema, aside from the obvious advice to avoid what aggravates the condition. Hand eczema is likely to be caused by household or industrial chemicals, rubber gloves, or rings. On the face, cosmetics could be the problem. Jewelry may touch off eczema on the neck, earlobes, fingers or wrists. Eczema under the arm could be due to irritating clothing. Eczema of the feet is often traced to some material in shoes.

Internal causes—viruses, yeast infection and the like—are harder to pin down. That's where nutrition may come in. Poor nutrition lowers the immunity; good nutrition gives it a boost.

Zinc Clears Up Eczema

Many nutrients are important to skin health. Zinc is one. Vitamins A, D and E—the fat-soluble vitamins—are also important. Vitamin C, like zinc, is essential to proper healing. And eczema sufferers have a lot of skin to heal.

Those nutrients make up the core of nutritional treatment of eczema by Jonathan V. Wright, M.D., author of *Dr. Wright's Book of Nutritional Therapy* (Rodale Press, 1979). In his medical practice in Kent,

Washington, Dr. Wright has used zinc-centered therapy to clear up over 40 cases of eczema in patients.

Although each individual case is different, Dr. Wright's zinc therapy basically starts at 50 milligrams, three times a day, plus 1,000 milligrams of vitamin C, twice a day. Added to that is a tablespoon of cod liver oil (containing the fat-soluble vitamins) during acute flareups. The program is then pared down to 25 milligrams of zinc a day, with 1,000 milligrams of vitamin C, plus cod liver oil in winter. In some cases, absorptive factors, such as low gastric (stomach) acidity or poor pancreatic enzyme activity, must be compensated for before zinc can take effect. Sometimes allergy screening is necessary to deal with possible irritants.

"Since there are no published studies that I know of concerning its treatment by zinc, I'd like to be particularly careful about the description of this skin problem that zinc helps," Dr. Wright says.

"One of the hallmarks of the condition is that it appears on the skin in front of the elbows and behind the knees. While it certainly may appear elsewhere (characteristically on the sides of the fingers, in the 'web' spaces, palms of the hands, wrists, forearms, further down the lower legs, and behind the ears), the [elbow and knee] regions are usually the first to appear and last to leave.

"In milder cases, the skin reddens and appears and feels rough," continues Dr. Wright. "As it worsens, scaliness of varying degrees develops as the skin peels off at varying rates. The redness worsens, becoming deeper and brighter. Frequently, in more severe cases, the skin will crack open, and the cracks won't heal. Sometimes bad cases will ooze fluid. Occasionally, eczema will become infected, although that is a complication, not an essential part of the problem.

"Frequently, atopic [allergic] eczema will come and go. In some it will clear completely between outbreaks; in others, it gets better and worse, but doesn't heal completely. Usually the worse the allergic involvement, the more resistant to healing. Most often, this is a problem of childhood, but it does appear occasionally in adults.

"Patience is essential to zinc-centered treatment of atopic eczema," emphasizes Dr. Wright. "Sometimes no improvement is seen for three to six weeks. Often, the problem is gone by three to four months, but I've seen it take six to eight months in some cases.

"In the past year or two, I've emphasized the use of essential fatty acids, along with zinc and vitamin C, in the treatment of atopic eczema. That seems to work just a little faster, and with fewer 'worsenings.' The essential fatty acids are contained in vegetable oils, such as safflower, sunflower, sesame and others. Very recently, research work has uncovered the zinc-essential fatty acid connection showing zinc to be crucial to the transformation of some of the nutritionally derived essential fatty acids to their active form," explains Dr. Wright.

Still another part of the answer to zinc's effectiveness may lie in a cell substance called RNA, says Dr. Wright. "Drs. Hsu and Anthony of Johns Hopkins University reported that zinc deficiency suppressed RNA synthesis in the skin but *not* in other organs (pancreas, liver, kidney, testes) in their experimental animal, the rat. RNA gives instructions for repairing protein tissues, such as skin, but can't do that when there is a zinc deficiency.

"Now obviously, rat results and people results are not always going to be the same," says Dr. Wright. "However, considering the human results with the use of zinc, this could be a large part of the answer.

"Whatever the reasons, zinc certainly works, especially if allergic and absorptive factors aren't neglected."

Now You See It, Now You Don't

On top of Dr. Wright's clinical experience, we've heard good reports from people who've stepped up their zinc intake in the face of disfiguring, drive-you-up-the-wall eczema.

A few months ago my dry, itching, sore facial skin sent me to a dermatologist. It didn't take him long to tell me that the condition was eczema. He prescribed a medicated cream and charged me $25. But it didn't help at all.

Then I remembered what I'd read about zinc and skin problems. I tried some zinc immediately (50 milligrams a day). Soon not one of those little blisters or pimples remained. I discontinued the cream and still my complexion was clear. I did run out of zinc and, sure enough, the eczema returned. When I resumed the zinc, my problem was gone again.

My wife had been suffering with eczema on her hands for a year, a bad case. Not one of several remedies helped at all.

She took zinc and the eczema cleared up dramatically in a week and was gone within the month. Amazing.

For many years I have had eczema on my hands. My condition became extremely aggravated during the time I was nursing my first baby. Although I tried various ways to treat my hands, nothing was really effective.

I started taking chelated zinc, 50 milligrams, three times a day. Within a month my hands showed a remarkable improvement.

I have continued to take the zinc. If I take less, my eczema reappears.

For years, I had been itching terribly, not being able to sleep nights. And for years, I'd been taking cortisone, which was prescribed to me by various dermatologists. But it hasn't helped me one bit.

Then one day I read that zinc is a skin healer. I went to a health food store, bought zinc tablets, and started taking them. In one week, my eczema cleared up, and now it's almost gone! At last, I'm relieved of the terrible itching that wouldn't let me sleep nights.

After having a problem with eczema on my neck for about a year and a half, I tried taking zinc supplements. I started with a 30-milligram dosage per day. In a little more than a week, the area that was infected was almost totally cleared up!

43

Boils

The Bible called them boils. Doctors call them furuncles. What-ever you call them, having miniature models of Mount St. Helens popping up here and there on your body every few weeks is no fun. Fortunately, keeping zinc levels up to par keeps boils from erupting in the first place.

A boil is a swollen, painful nodule caused by inflammation between the skin and sub-skin tissues. Boils crop up most often on the neck and buttocks, although they may erupt wherever friction, irritation, or a scratch or break in the skin allows bacteria in. A specific type of bacteria (staphylococci) is accountable. The problems start when those germs find their way underneath the surface through a tiny break or abrasion.

After entering the skin, the infection settles into the hair follicles or sebaceous (oil) glands. The swelling begins.

To combat the infection, a mass of leukocytes (disease-fighting white blood cells) speed to the site of the boil and attack the invading bacteria. At that point, healing may take one of two directions. The body's defense may immediately and successfully overcome the invaders so that the boil subsides by itself. Or some bacteria and leukocytes die in combat, leaving behind a watery liquid and pus. The pus may build up pressure against the skin—causing pain—to the point where the dome ruptures, drains and finally heals.

Obviously, the boil that heals quickly on its own is the best kind. Not all do. And some people get boils again and again. Standard treatment for repeated outbreaks is lancing, plus applied and oral antibiotics. But that doesn't keep new ones from sprouting.

While even otherwise healthy people can get boils, more often than not they're a sign of low resistance, poor nutrition—or both.

Zinc Keeps Boils from Erupting

Dr. Isser Brody, a dermatologist at the General Hospital in Eskilstuna, Sweden, found that 15 of his patients with recurrent boils had low blood levels of zinc. Boils had beleaguered them for three to ten years, appearing one or more times a month. Boils sprang up just about everywhere except on their arms or lower legs—groin, thighs, buttocks, abdomen, breasts, face and neck.

The patients were divided into two groups. In the first, four men and three women were given standard boil treatment—incision of the lump plus antibiotic therapy. But during the next three months, new boils appeared. It was a losing battle.

The other eight patients (four men and four women) took zinc sulfate (45 milligrams, three times a day) and did much better. Those patients were followed for three months, and one was followed for seven. In all eight, blood levels of zinc rose to normal within the first month. Existing boils disappeared. And best of all, no new boils erupted (*Lancet,* December 24 & 31, 1977).

Judging by zinc's track record for fighting inflammation and skin problems of other kinds, it's not surprising to see the mineral boost resistance to this type of infection.

44

Body Odor

Everyone smells less than fragrant at one time or another. Maybe you got dressed in a hurry and forgot to put on deodorant. Or tried a new brand that didn't live up to its claims. Or returned from jogging to find the plumber had dismantled your shower. Sometimes body odor just can't be helped.

For some people, though, body odor defies all control. No amount of bathing or expensive roll-ons will stifle the odor. The problem goes below the surface.

Zinc and Magnesium for Our Sweet-Smelling Selves

Body odors are related to the body's total inner health, and that includes nutrition. Zinc and magnesium seem to be the two key minerals in keeping us smelling fresh as a daisy under all but the most grueling circumstances.

B. F. Hart, M.D., a physician in Fort Lauderdale, Florida, has found that magnesium, when given with zinc and two B vitamins (B_6 and para-aminobenzoic acid, or PABA) can effectively control offensive body odors and breath odors. The nutrients seem to act as waste scavengers, removing substances that give off acrid odors in the body. Metabolic cleanup takes about five days, says Dr. Hart.

One dermatologist also hit upon zinc's deodorant powers and reported his experience to a medical journal:

"About two years ago, I saw a patient who was being given 220 milligrams of oral zinc sulfate (equivalent to 50 milligrams of elemental zinc) three times daily by his surgeon as part of the management of recurrent leg ulcers. This observant gentleman noted that while he was taking zinc there was a marked reduction in [underarm] perspiration odor. This problem, which had been most distressing to him for most of his adult life, returned within days after the zinc was discontinued. When he again started taking the capsules, the odor again markedly diminished (confirmed by his wife).

"Based on this observation, I have given zinc sulfate to five other persons, with uniformly good results. Most responded to daily doses as low as 20 milligrams of elemental zinc. All had tried a wide variety of deodorants and antiperspirants without success. This report is submitted in hope of helping other unfortunate persons who suffer from socially incapacitating perspiration odor," says Morton D. Scribner, M.D., of Arcadia, California (*Archives of Dermatology*, September, 1977).

People who've read about zinc's power to rub out body odors decided to try it for themselves. Here are some of their results, as reported to *Prevention* magazine's "Mailbag":

> Having read about the wonders of zinc, I recommended 30 milligrams a day to my son, who has had a persistent body odor problem for years. Five minutes after he would wash twice and apply deodorant, he would still offend on a hot day.
>
> Imagine his complete delight when within *one day* we could all notice a difference! At the end of a week he cut the lawn in 80° temperature and we could detect no offensive odor about him! It seems like a modern-day miracle to him.

Another person told us:

> I purchased some zinc to find out for myself if this would really check my own problem. I had tried one of the highest-priced deodorants on the market but that did not even work and the thought of applying high-powered chemicals to my skin didn't appeal to me.
>
> The first day after taking zinc I could tell the difference! On the second day, even after jogging, there was no body odor. It was

terrific! Because zinc worked so well for me, I urged my brother to take 30 milligrams a day. His body odor was also checked.

Sometimes body odor results from medical treatment that upsets our chemical balance:

> About two years ago, I underwent chemotherapy. Besides all the usual upsetting side effects, I also had a terrible body odor.
>
> Because of all the chemicals going into my body, I increased my vitamin and mineral intakes. Also, after reading about zinc, I decided to take ten milligrams three times a day. I wasn't looking for anything specific, I just thought the zinc might help in healing my body.
>
> Within a month, the terrible body odor disappeared. Just to make sure it was the zinc that helped, I stopped taking it and again within two weeks the odor was back.

When excessive sweating is part of the problem, zinc may also help:

> I have been taking zinc tablets for three weeks now, and my excessive perspiration problem has been more than cut in half. Also, I no longer suffer from odors on my body and clothing.

Going one step further, one concerned mother decided to see if zinc would help her ten-year-old son's hair and scalp odor:

> Within the past few years, he developed a severe case of this embarrassing odor. I tried a variety of shampoos and scalp treatments, yet his hair always smelled sweaty and dirty (even while wet after shampooing). Naturally, he was extremely self-conscious about it.
>
> I started giving him 40 milligrams of zinc daily and two days later there was only a trace of the devastating odor. After a week, I'm delighted to report that his hair smells fresh and clean.

Magnesium Helps Too

Jonathan V. Wright, M.D., a practitioner in Kent, Washington, has achieved similar results in relieving body odor with magnesium. And the mineral's deodorant strength isn't confined to only extreme cases.

"I find that in just about any case [of body odor] magnesium can lessen the odor. And there's a particular sort of smell associated with magnesium deficiency that I am able to identify. I usually get it right."

The scientific proof for all this?

Unfortunately, Dr. Wright says, researchers have generally ignored the nation's body odor. "You just can't come up with the research grant funds for something like that. It's like dandruff."

CHAPTER

45

Iron Deficiency Anemia

Iron deficiency anemia is one of the most frequently occurring health problems in the world. At the same time, it's also frequently overlooked. Yet it's one of the easiest to correct—and prevent.

Iron deficiency anemia is not actually a disease, but rather a sign that something is wrong. By definition, iron deficiency anemia is a drop in the quality or number of circulating red blood cells. That is, as red blood cells emerge from the bone marrow, they're misshapen or oversized. Or there's a sparse distribution of hemoglobin (the blood's oxygen-transporting molecule) in circulation. Either of those changes seriously hinders the ability of blood to take up oxygen and deliver it to body tissues—literally suffocating body cells.

Almost any system can be affected, and the symptoms bear that out. Fatigue is the most common complaint, but effects can range from weakness and dizziness, to headaches, itching, sore tongue, and brittle or ridged fingernails—plus a whole host of other complaints. Clumsiness. Difficulty walking. Confusion. Apathy. Loss of appetite.

Because many of those complaints are commonly accepted as an inevitable part of aging, they're often ignored in the elderly. Older people either shrug off their discomfort or hesitate to bring it up, figuring they're "just getting old." Women who drag themselves to their doctors are often told "it's just your nerves." And that's a shame, because correcting the problem could very well restore the anemic person to his or her rightfully alert and energetic self.

Iron on the Seesaw of Blood Balance

Both bone marrow and circulating hemoglobin rely on iron to keep red blood cells growing normally and oxygen flowing to tissues. Our bodies each contain about four or five grams (about ⅙ ounce) of iron at any one time. Most of it is involved in some aspect of red blood cell activity.

The equilibrium between intake and outgo of iron is balanced like a metabolic seesaw: ample intake from iron-rich foods compensates for normal everyday losses through skin, sweat, urine and the gastrointestinal (GI) tract. A little is set aside for storage, also. To help keep that balance steady, the body learns to compensate for any slight dips in intake or small depletion of body stores by stepping up absorption. The body hustles to keep cells from suffocating—up to a point. Beyond that, very low intake—or heavy or long-term blood loss—can upset the balance. If either occurs, anemia is almost certain.

Sometimes bone marrow disturbances, red blood cell destruction, or decreased absorption—due to other underlying disease—may cause iron deficiency anemia. But more often than not, low intake or heavy blood loss is the problem.

Even though iron deficiency anemia is one of the most common problems around, it's also very insidious. A person could have it for years and not realize it. The symptoms are so common and varied that they could indicate a number of other disorders. Tender bones, swollen ankles and angina may be partially due to iron deficiency anemia—or signal some other disease, like congestive heart failure.

On the other hand, fatigue, headaches and loss of appetite are precisely the kind of complaints that people might hesitate to mention for fear their discomforts will be dismissed as groundless—or exaggerations. Or blamed on old age. That's especially true for women and the elderly, two groups of people most likely to develop anemia.

Testing for Iron Status

Three easy blood tests—all performed from a finger-prick sample—can tell your doctor a lot. Special features in blood help rule out or confirm whether your troubles are rooted in anemia.

Serum (blood) iron is normally 60 to 180 milligrams per 100 milliliters of blood. There's some dickering over just how low your serum iron has to fall before you're declared officially iron-deficient. It's somewhere around 12 milligrams per 100 milliliters. At any rate, it varies considerably during the day so it's best if the sample is taken before breakfast.

Another item to look for is total iron-binding capacity—about 300 to 360 micrograms per milliliter (or 220 to 420 milligrams per decaliter). The test will also measure transferrin, the protein that carries circulating iron. Normally, transferrin is two-thirds saturated with iron. Undersaturation usually indicates iron deficiency.

Almost all iron-bound transferrin is rapidly taken up by bone marrow to synthesize hemoglobin, so the best index of total body iron is bone marrow. There iron is stored up in a colorless protein called ferritin. Bone marrow is a little more trouble to sample, though, and only necessary in difficult cases. Otherwise, serum iron is close enough.

Low Iron, Poor Health

Like most tests, blood values are interpreted in terms of arbitrary numbers dividing the "normal" from the "abnormal." What "abnormal" values really reflect, though, is a range of iron-deficient states:

During the first stage of deficiency, the blood test may appear perfectly normal, even though iron stores are run down. But perhaps it takes a little extra push to get out of bed in the morning. Or your appetite's dropped off. You may not feel sick, but on the other hand, you're not quite yourself anymore. That could go on for years.

At stage two, there are some abnormalities in blood. Iron is low, but without outright anemia. Perhaps you feel depressed or confused for no apparent reason.

At stage three—the only stage a blood test can confirm without question—iron deficiency is severe enough to produce recognizable anemia. Most likely, fatigue is undeniable. In severe cases, changes take place in the tongue, nails, mouth and stomach. Fingernails grow thin, ridged or spoon-shaped. The tongue becomes smooth and glossy, or reddened. Swallowing may be difficult. Indigestion—similar to that felt after overeating—may result from inflammation of the stomach (gastritis).

Some of those effects are the direct result of body tissues deprived of oxygen. But evidence also indicates that it's depletion of iron-containing enzymes rather than hemoglobin that's responsible for the fatigue, weakness and loss of appetite that are so common in anemia. Studies in rats show that low enzyme activity due to low iron may produce skeletal muscle malfunction, causing weakness. And as might be expected, enzymes that do not contain iron but require it to function at their best are also affected. And a more subtle but nonetheless important effect is that the manufacture of DNA (the molecule that gives orders for cell division and repair) may be disturbed.

Immunity Suffers

One far-reaching effect of iron deficiency anemia may be a slack immune system that leaves you wide open to bacterial infection, viruses and other disease. Researchers at India's National Institute of Nutrition found that anemic people have lowered cell immunity in general. Also, leukocytes (germ-fighting white blood cells) are stripped of much of their bacteria-killing power. Drs. Bhaskaram, Prasad and Krishnamachari drew blood samples from 13 anemic children and slipped the blood cells into test tubes, then introduced a specific strain of bacteria. Leukocytes had a hard time fighting the germs. Each child then received 180 milligrams of iron daily, as ferrous sulfate (60 milligrams, three times a day) for two months. Blood cells were again sampled and challenged with bacteria.

In a second group of ten anemic children, blood cells were also challenged before and after intramuscular injections of 100 milligrams of iron. (Injections work faster than oral supplements, so the dosage was lower.) There was no other treatment in either group. The children were given no special diet.

Both groups showed clear improvement in blood cell immunity and ability to fight off bacteria after iron supplements. "These results point to a specific role for iron deficiency in altering immunologic status," say the researchers (*Lancet,* May 7, 1977).

So while iron may not be the only factor in strong immune response, it's certainly an important one.

Pinning Down Iron Losses

The first and immediate step to correct iron deficiency is to find out what's causing the problem. Low intake? Hidden losses? While underlying disease must not be ruled out, in most cases it's not the main cause.

Poor Diet

In younger people, crash dieting, junk food binges, or simply poor food choices are often to blame, especially when superimposed on increased demands of growth.

In older people, low intake could be an indirect result of the disorder itself, in a roundabout way. Weakness, apathy and loss of appetite can lead to self-neglect and poor eating habits, further lowering iron intake. It's a vicious cycle. At age 60, chances of developing anemia double, especially in people housebound or living alone. Also, iron absorption and hemoglobin production tend to drop off as we age, so older people are very susceptible. One medical doctor says, "The prevention and early detection of anemia can be aided by insuring that elderly people receive an adequate diet and have regular medical supervision" (*Geriatrics,* December, 1977).

"An adequate diet" for young or old means plenty of iron-rich foods.

Apricots. Blackstrap molasses. Brewer's yeast. Green leafy vegetables. Nuts, legumes and seeds. Meat—especially liver and other organ meats. Wheat germ and other whole grain foods. Plus plenty of vitamin C sources—fruits, peppers and greens—to boost iron absorption.

The other thing to look for is blood loss. Women of childbearing age don't have to look too far. Heavy menstrual periods, repeated or closely spaced pregnancies, or excessive blood loss during labor and childbirth sap blood and iron from body stores.

Menstrual Periods

Doctors shouldn't hesitate to suspect iron deficiency anemia in women during their reproductive years (teens through menopause). Blood tests may not even be necessary, nor search for other disease. "Iron deficiency is so often the culprit in these patients that this is the one situation in which I would initiate a therapeutic trial of iron without further investigation," says Dorothea Zucker-Franklin, M.D., professor of medicine at New York University School of Medicine (*Consultant,* April, 1978).

Even women just embarking on menopause may have irregular bouts of heavy or prolonged bleeding—enough of a drain to still make them vulnerable to anemia.

"I believe the physician may safely accept menstruation or dietary deficiency as a cause of iron deficiency in otherwise healthy [women]," says Joseph R. Morrisey, M.D., associate professor of family medicine, University of Western Ontario, London, Canada.

Pregnancy

Pregnancy places heavy demands on iron stores. Not only is a lot of iron shunted to the growing baby, especially during the last few months, but an increase in body fluid tends to dilute hemoglobin. Low iron is the net result.

In the past, obstetricians recognized that fact and routinely pre-scribed iron supplements for pregnant women. Taking a step backwards now, it's no longer routine. "They prefer to wait until anemia appears, and then attempt to correct it," remarks Dr. Morrisey. That's in spite of the fact that it's difficult to raise hemoglobin by oral iron late in pregnancy. What's more, iron deficiency anemia is frequently complicated by folate (a B vitamin) deficiency. Dr. Morrisey feels that not providing iron to pregnant women is foolish. "I feel that the woman with the lower hemoglobin level is at much greater risk of serious [consequences] should a [post-birth] hemorrhage occur. . . . I still prescribe it routinely" (*The Female Patient,* December, 1979).

During breastfeeding, iron is secreted with milk. Losses to a nursing mother probably equal about what she would lose with menstrual flow. Unless iron is prescribed to replace the amount lost during pregnancy, childbirth and breastfeeding, iron deficiency anemia will develop.

Hemorrhoids, Ulcers and Aspirin: Other Causes of Iron Loss

In men, the most common cause for increased blood—and iron—loss is hemorrhoids. But either sex can be affected. Other possible causes in anyone are peptic ulcer, surgery (especially stomach surgery), hiatal hernia, diverticular disease—even frequent nosebleeds or voluntary blood donations. All call for extra iron to replace losses.

Aspirin can cause internal bleeding and slow blood clotting, thereby causing easily overlooked blood losses in heavy users. Aspirin and other analgesic (pain-relieving) drugs are often taken daily to ease the inflammation of rheumatoid arthritis, in which case iron deficiency should be suspected. Other uses of aspirin are harder to justify and should be avoided. "Aspirin taken to relieve hangovers, insomnia and anxiety is especially likely to exaggerate GI blood loss, both through aspirin's local corrosive effect and its effect on platelet function," says Robert H. Kough, M.D., in an article on dealing with iron deficiency anemia (*Modern Medicine,* July 15-August 15, 1980).

If your doctor doesn't inquire about any of those circumstances—history of surgery, menstrual troubles, even blood in your stools—be sure to volunteer the information. Iron deficiency anemia is hardest to diagnose in otherwise healthy adults.

Building Strong Blood

Once iron deficiency anemia has been established, iron stores need to be replenished at once. Standard treatment for adults is 180 to 200 milligrams a day, in the ferrous form. That's the most easily absorbed. Ferrous sulfate or ferrous gluconate are the two most commonly used: one tablet of 60 milligrams, three times a day, between meals. Iron supplements are absorbed best when the stomach is empty. Occasionally, however, doses that large will cause constipation or other gastrointestinal discomfort. That can be helped by taking supplements with meals, although absorption is cut down. Dividing dosage into three intervals also minimizes those effects. In most people, iron supplements are well tolerated.

Slow-release supplements, designed to combat upset stomach in sensitive patients, are available. They're taken once a day. That may be more convenient for some people, but absorption is not guaranteed because the pill bypasses the duodenum (lower part of the stomach), the most active site of iron absorption.

"Only rarely do patients fail to respond to [iron] therapy," says Dr.

Zucker-Franklin. Blood levels of iron are the first to bounce back to normal, within a week or two to as long as two months. Bone marrow iron takes longer to build up again. Total therapy runs about six months.

Of course, it goes without saying that a high-iron diet plays a big role in preventing a recurrence. And it's a must for prevention. Most men need at least 10 milligrams of iron a day; most women, 18 or more. For men, that means the equivalent of 4 ounces of beef liver a day. Or 2 cups of raisins. Or 2 pounds of haddock or cod. *Every day.* For women, it means the equivalent of over 7 ounces of liver every day. Or 3½ cups of raisins. Or over 3½ pounds of haddock or cod. Clearly, iron supplements provide an easier way to bridge the gap between what you eat and what you need.

CHAPTER

46

Fatigue

At one time or another, each of us feels tired. After a hectic day at the office. Up all night with a sick child. Rushing to meet a deadline.

Normally, we bounce back after a day or so of rest. Sometimes, though, fatigue seems to linger. We drag ourselves around like we've got a lead ball chained to our ankles. No matter how long we sleep, we're more tired when we wake up than when we went to bed. Or we come home from work and collapse when our friends go out to jog or swim laps. Meanwhile, just the thought of cooking supper or doing the laundry makes us tired.

That's more than just discouraging. It can be downright depressing.

Chronic fatigue drags more people to their doctors than any other problem. One medical columnist writes, "If I were to choose the one most common complaint I've heard from patients, it would be 'I'm tired.' People suffer from pain, cough, nervousness, headaches and innumerable other disagreeable sensations, but fatigue leads the list."

Sometimes fatigue is a symptom of disease. But in 80 percent of the cases, there's nothing physically wrong with the ever-weary people—at least according to x-rays and lab tests.

Or is there?

Disease is but one of a number of possible causes. Besides lack of exercise and side effects of various drugs, faulty nutrition can cause fatigue. Overeating or crash dieting can do it. And while any overall nutritional deficiency is likely to slow you down, certain minerals—magnesium, potassium and iron—are particularly important.

Cross Fatigue off Your Schedule

Could a teary, depressed and irritable housewife be nothing more than the victim of a potassium deficiency? Yes. One physician dubbed the problem "The Housewife Syndrome." But it could very easily apply to men and women holding jobs outside the home. It goes something like this:

Twenty pounds of laundry, but you don't have an ounce of strength. You've got to pick the kids up from school at 3:00, have dinner ready by 5:00, a PTA meeting at 7:00. But you can hardly wait till 11:00 so you can finally go to sleep.

Add to that a job outside the home, and life is a chore, and another chore, and another.

Potassium and Magnesium for Peak Energy

If you can't take any more, check to see if your diet provides enough potassium—and magnesium.

Tiredness is hard to define. But, in many cases, it means tired *muscles*—muscles that feel leaden or drained of energy. A lack of magnesium, which helps muscles contract, can cause that tiredness. So can a lack of potassium.

A doctor chose 100 of her chronically fatigued patients—84 women and 16 men, 1 in 5 of whom held full or parttime jobs. Some traveled a lot. She put them on a supplementary program of potassium and magnesium. Of the 100, 87 improved.

"The change was startling," writes Palma Formica, M.D., of Old Bridge, New Jersey. "They had become alert, cheerful, animated and energetic and walked with a lively step. They stated that sleep refreshed them as it had not done for months. Some said they could get along on 6 hours sleep at night, whereas formerly they had not felt rested on 12 or more. Morning exhaustion had completely subsided.

"Almost all patients have undertaken new activities," she notes. "Six who had not worked outside the home before obtained parttime jobs. Two of the pregnant patients continued to work for a time. Several of the husbands called and expressed appreciation of the physical improvement and consequent increase in emotional well-being of their wives.

"Four of the men reported that they had started repairs on their houses, which they had been unable to do before, one has obtained an additional job, and two have assumed new civic duties. Within ten days the president of the local fire company was commuting daily to his demanding position and also performing firefighting services as required without the exhaustion he had suffered before."

Some of those people had had chronic fatigue for over two years. Yet it took only five to six weeks of magnesium and potassium therapy to clear up their problem (*Current Therapeutic Research,* March, 1962).

Magnesium sparks more chemical reactions in the body than any other mineral. In a severe deficiency, the whole body suffers. You stumble instead of walk, feel depressed and have heart spasms. Doctors are trained to recognize those and over 30 other symptoms of a severe deficiency. But they aren't trained to recognize a *mild* deficiency of magnesium. It has only one noticeable symptom—chronic fatigue.

"A deficiency of magnesium is a common cause of fatigue," says Ray Wunderlich, M.D., of St. Petersburg, Florida.

But that fatigue can easily be cured. In addition to Dr. Formica's report is a study of 200 men and women who were tired during the day and were given magnesium. In all but two cases, waking tiredness disappeared (*Second International Symposium on Magnesium,* June, 1976).

Potassium deficiency is a well-known hazard among long-distance runners and professional athletes. The mineral helps to cool muscles, and hours of exertion use it up. If it's not replaced, the result is chronic fatigue—even for a highly trained athlete. "When you lack potassium," says Gabe Mirkin, M.D., runner of marathons and coauthor of *The Sportsmedicine Book* (Little, Brown, 1978), "you feel tired, weak and irritable."

But a potassium deficiency and the weakness that goes with it aren't limited to athletes. In one study, researchers randomly selected a group of people and measured their potassium intake. Those people with a deficient intake of potassium—60 percent of the men and 40 percent of the women in the study—had a weaker grip than those with a normal intake. And as potassium intake decreased, muscular strength decreased (*Journal of the American Medical Association,* October 6, 1979).

You could probably put up with a few days of weakness. But after a few *months* you feel terrible. "In chronic potassium deficit," writes a researcher who studied the mineral, "muscular weakness may persist for many months and be interpreted as being due to emotional disability" (*Minnesota Medicine,* June, 1965).

Iron Boosts Work Capacity

Not all cases of chronic fatigue are caused by a lack of potassium and magnesium. In fact, a good many are caused by a lack of iron.

Iron helps form hemoglobin, the substance in red blood cells that carries oxygen from your lungs to the rest of your body. If that oxygen supply is reduced, you have apathy, tiredness and irritability—the symptoms of iron deficiency anemia.

But you can be iron deficient without anemia. "A deficiency of iron may be present when blood hemoglobin falls within normal limits," says Dr. Wunderlich. "This syndrome of iron deficiency without anemia," he continues, "is an exceedingly important cause of fatigue."

Iron deficiency creeps up on you. Menstrual periods drain iron. Pregnancies sap it. Reducing diets cut down your intake. Before you know it, every cell of your body is dragging.

One study shows just how slow you go compared to someone who's not iron deficient. Researchers studied the "physical work capacity" of 75 women, some anemic, some not. The anemic women could stay on a treadmill an average of eight minutes less than the nonanemic group. None of the anemic women could perform under "highest work load" conditions. All of the nonanemic group could. During a work test, the heartbeat of those with anemia rose to an average of 176 per minute; for nonanemics, heartbeat rose to just 130. Levels of lactate, a chemical in the muscles that is linked to fatigue, were almost twice as high in the anemic group (*American Journal of Clinical Nutrition,* June, 1977).

Relief from iron deficiency-induced fatigue is simple. Replace the iron.

Workers on an Indonesian rubber plantation were paid by productivity, and researchers found that those who were anemic earned the least. But after two months of iron supplementation, the previously anemic workers had normal levels of iron and earned the same amount as those free from anemia (*American Journal of Clinical Nutrition,* April, 1979).

What's more, extra iron may improve work performance even in the absence of anemia, according to researcher Per Ericsson at the departments of medicine and clinical physiology, University Hospital, Uppsala, Sweden. A group of healthy people aged 58 to 71 took 120 milligrams of iron a day for three months. Work capacity—measured by how long they could ride on a bicyclelike machine—went up by 4 percent in the men and by 12 percent in the women (*Acta Medica Scandinavica,* vol. 188, 1970).

A bachelor who overcame fatigue by upgrading his mineral nutrition wrote to tell us:

> Over the past couple of years, I've been a victim of chronic fatigue. This is due in part to my job. Currently I work for the *Philadelphia Inquirer* as a driver-delivery man. Between my hours (8 P.M. to 5 A.M.) and the nature of the job, I've found getting proper rest sometimes impossible. In addition to my job, I'm very active athletically. It's not unusual for me to jog four or

five times a week, between two to six miles at a time. On top of all that, I'm a single 28-year-old bachelor living alone, responsible for keeping my apartment, cooking and doing laundry.

To help combat some of my eating deficiencies, I'd been taking selected vitamins and minerals. However, potassium and iron were not among them. Well, since adding those two to my daily intake, I've felt totally rejuvenated. I feel physically stronger and mentally clearer. I'm sleeping sounder and feeling refreshed when awakening. In the past I could be in bed nine or ten hours and still arise tired.

Of course, the *best* way to boost potassium intake is through diet. Apricots, bananas, beef, blackstrap molasses, chicken, halibut, oranges, potatoes and seeds are some of the richest sources. For a more complete list of potassium-rich foods, see chapter 6, Potassium.

47

Muscle Cramps

Calcium for Knotted Muscles, Painful Cramps and Growing Pains

Besides the heart, there are over 100 muscles in the body. Any one of them could knot up. What can you do about it?

As far back as 1944, research indicated that calcium can go a long way in relieving cramps. In that year, Elizabeth Martin, M.D., reported a study in which 79 of 112 young children were completely relieved of "growing pains"—the nighttime cramps that can have a young child kicking and screaming—with either calcium phosphate or bone meal (*Canadian Medical Association Journal,* June, 1944).

Dr. Martin gave her pregnant patients calcium supplements. None of those women suffered the usual aching legs or nocturnal cramps that are so common in pregnancy. Dr. Martin noted that while all the women were spared leg cramps and had healthy babies, the babies of the mothers who got bone meal had exceptionally long silky hair and long beautifully formed fingernails. Perhaps that finding led her to favor bone meal as the calcium-containing supplement of choice.

One person told us, "My mother and I have for years been plagued by terrible cramps in our feet. I started taking calcium supplements about four months ago and have not had a cramp since."

No one really knows why or how calcium works for leg cramps. In the November, 1975, issue of *Postgraduate Medicine,* a physician queried the magazine, "Why does this therapy appear to work in many patients in whom there is no obvious calcium deficiency and in whom the results are too long-standing to be a placebo effect?" The answer: "There is no metabolic reason why calcium in low dosages should prevent leg cramps."

Metabolic reason or not, calcium most certainly *does* prevent leg cramps, as well as other types of cramps. The Calcium Research Project, conducted by *Prevention* magazine in 1977, in which readers reported on calcium for arthritis, turned up 1,653 reports of calcium associated with relief from muscle spasms or cramps.

Mrs. N.C., 66, of Houston, Texas, reported that calcium relieved cramping in the calves, one of the most common conditions reported to be overcome with calcium. At age 60, she said, she retired from nursing and went into selling. She had to stand on hard floors for long hours on end, causing a great deal of pain and cramping in her legs at night. She began taking one dolomite tablet before each meal and another at bedtime, which "has made a new woman out of me."

Mrs. H.B., of southern California, said that following a stroke in 1959, "I began getting muscle spasms in my spinal curvature, due to damaged nerves at the base of my brain. I had drugs and painkillers constantly, costing $100 to $150 per month. . . . Within six months after starting to take dolomite, bone meal and calcium, I was able to stop taking drugs and traction treatments and have not had any muscle spasms nor calcium spikes on my spinal curvature.

"I had spinal curvature x-rays two years ago and much to my surprise and the surprise of my neurologist, there were no calcium spikes. No wonder there was no more pain."

Mrs. C.D.T., of Maryland, said that following six weeks of studying five hours a day for her Ph.D. preliminary examinations, she was in a constant state of muscle spasm. She had had similar problems before, though not so bad, and her doctor had told her the spasms were a result of arthritis in her lower spine.

"By spring of 1975 I could not get down on the floor, or if I did, I could not get up without assistance or extreme pain. I could not lift my right leg except by picking it up with my hands. Muscle spasms in legs and buttocks replaced climax during sex. I could not stand up straight. The contractions were persistent and began to extend to the upper back. I do not exaggerate when I say I was in writhing agony!

"I made a formal list of my symptoms which I submitted to my physician in April, telling him at that time how depressed I was feeling and how wearing it was to be in constant pain. He barely glanced at the list, and made no further comment than 'Hmmm, a typical clinical case of arthritis. Let's file your list in your chart, so that we can compare how you are now with how you'll be two years from now.' Then he wrote me a prescription for an anti-inflammatory drug which I refused to take in case I would be worse in two years and might need it more then."

Mrs. C.D.T. proceeded to do a lot of detective work, which included having her serum calcium measured, carefully observing her body sensations under different conditions, reading and reflecting. Two of numerous clues told her she needed calcium: any kind of moderate exertion caused her muscles to tremble; and a statement in a book by Dr. Roger Williams said that people in an anxiety state may need five times the calcium required by the normal person, as their calcium can become bound up in the form of calcium lactate. While she did not consider herself to be exactly in an anxiety state, she did recognize the fact that she was an "anxious person."

She began taking 640 to 800 milligrams a day of calcium in the form of bone meal. Significantly, she had no relief for the first two months. Following that, however, during an overseas vacation, she wrote, "I took advantage of the wonderful dairy products available in the countries I visited. My lunches consisted of much cheese, for one thing, and in addition, I was taking up to a quart of milk and yogurt per day. The night before I came home I was free of all symptoms which had been bothering me for eight years, and I am still comfortable two years later."

While a nutritionist might say that all that milk, yogurt and cheese she was eating—in addition to the bone meal tablets she kept taking—probably did the trick by raising her calcium intake to over 2,000 milligrams a day, a psychologist might say it was the three weeks in Europe that did the trick. A holistically oriented physician would say that *both* probably played important roles in bringing about her relief.

Calcium Quells Menstrual Cramps and Distress for Many

And good news for millions of women—calcium may prevent menstrual cramps and distress, in addition to back and leg spasms. One woman from Delaware said, "Calcium relieves and prevents the leg cramps that my nine-year-old gets," and added that extra calcium has also "completely eliminated" her own severe premenstrual cramps.

Another woman told us, "Even though after having two babies I was still plagued with cramps, calcium has now set me completely free of drugs. I double or triple my daily intake of calcium as soon as I feel the tension mounting the day before my period starts."

All in all, improvement or total relief of menstrual cramping and distress was reported by 293 women, about 10 percent of the total number of Calcium Research Project respondents. Mrs. A.G., of Phoenix, Arizona, remarked, "For ten years, I took birth control pills to avoid the terrible menstrual cramps that sent me to bed every month since I began menstruating. But I was afraid of the Pill, so I tried calcium. Now I have absolutely no incapacitating menstrual cramps." She reported taking 1,000 milligrams a day in the form of calcium carbonate, along with moderate amounts of other vitamins and 500 milligrams of magnesium a day.

A letter from Mrs. R.F., 37, also of Arizona, reveals an interesting connection between menstrual cramps and muscle spasms in other parts of the body. "I had hard menstrual cramps, lasting two or three days; premenstrual tension and bloating. On the first day of menstruation I always felt as if my brain wasn't really functioning. I was in a fog. Also, I had arm cramps sometimes going from my little fingertip to my shoulder and all the way down my spine. These arm cramps awakened me almost every night." After taking 1,800 milligrams of calcium daily in the form of bone meal, Mrs. R.F. reported that, "All conditions have been completely eliminated."

48

Arthritis

Calcium for Corroded Joints

There is good reason to believe that many cases of what people believe to be arthritis are actually caused in large part by a calcium deficiency. Certainly, a calcium deficiency does not cause inflammation of the joints. But what seems to happen is that the inflammation causes a local erosion of calcium, and in some, but not all, cases, a major part of the pain and even lack of mobility is caused by that calcium loss.

One of the many people who suffer arthritis and who tried calcium on their own told us:

> My health was always good, except for arthritis of the hip of five years' duration, with agonizing, gnawing pain. Much of that time I had to walk with a cane, could not carry anything heavy, and literally crawled up stairs, holding on to the banisters with both hands.

I was told by the M.D.'s that I'd have to learn to "live with it."
After six months of calcium, the pain vanished completely, and had not returned. My health is excellent—my back's straight and very strong, and I can *run* up stairs.

A coincidence? The woman herself considered the possibility that her astonishing recovery may have had little or nothing to do with the fact that she had begun taking 1,200 to 1,500 milligrams of calcium a day (in the form of bone meal and dolomite), plus some vitamin D, eight years ago. This is how she put it:

I have often wondered if I'd had a "spontaneous remission" of arthritis, but I'm very, very strongly of the opinion that it has been due to the calcium I've taken religiously for the past eight years.

That woman's letter was one of 3,500 responses sent in by people participating in the Calcium Research Project, a survey conducted by *Prevention* magazine in 1977. A few numbers from that project may be of interest to you. Of those 3,500 responses received, some had to be discounted because the information provided was not complete. Of the 2,959 responses that could be tabulated, 1,379 said that bone pain had been either relieved or abolished after taking calcium. With nearly half of the respondents reporting that effect, the chances are that the woman just mentioned was on the right track in thinking that the calcium did in fact help her aching joints.

Most doctors, the survey revealed, are not enthusiastic about supplements. A typical letter along that line came from a woman from Long Beach, New York, who said that after taking bone meal and dolomite, she noticed that the arthritis she had suffered from for many years, along with several other problems, including bad nerves and muscle tension, improved considerably after she began taking about 1,200 milligrams of calcium and a wide range of other vitamins and minerals.

"I can notice there's been very much less pain and no swelling in the knees, which I used to have," she pointed out. She then said that about a year ago, she fell down ten steps and took a three-point landing on a cement floor, which gave her cuts and severe bruises—but no broken bones. When she went to the doctor, she related, he was surprised that she had not broken any bones. But when she said that she attributed that fact to her having taken bone meal and dolomite, her doctor "just laughed and said, 'Oh, you and your minerals and vitamins!' "

Then, she added: "I can't understand why he couldn't see that there must have been *something* preventing a woman, 77 then and arthritic, from breaking a bone. Well, as my grandmother used to say, 'There's none so blind as those who refuse to see.' "

One reason for passing along these stories is that they're perfectly typical of many, many other stories that came in via the Calcium Research Project. Should *you* try calcium for your arthritis? You decide. There are so many other reasons—perfectly solid, proven reasons—for taking calcium, that the idea makes sense. So while we can't point to scientific studies of calcium's role in arthritis, it's difficult to ignore the possibility that calcium will improve some cases of arthritis.

At this point, you're probably wondering how or why calcium helps arthritis, at least in some cases. We don't have that answer. We can only suggest that in many cases, the pain and stiffness is not a result of some mysterious kind of degeneration but simply the result of too much calcium having been withdrawn from the bones through the years in order to keep blood levels of this vital mineral at the required level. What's more, there's reason to suspect that the "calcium deposits" that sometimes accompany joint problems are associated *not* with too much calcium, but rather too little. What may be happening is that the calcium withdrawn from the bones for some reason has a tendency to pile up in the wrong places. It is surely one of the ironies of physiology that many people with calcium deposits report greatly improved joint mobility after taking in more calcium.

We'd like to share one last calcium/arthritis story with you. Mrs. V.M., 56, of Carmel Valley, California, wrote:

> Two years ago I was literally crippled. My troubles started at 53, with pains in my back, neck, elbows and shoulders. I went to one of our leading orthopedic doctors and x-rays revealed arthritis and osteoporosis. My left arm and hand were completely numb.
>
> The doctor injected me with cortisone on several visits. Finally I was referred to a neurologist who ordered more x-rays, a brain scan and a complete skull series, as he had found diminished sensation on the entire left side. All tests were normal, though, except the arthritis. They fitted me with an orthopedic back brace, my right arm was put in a sling, and I was given a Philadelphia collar for my neck. I was forced to quit work and go on Disability Social Security.
>
> We were fortunate to have a young orthopedic surgeon come to this area. As I felt things could not get worse, I went to see him. More x-rays. Three days later, he called me to his office and—now what I call the "miracle"—he ordered 750 milligrams of calcium three times daily, plus 500 milligrams of vitamin C and 500 milligrams niacinamide [a B vitamin], plus at least a quart of milk daily with a high-calcium diet.
>
> I was advised how to position myself for sleep (the hardest part, as I had been a stomach sleeper). The first month I discarded the back brace and sling and used a soft collar for another month. The only pain I have now is occasionally in my

right elbow. I exercise and can do anything from turning cart-
wheels to using a trapeze bar. I returned to work (full duty)
October 1, 1976.

Copper, Too, May Help Weather Arthritis

From time to time, the old folk notion that wearing a copper
bracelet will reduce arthritic pain resurfaces—with or without a scientific
theory to back it. One biochemist, Helmar Dollwet, Ph.D., at the University of Akron in Ohio, believes there's something to the idea. He's found
that copper from such a bracelet reacts with chemicals in the skin to
produce both anesthetic and anti-inflammatory substances. If absorbed,
says Dr. Dollwet, those substances could circulate through the bloodstream
to the affected joints—thereby relieving pain. Moreover, the copper itself
may find its way to the joints and have a similar effect. The medical establishment, though, persistently dismisses such claims as old wives' tales.

Copper bracelets or not, though, *dietary* copper just might relieve
arthritic flareups—from the inside out. That is, copper may maximize the
body's natural response to the painful inflammation of arthritis.

When food is digested, copper is bound up (or chelated) to other
substances to form copper complexes, active forms of the mineral. Some
copper circulates, some is stored in the liver. In the event of disease—such
as arthritis—the body releases stored copper complexes, raising blood
copper levels two- to threefold.

And not without good reason. Apparently, the dramatic increase
in copper complexes meets some increased physiological demands of the
disease. John R. J. Sorenson, Ph.D., an associate professor of medicinal
chemistry at the University of Arkansas Medical Sciences Campus in Little
Rock, noticed that in 153 people with arthritis-like diseases (including
rheumatoid arthritis and lupus erythematosis), copper levels rose and fell
with flareups and remissions of the disease.

He also noted that giving copper acetate to animals with arthritis
was an effective way to treat the inflammation. Dr. Sorenson put two and
two together and figured that the rise in copper complexes must be the
body's way of dealing directly with the inflammation, probably through
copper-containing enzymes.

Antiarthritis drugs, like aspirin, work in the same way, prompting
the formation of copper complexes in the blood, which in turn go to work
against inflammation. The problem is, those drugs can cause stomach
ulcers and gastrointestinal distress, especially if taken in the large and
frequent doses needed to trigger the anti-inflammatory response.

So why not just use copper compounds? reasons Dr. Sorenson.
Copper compounds not only are nonirritating, but they actually heal or
head off stomach ulcers, doubling their potential value as antiarthritics.

"If copper complexes have increased anti-inflammatory . . . activities and do not cause gastrointestinal irritation or other toxicities associated with the currently used drugs, they would offer more effective and less toxic therapy of arthritis . . ." concludes Dr. Sorenson (*Journal of Applied Nutrition,* April, 1980).

For Some, It's Zinc to the Rescue

Zinc, too, may relieve arthritis. Reduced pain and swelling, plus marked improvement in joint mobility and grip strength followed treatment with zinc supplements in one notable study conducted by researchers at the Finsen Institute and University of Copenhagen in Denmark. Twenty-four people with psoriatic arthritis (a type of rheumatoid arthritis accompanied by the skin disease psoriasis) were treated with zinc sulfate (220 milligrams, three times a day). In the first part of the trial, 11 people were given zinc for six weeks, followed by six weeks of a placebo (a do-nothing pill). The rest were treated with placebo first, then zinc.

After that, the first 11 patients were continued on zinc for six months. Throughout the course of the study, the researchers regularly measured changes in wrist and finger joints (the areas most severely affected by that type of arthritis). In most, stiff joints once again became mobile and useful. Grip strengthened. Swelling went down. Pain and morning stiffness all but disappeared.

But the arthritic patients didn't need clinical tests to tell them all that: they felt definite improvement. Need for aspirin and other painkillers fell. What's more, improvement was greatest in those who continued zinc therapy for six months.

The authors of the study credit the success of that therapy to zinc's known abilities to reduce inflammation through the immune system. And because blood levels were normal at the start of the study and rose with supplementation, say the authors, there doesn't necessarily have to be an actual zinc deficiency for zinc to work. They wrap up their report by saying, "It seems fair to conclude that oral treatment with zinc sulphate might prove valuable in the treatment of psoriatic arthritis" (*British Journal of Dermatology,* October, 1980).

49

Bruxism
(Teeth Clenching)

Unclench Your Teeth with Calcium

Teeth grinding or clenching—called bruxism—is more than an unpleasant habit. A Swiss dental scientist, Peter Schaerer of Bern, says that people who clench their teeth during sleep or during a "confrontation" can cause damage to the teeth, gums, jaw joint and muscles (*Journal of the American Dental Association,* January, 1971).

According to Emanuel Cheraskin, M.D., D.M.D., and W. Marshall Ringsdorf, Jr., D.M.D., of the University of Alabama School of Dentistry, bruxism is a nutritional problem that can be relieved with increased daily supplies of calcium and one particular B vitamin, pantothenate. (Pantothenate is also known as pantothenic acid or calcium pantothenate, and is found in beef liver, broccoli, brown rice, eggs, mushrooms, rolled oats, roasted peanuts, trout and wheat germ.)

Drs. Ringsdorf and Cheraskin did a nutritional survey of a group of people, some of whom were bruxists (teeth gnashers). Those without bruxism recorded higher levels of calcium and pantothenate intake. A year later—after dietary instruction—the entire group was surveyed again. This time the doctors found that those bruxists who had significantly increased their intake of calcium and pantothenate were no longer teeth gnashers (*Dental Survey,* December, 1970).

CHAPTER

50

Periodontal (Gum) Disease

Calcium for the Silent Tooth Destroyer

Calcium can do for the teeth and jawbone that supports them what it does for the large bones of your legs and arms and the vertebrae of your back. In fact, even for the estimated 20 million or more Americans who have lost all their teeth, there is impressive evidence that some relatively simple dietary changes—including the addition of a daily calcium supplement—could prevent some of the denture problems that are so common among them. And even more important, such measures, if applied early enough, might very well lower the chances that you'll ever lose your teeth at all.

Over and above a sound jawbone, you need sound gums. The most serious and widespread problem affecting the gums is periodontal disease—a

410

chronic, progressive inflammation and infection of the gum tissue and underlying jawbone. Most medical researchers believe that the disease is caused by residual food, bacteria and tartar deposits that collect in the tiny crevices between the gums and the necks of the teeth. As the bacterial infection spreads deeper into the periodontal tissue surrounding the jaw-tooth connection, the jawbone itself begins to shrink around the pockets until teeth loosen and fall out. An estimated 75 percent of the adult U.S. population suffers from some degree of periodontal disease, and it is the leading tooth destroyer among the middle-aged and older.

Keeping the teeth and gums clean and free of sticky plaque, or film, which can harbor harmful bacteria, is essential. Careful, effective brushing (particularly at the gum line) along with daily between-the-teeth cleaning with dental floss is the backbone of a preventive program. But sound nutritional habits can play a critical role. While vitamin C and the B vitamin folate have been shown to play an important part in resisting bacterial growth and gum sponginess, calcium may also be very important.

While most periodontal researchers focus on ways to cope with the onslaught of plaque at the gum line, others are working at the problem from an entirely different angle. In a major study reported in *Cornell Veterinarian* (January, 1972), Lennart Krook, D.V.M., Ph.D., and several associates proposed that the real problem in tooth loss is a shrinking jawbone brought on by a calcium-deficient diet. Examining ten people with periodontal disease, they discovered that nine had estimated daily calcium intakes of 400 milligrams or less—far below the Recommended Dietary Allowance of 800 milligrams.

When the patients were given 500 milligrams of supplemental calcium twice a day for six months, remarkable reversals in the disease process were noted. "All patients had gingivitis [gum inflammation] and bleeding at the start," the researchers write. "After treatment, inflammation was improved in all cases and absent in three. Calculus [mineral deposits] was reduced in half the cases. Pockets along the root were recorded in eight patients before the study. Pocket depth was reduced in all cases after treatment. Tooth mobility was likewise recorded in eight patients. It was reduced in seven patients, and in one there was no mobility after treatment." In other words, the teeth were more firmly fastened in their sockets.

Of special interest was the fact that x-rays taken after calcium supplementation showed the appearance of new bone in the jaw. Instead of continuing to shrink away from the teeth, the jawbone was actually laying down new growth.

"The improvement in amount of alveolar [jaw] bone was remarkable, considering the relatively short period of treatment," the researchers stressed.

How to Keep Your Teeth Even After You Lose Them

You may have seen many commercials like this on television over the years:

The whole clan has gathered for a traditional family picnic—hamburgers, potato salad, corn on the cob . . . the whole works. Everyone's enjoying the food with gusto except a certain middle-aged denture wearer whose eating adventures are obviously not what they used to be. In fact, he's been reduced to *cutting* his corn off the cob with a knife before eating it, or else risking the embarrassment of losing his ill-fitting dentures in a mismatched tussle with the cob.

The ad goes on to suggest that a certain brand of denture adhesive could solve this person's chomping problems overnight, and thus restore the forbidden pleasures of not only corn on the cob, but steaks, apples and a host of other hard-to-bite foods.

It's true that for most people who have lost their natural teeth, wearing dentures is no picnic. Even the best false teeth are woefully inefficient and clumsy, compared with the set nature provided us with. Add the hassle of irritation and friction caused by poor fit, and the experience of trying to adjust to your dentures can become a continuing nightmare.

But adhesive pastes and glues aren't necessarily the answer. (In fact, the Federal Trade Commission now prohibits the kind of ad claims described above, because it feels they are unrealistic.)

Better-Fitting Dentures

That's where calcium comes in. Evidence that calcium supplements and other nutritional changes can make dentures less of a problem should be of special interest to those who shell out hundreds of dollars for artificial teeth that just aren't working out the way they expected.

According to Emanuel Cheraskin, M.D., D.M.D., and W. Marshall Ringsdorf, Jr., D.M.D., "Recent evidence indicates that denture failure is a much too frequent result in the patient with complete dentures. In these surveys, dissatisfaction with dentures ranged from 15 percent to 45 percent of the studied samples. Of the 22.6 million denture wearers identified by the 1971 national health interview survey, almost 30 percent 'thought their dentures needed refitting or that they needed new dentures' " (*Journal of the American Dental Association,* January, 1976).

Part of the problem is the bony ridge or foundation upon which those dentures are supposedly anchored. "In a great percentage of denture wearers, the jawbone keeps shrinking away," said Kenneth E. Wical, D.D.S., chairperson of the removable prosthodontics department at Loma Linda University School of Dentistry in Loma Linda, California. "Some dentists accept this shrinkage as normal, but it probably isn't normal at all.

"As the jawbone grows smaller, it becomes more difficult for people to wear their dentures," Dr. Wical told us. "Some have gradually lost half of their original jawbone or even more. Eventually they reach the point where they can no longer wear their dentures. There's nothing left for the dentures to fit around! Denture adhesive makers capitalize on this. It's directly related."

Extra calcium can apparently slow that whole process down, however. "Back in 1974, we did a study involving a group of patients with dentures," Dr. Wical told us. "We found that those with good underlying bone had a daily dietary intake of about 900 milligrams of calcium. Those with jawbone problems were only getting about 500 milligrams of calcium."

In a newer study, Dr. Wical and a co-worker divided a group of 46 denture patients into two groups. All had had several teeth pulled, followed by the immediate placement of dentures. For the next year, half received supplements that provided a total of 750 milligrams of calcium and 375 units of vitamin D daily. ("Adequate vitamin D is absolutely essential for absorption and metabolism of calcium," the two researchers remind us.) The other group received a nontherapeutic placebo tablet.

During the course of the study, x-ray pictures of the patients' jaws were made, and the degree of bone loss—what the scientists call alveolar bone resorption—was recorded and compared. The results were quite significant. At the end of the year, the people taking calcium had lost 34 percent less of their upper jaws and 39 percent less of their lower jaws than the unsupplemented group—"an average difference of 36 percent less resorption when both dental arches are considered" (*Journal of Prosthetic Dentistry*, January, 1979).

The Right Kind of Diet for Life-Long Teeth

Dr. Wical and his researchers found another important dietary variable besides total calcium intake: the *ratio* of another mineral, phosphorus, to calcium. As levels of phosphorus rise, thus increasing the phosphorus:calcium ratio, jawbone resorption seems to speed up. On the other hand, five people in the unsupplemented group whose bone retention figures compared quite favorably with the supplemented group had relatively low phosphorus:calcium ratios.

As a result, the authors conclude, "For patients who demonstrated severe or rapid alveolar bone loss and whose dietary history suggests a low calcium intake and/or high phosphorus intake, we believe that calcium and vitamin D supplementation will help to increase the resistance of the bone to both mechanical and biochemical stresses."

We asked Dr. Wical if there were other dietary changes a person might wish to make. "The problem with certain types of food is there's such an imbalance of phosphorus," he told us. "The ideal ratio is about 1:1. But in meat, for example, the ratio is 20:1. That's a tremendous imbalance. Refined cereal products are about 6:1, and potatoes 5:1.

"What we find over and over again is that meat, bread and potato eaters are the ones who experience this bone loss problem. Also, soft drinks contain large amounts of phosphorus in the form of phosphoric acid. That's another problem with the American diet. Teenage girls, for instance, often seem to exist on soft drinks and little else. As a consequence, we're finding that people are starting to lose bone very early in life.

"The phosphorus:calcium ratio of the average U.S. diet is approximately 2½:1, instead of the ideal 1:1," Dr. Wical said. "We see the results of this imbalance every day in the dental clinic."

For those reasons, he added, "Denture wearers who take calcium supplements may have an advantage in the long run, particularly if their diet would otherwise be low in calcium." What would be a good source of calcium to take? "Bone meal has a favorable phosphorus:calcium ratio [approximately 1:2], but it does add some additional phosphorus to the diet," Dr. Wical said. "It's all right for people who are presently consuming only moderate levels of phosphorus.

"But for our patients, especially those with high phosphorus intake, we recommend a phosphorus-free calcium and magnesium supplement like dolomite. We've found that patients who are short of the one mineral are almost invariably short of the other as well, so it's a good combination.

"I presently feel very strongly that periodontal patients [as well as denture wearers] should be taking calcium supplements," Dr. Wical told us. "It's the same disease, the same problem. There's no question in my mind that the bone loss is the same—whether you have your teeth or not."

51

Multiple Sclerosis

Calcium is necessary for the proper transmission of messages along the body's nervous system, and at the critical control points where nerves and muscles meet. Calcium plays an important role in muscle contraction, both in relaying the command impulses from nerve to muscle, and in the actual contraction of the muscle itself.

Does a Lack of Calcium Set the Stage for Nerve and Muscle Problems?

Calcium is important not only to the way nerves themselves actually work, but to the way they are put together as well. And some scientists believe that the damage done when nerve cells form without sufficient calcium is the best explanation for the development of the incurable nerve disease, multiple sclerosis, or MS.

Paul Goldberg, Ph.D., a research scientist with the Polaroid Corporation, has found an intriguing correlation between the incidence of multiple sclerosis in different parts of the world and the amount of sunlight that falls on those regions (*International Journal of Environmental Studies,* vol. 6, 1974). As you know, vitamin D is necessary for the proper absorption of calcium, and one of the best sources of vitamin D is sunlight. Dr. Goldberg applied statistical analysis to a number of previous studies and found that the more sunlight an area received, the lower was its rate of multiple sclerosis. The risk of developing multiple sclerosis is highest in the northern latitudes of Europe and North America, and decreases to a low rate as you approach the equator. Interestingly enough, Dr. Goldberg's observation coincides with the fact that zoo animals originating in sunny equatorial regions needed vitamin D supplements to stay healthy in foggy England, which we will discuss in the upcoming chapter, Osteomalacia.

In Switzerland, Dr. Goldberg points out, the rate of multiple sclerosis in various regions differs according to the altitude rather than the latitude. But, as the rate of MS varies with the altitude, so does the amount of shorter wavelength radiation that reaches the ground through the atmosphere. It's the shorter wavelength radiation that causes the formation of vitamin D in the skin. So, Dr. Goldberg believes, the higher you live on the mountainside, the more shortwave radiation you receive, the more vitamin D your skin forms, the more calcium your intestines absorb, and the lower your risk of multiple sclerosis.

MS, a Tie-in with Tooth Decay

William Craelius, Ph.D., a biologist at Lafayette College in Pennsylvania, discovered further evidence of a connection between calcium deficiency and multiple sclerosis when he compared the rates of tooth decay and MS in different populations (*Journal of Epidemiology and Community Health,* vol. 32, no. 3, 1978). When Dr. Craelius looked at statistics for Australia and the United States, the pattern was clear—the higher the rate of tooth decay in a particular area, the higher the number of deaths from multiple sclerosis.

Tooth decay is lower among poor Americans than among the rich, lower among Chinese immigrants to England than among English natives, lower among blacks than whites, lower among men than women. The rate of tooth decay is higher during pregnancy. In all those groups, the incidence of multiple sclerosis seems to follow the incidence of tooth decay. Wherever one is high, so is the other. It's as if the same thing that makes for healthy teeth also protects the body against multiple sclerosis.

Drs. Craelius and Goldberg believe the "X factor" here is calcium. Multiple sclerosis is characterized by destruction of myelin, the fatlike substance that surrounds and protects nerve fibers. Calcium is known to speed the production of one of the key constituents of myelin. That fact, plus the general importance of calcium in holding cells together, led Dr. Goldberg to conclude that a lack of calcium in a child's critical growth years could irreparably weaken the myelin structure, and increase the risk of multiple sclerosis later in life.

Dr. Craelius has done work that supports that hypothesis (*Neuroscience Abstracts*, 1978). "We removed the spinal cord from a chicken embryo," he told us, "and placed it in a medium where it would continue to grow and we could observe its development. We grew the myelin for several weeks in a medium that was only slightly deficient in calcium. When we looked at the myelin under an electron microscope, we thought that it was not as complete, not as mature as it would be normally."

52

Osteomalacia

Weak Bones from a Sunshine Deficiency

Although calcium is the first consideration in building and keeping strong bones, our bodies cannot use calcium without vitamin D. The amount of vitamin D we get determines how much calcium is absorbed and used. When people do not get enough vitamin D, they may experience a decrease in bone density which causes the pain, tenderness and muscular weakness of osteomalacia, or adult rickets.

Vitamin D is rare in foods. Its primary source is sunlight. As much as 84 percent of the vitamin D in the blood is produced from the skin's reaction to the sun, report J. G. Haddad and T. J. Hahn in *Aviation, Space and Environmental Medicine* (June, 1976). The summer sun is an excellent source of vitamin D, but in winter that source is greatly diminished. And a lack of vitamin D helps to lead to a calcium deficiency.

Studies show that bones are weakest and most likely to break in winter and spring. The days are short, sunlight (and hence vitamin D) is scarce, and calcium in the body is low.

In examining thigh fractures in 134 patients, researchers in Leeds, England, found calcium was at its lowest from February to April. The calcium level was highest from August to October. Bone density was least from April to June and greatest from October to December (*Lancet,* July, 1974). So bones are at their best at the end of the summer and weakest at the end of winter.

That problem has been particularly well documented in Great Britain, where sunshine is often sparse. Even monkeys at the London Zoo develop osteomalacia after they leave sunny Africa for the fog-ridden shores of London. Reptiles, birds and mammals from the equator are all subject to vitamin D deficiency at the zoo, and must be given vitamin supplements to remain healthy.

Do you need to take vitamin D supplements? Maybe you do and maybe you don't. A study of 110 children and 11 adults in England produced evidence that in winter, vitamin D levels are determined more by previous exposure to the summer sun than by dietary intake of vitamin D. Levels of vitamin D in the blood were higher in children who had been on vacation at the seashore the previous summer than in those who remained home that year (*British Medical Journal,* January, 1979).

While basking at the seashore may be an excellent way to build up vitamin D in young people and middle-aged adults, older folks may have to rely on supplements the year round for their vitamin D. In a study of 62 elderly patients, ranging in age from 65 to 95, sunlight appeared to have no effect on vitamin D levels in their blood. The levels *did* increase, however, after the patients were given vitamin D supplements. The study concludes that older people may benefit more from taking vitamin D supplements than from depending too much on sunshine (*Gerontology,* vol. 24, 1978). Of course, taking *too much* vitamin D can bring problems of its own, so anyone using that vitamin should be cautious about dosage. The Recommended Dietary Allowance for vitamin D is 400 I.U.

CHAPTER

53

Paget's Disease

New Hope for Pain of Severe Bone Disease

Paget's disease is a rare, painful degeneration of the bones. Doctors don't know what causes Paget's disease, although it sometimes runs in families. Any bone in the body may be affected, but the most common sites are the long bones of the legs, the lower spine, the pelvis and the skull. In the early stages of the disease, calcium is removed from the bones, softening them. In later stages, the bones begin to grow again. But somehow the new growth is distorted. The bones remain soft and become abnormally thick.

Deep, dull, aching bone pain is the most common symptom. If the deformity is in the skull, headache may occur. Deafness and blindness can result if a deformed bone in the skull presses on a nerve. When leg bones are affected, the legs become bowed under the weight of the body.

Until a few years ago, there was no effective treatment for Paget's disease, although doctors tried several drugs and therapies, including x-rays. Then it was discovered that calcitonin, a hormone secreted by the thyroid gland, relieved pain when given by injection. Unfortunately, the treatment is extremely expensive. A year's treatment with calcitonin can cost thousands of dollars. The drug also produces nausea in many people, and may be the cause of allergic reactions.

But now a safe, effective, low-cost treatment has been developed by an Australian physician. Dr. R. A. Evans, Repatriation General Hospital, Concord, New South Wales, successfully used calcium supplements and a combination of medications designed to keep blood levels of calcium high in nine sufferers of Paget's disease.

Searching for an alternative to expensive, hazardous drug treatment, Dr. Evans decided to try to raise the blood level of calcium in people with Paget's disease. To do that, he gave them from 500 to 1,000 milligrams of calcium three times a day between meals, an antacid tablet with meals to keep phosphorus from interfering with calcium absorption, and a drug to keep calcium from being excreted in the urine. The treatment went on for 200 days.

In Dr. Evans's words, "Bone pain subsided or was considerably reduced in eight of the nine patients after a period of 20 to 70 days. . . . Two female patients who were invalids prior to commencing therapy were able to return to light household duties. There were no serious side effects."

Dr. Evans believes the treatment works by stimulating the body's natural secretion of calcitonin, which the thyroid gland secretes when blood levels of calcium rise. Biochemical tests performed by Dr. Evans confirmed that his patients were not merely experiencing a "placebo response" to the treatment.

Dr. Evans goes on to say that "The regimen described here costs approximately 2 percent [of the usual drug treatment] and can be made still cheaper by the use of simpler forms of the drugs. . . . In view of the extremely low cost of this drug combination and its lack of side effects, it is suggested it be considered as a treatment for Paget's disease of bone" (*Australian and New Zealand Journal of Medicine,* June, 1977).

CHAPTER

54

Loss of Taste

"Basically," says Robert Henkin, M.D., "we're the taste and smell doctors."

Dr. Henkin runs the Center for Molecular Nutrition and Sensory Disorders at Georgetown University Medical Center in Washington, D.C. He has been seeing patients with taste and smell problems at the Georgetown clinic since 1975, and before that at the National Institutes of Health in Bethesda, Maryland. Thirty to 40 patients with loss of taste or smell come into his clinic each week.

Those patients are not alone in their complaint, Dr. Henkin told us. "There are probably 10 million people in the United States who have taste problems. That's about as many as have diabetes." One-third of those people, Dr. Henkin believes, may be suffering from zinc deficiency.

The scientific name for taste loss is hypogeusia (pronounced "hi-po-GU-ze-ah"). Actually, Dr. Henkin told us, hypogeusia is not itself a disease. "Hypogeusia is a symptom which occurs in a whole slew of diseases. A lot of people who have a lot of different diseases have hypogeusia. Zinc deficiency is one cause of hypogeusia, but there are many different causes."

For example, we all know taste loss can accompany a bad cold.

Nutritional factors may also be involved in hypogeusia. "Copper deficiency can influence it [taste perception], vitamin A deficiency can influence it, as well as vitamin B_{12} deficiency and vitamin B_6 deficiency," Dr. Henkin said. "It's a very active system, and many vitamins and minerals impinge upon it in different ways.

"In terms of taste and zinc there has been real confusion in the past. The confusion relates to the fact that, by analogy, although a horse is a four-legged animal, all four-legged animals aren't horses. People who are zinc deficient almost uniformly have taste problems, but there are a lot of people who have taste loss who don't have any problem with zinc. Our data suggest that one-third of the people who have taste loss are zinc deficient. Of course, if there are 10 million people in the United States with taste loss, that's still an awful lot of people."

How Zinc Works

In a recent study, Allan Shatzman, Ph.D., a biochemist associated with the taste center, and Dr. Henkin set out to conclusively demonstrate the effects of zinc therapy on taste loss, and the way zinc was working. "This was a lot of work," Dr. Henkin said. "Looking at just one patient requires a lot of effort, which is why we reported only one case, but he is representative of a number of cases we've handled."

Each day of the study, samples of the patient's saliva were collected from the parotid gland (which secretes the majority of the protein found in saliva) and analyzed for their content of zinc and gustin. "Gustin is a salivary protein," Dr. Henkin explained, "the major zinc-containing protein in saliva. Seventy-five to 80 percent of the zinc in saliva is bound to this protein."

The patient's saliva was compared with saliva from normal, healthy people. Both the healthy saliva and the saliva taken from the patient with taste loss were first broken down into separate components, or fractions, as the scientists call them, of the whole saliva from the parotid gland. "In normal people, and with patients with hypogeusia, all these fractions are about the same, except for fraction II," Dr. Shatzman told us. "Fraction II is the fraction of saliva that contains gustin, the zinc-containing protein. We could clearly see that something was going on in fraction II of the saliva."

While the zinc content of all the saliva of patients with taste loss may be about half the normal amount, the deficiency is particularly acute in fraction II of the saliva. There the levels of gustin and zinc are as low as *one-fifth* of normal. All signs point to gustin, and the zinc it contains, as crucial factors in normal taste.

That suspicion was confirmed when the test patient was given zinc supplements. As the treatment with zinc went on, the levels of zinc and gustin in the patient's saliva increased, and his ability to taste improved dramatically. By the ninth day of treatment the zinc and gustin levels had reached a peak, and taste returned to normal several days later.

"The patient reached a maximum ability to taste on day 12," Dr. Shatzman told us. "The return to normal taste followed by 3 days the return to normal biochemistry in the saliva. That makes sense if you believe gustin has something to do with maintaining normal taste buds, because you have to have a return to normal taste bud anatomy and biochemistry before you can have normal taste. It makes sense that there's a lag period."

Dr. Henkin believes that while this evidence indicates that zinc works to maintain the sense of taste directly in the mouth, zinc may also affect taste centers in the brain where information from taste buds is received and processed. However, he said, "the majority of patients we see who have taste problems have biochemical problems that are influenced by changes in saliva or the taste buds directly, not in the brain."

Though a change in diet helps correct the taste problems of many of Dr. Henkin's patients, he believes that the original cause of their problems is not an inadequate diet but the way they absorb the food they eat. "These people are probably taking in the same amount of zinc as you or I, but they don't absorb it properly," he told us. Unpredictable idiosyncrasies in the way their bodies work require that they take in more zinc than others.

Pregnant Women Need More Zinc

When normal foods or beverages begin to taste or smell unpleasant to a pregnant woman, it could indicate an increased loss of zinc from the body. Zinc is transferred to the fetus in substantial amounts. Copper is also transferred, but to a lesser degree. Deficiency in these minerals can cause symptoms ranging from cravings to loss of appetite, changes in eating habits, and unpleasant taste and smell sensations in familiar (and ordinarily acceptable) foods and beverages. All this explains why the Recommended Dietary Allowance (RDA) of zinc for pregnant women is now set at 25 milligrams daily, nearly 50 percent higher than for nonpregnant women. It is sometimes startling how quickly these abnormal sensations are corrected by appropriate supplements of the mineral.

Dull Taste Means Bad Diet?

Even considered in terms of the government's Recommended Dietary Allowances, which set the adult zinc requirement at 15 milligrams a day, great portions of the American population are not getting enough zinc to meet their needs. The typical American is believed to consume between 10 and 15 milligrams of zinc a day. That means the typical American is marginally zinc deficient, even by the government's low standards. Among older people, zinc intake is often less than two-thirds of the RDA. Older people, not surprisingly, also commonly suffer taste loss.

What this wholesale deadening of the nation's taste buds does to our cuisine is anyone's guess. Would it be harder for people to wolf down fast foods if they could actually taste what they were eating? Are some people's palates so dull that they *can't* do anything more subtle than distinguish between pretzels and cotton candy? Is that why blatant seasonings like salt and sugar dominate our preparation of food?

Could be. Zinc has been tested recently on ordinary, "healthy" people who show no overt signs of zinc deficiency, with some interesting results. A study of young women reviewed their zinc status by analyzing their blood, saliva, hair and diet. Their zinc status was judged to be normal, and they were given different concentrations of zinc supplements. There was no change in the women's ability to detect three of the four basic tastes—sourness, bitterness and saltiness. But for women receiving 50 milligrams of zinc a day, there was a significant increase in their ability to taste sweetness (*Federation Proceedings,* March 1, 1980, abstract no. 2038).

Another study recorded an improvement in older people's ability to taste sweetness with zinc supplementation, plus an improvement in the ability to taste salt. But the improvements were not statistically significant—perhaps, the authors of the study speculated, because the people were receiving only 15 milligrams of zinc supplements a day (*American Journal of Clinical Nutrition,* April, 1978).

In any case, the interesting thing about those two studies is the improvement in the ability to taste sweets recorded in both. The more sensitive you are to sweetness, the less sugar you need to eat to achieve the same taste. Getting adequate zinc might be one way to cut back our intake of sugar.

That means eating foods like eggs, fish, green beans, lima beans, nuts and whole grain products, all good sources of zinc. It means taking zinc supplements if necessary. Eating, after all, was meant to be one of the true pleasures of life, not just something you do after the evening news and before prime time TV. Without sharp taste, good, healthy, enjoyable eating is impossible.

55

Prostate
Trouble

Among men 40 years of age and over, some kind of prostate problem is nearly epidemic—an estimated 12 million men in the United States alone can attest to that personally. Among American men over 60, the likelihood of suffering from an enlarged prostate gland is even greater, increasing to nearly 95 percent by age 85. And perhaps most disturbing is the increasing rise in deaths from prostate cancer—over 18,000 American men each year.

What is this troublesome gland and why is it such a problem?

The prostate gland is an accessory organ of the male reproductive system, whose only known function is to produce the lubricating fluid that transports sperm cells out of the body. (That's why the prostate has been proverbially associated with sex.) The gland rests just below the bladder and completely surrounds the bladder's narrow neck called the urethra, the tube that moves liquid waste out of the body. Healthy, the prostate is about the size of a walnut. Diseased, it grows and can reach the size of an orange.

That's the essential problem in the most common kind of prostate trouble—benign prostate hypertrophy (BPH for short), which means simply a noncancerous enlargement of the prostate. Picture the urethra as a garden hose. The enlarged prostate can pinch off the urethra, interfering with urination. The symptoms are increased need to urinate, a burning pain, false starts, dribbling and inability to void the bladder.

The other two major kinds of prostate trouble—prostatitis, an inflammation of the prostate, and prostate cancer—usually show the same symptoms.

All these kinds of prostate trouble can be treated. Antibiotic therapy for bacterial prostatitis, and surgical removal of all or part of the prostate for both BPH and prostate cancer are the commonest treatments. These are still the only reliably tested treatments for the major prostate diseases. Yet each has its difficulties, risks and failures. So it's well worth considering what can be done to *prevent* prostate trouble before it starts. Fortunately, there are several promising leads.

Zinc, Fat and the Prostate

The prostate wasn't always so troublesome. According to one prostate researcher, Erik Ask-Upmark, M.D., of the department of medicine at Sweden's University of Uppsala, prostate disease "represents a relatively new pathologic entity. When I was studying medicine, one heard of its existence, but chiefly as a . . . curiosity" (*Grana Palynologica*, vol. 2, no. 2, 1960). Apparently, in our century some basic change has come about that has made alarmingly common what was once a rare disease. There is evidence to indicate that this basic change has to do with the way we Westerners now eat.

For one, high-fat diets may be to blame for BPH. That's the indication of studies by Carl P. Schaffner, Ph.D., professor of microbial chemistry at Rutgers University. Man's best friend shares man's prostate problem, and Dr. Schaffner discovered that by reducing cholesterol levels in aged dogs, he was also able to reduce the size of the animals' enlarged prostates (*Proceedings of the National Academy of Sciences,* August, 1968).

Another study, reported to the American Urological Association in 1976, using autopsied *human* prostates, corroborates the possibly harmful effect of high cholesterol levels on prostate disease. Camille Mallouh, M.D., chief of urology at Metropolitan Hospital, New York, examined 100 prostates from men of all ages and found an 80 percent higher cholesterol content in prostates with BPH.

There may be a link between BPH and prostate cancer. In a study involving almost 1,200 case histories, researchers from the department of epidemiology at Johns Hopkins University and the department of biostatistics at Roswell Park Memorial Institute discovered an almost four times greater risk for prostate cancer among cases of BPH. They estimate that in countries where males have long life expectancies, 43 percent of the cases of prostate cancer could be attributed to BPH (*Lancet,* July 20, 1974).

Risk from Fatty Foods

The link between BPH and prostate cancer may involve high fat levels in our food. Observing that rural, black South Africans—who eat a low-fat, whole food diet—are a low-risk group for prostate cancer, Peter Hill, Ph.D., of the American Health Foundation in New York City, conducted a study to test whether diet was responsible for their relative immunity.

Dr. Hill and his associates placed a group of black South African volunteers on a typical Western diet with lots of fats and meats. At the same time, a group of North American volunteers, blacks and whites, were put on a low-fat diet. To determine the potential effect of these diets on inducing prostate cancer, Dr. Hill tested for diet-induced hormonal changes that are associated with the development of prostate cancer.

"By changing diet, you can change hormonal metabolism," explains Dr. Hill, "and prostatic cancer seems to be a hormonally associated disease."

After three weeks, Dr. Hill found that the South Africans eating the Western diet were excreting notably more hormones, while the reverse occurred with the North Americans eating the low-fat diet. The metabolic profile of the North Americans now resembled that of the low-risk group (*Cancer Research,* December, 1979).

"This study is a preliminary indication that a low-fat diet is one of the factors that can lower the risk of prostatic cancer," Dr. Hill told us. "By reducing total calorie intake, and substituting fruit and vegetable calories for animal calories, a high-risk prostatic cancer group was switched to a low-risk one."

Zinc for Prostate Problems

But if those who suffer from prostate diseases have too much fat in their diets, one nutrient they apparently have too little of is zinc.

That zinc is somehow essential to the health of the prostate gland has been known for about 50 years. Normally, there is an extraordinary concentration of zinc in healthy human prostatic fluid (the fluid that transports sperm cells)—seven milligrams per gram of fluid. But zinc is also one of the nutrients hardest hit by food processing.

A cooperative study by the Chicago Medical School, Cook County Hospital, Hektoen Institute for Medical Research and Mt. Sinai Medical Center in Chicago checked prostate zinc levels in 265 healthy men of various ages. Researchers found that 7 percent of the men had low prostate and semen zinc levels, and that 30 percent more were borderline cases. In other words, more than 1 out of every 3 men didn't have an adequate amount of zinc in the prostate.

An extensive study led by Irving M. Bush, M.D., of Chicago's Cook County Hospital, has dramatically shown the healthy prostate's reliance on zinc. Dr. Bush and his associates discovered that zinc levels drop when disease strikes the gland. They found that patients with chronic prostatitis generally suffer from low levels of zinc in both prostate and semen. And they found that patients with prostate cancer also have similar low zinc levels.

Encouraged by these findings, Dr. Bush started treating 755 patients suffering from various prostate complaints with zinc supplements. In 1974 at a national convention of the American Medical Association, he reported his results.

Symptoms Were Relieved

Nineteen patients with BPH received 34 milligrams of oral zinc a day for two months and were then placed on a long-term program of 11 to 23 milligrams daily. Lab tests revealed gains in semen levels of the mineral. But more important, all 19 patients reported an easing of the painful symptoms and, on examination, all but 5 of them did in fact show a decrease in prostate size.

The effect of zinc therapy on patients suffering from infectious prostatitis is even more impressive. Two hundred patients were given between 11 and 34 milligrams of zinc per day for up to 16 weeks. They all registered higher semen levels of zinc. And 70 percent reported relief of their symptoms.

Although, according to Dr. Bush, zinc therapy isn't ready to replace the conventional treatments of most prostate disorders, such evidence does help explain why so many who've taken zinc have seemingly been helped.

"For 23 years I was afflicted with chronic prostatitis, requiring a visit to a urologist every five weeks for a prostate massage," a Florida man told us.

Then he tried zinc supplements. "I started taking 50 milligrams a day for a month, then dropped to 20 milligrams a day ever since. In about three months the inflammation was gone, and it was apparent that a developing hypertrophy [enlargement] was reversing itself, and continued on that course for about a year.

"I haven't had to see a urologist in over two years, and then only for a check to make sure all was well. The doctor agreed that he had heard about the research on zinc's effectiveness—but it had never occurred to him to tell me about it!"

Combining adequate amounts of zinc with a low-fat, high-fiber diet certainly can't hurt and might very well help men who are entering the high-risk age for prostate problems. With prostate diseases, as with all disease, prevention is undoubtedly the best policy.

CHAPTER

56

Impotence

Oysters don't seem to have much in common with a rhinoceros horn or bird's nest soup. Yet, legendary folklore has it that all three are aphrodisiacs able to put a man's sex drive in high gear.

We can't vouch for the latter two remedies. But there does appear to be a sound scientific basis for the shellfish's reputation. Oysters, though not all loaded with pearls, mind you, are filled with something else that just might add a new luster to your love life.

That something is zinc, recently recognized for its key role in sexual development. Zinc deficiency will likely impair sexual growth and maturation, because this mineral appears to be essential for the metabolism of a primary male hormone called testosterone.

Sex Glands Depend on Zinc

About 15 years ago, a group of adolescent boys in Egypt, who were both physically and sexually retarded, were found to have poor diets in general, and to be specifically deficient in iron and zinc. When fed a good diet, the youths grew an average of two inches a year. Those who received a good diet plus iron supplements grew about three inches. Those who also received zinc grew *five* inches. But more to our point, with zinc, sexual maturity developed much more rapidly. A few years later, in Iran, a similar group of youths were also found to respond much better to a good diet plus zinc than to a good diet alone, developing sexual maturity more than three times as quickly.

For some years, these results seemed to be little more than medical curiosities. After all, how many sexually retarded dwarfs do you know?

It *was* known that there's a very high concentration of zinc in the male sexual organs, including the prostate gland. But there was a kind of assumption that if the organs had already developed in a physically normal manner, there was nothing much that zinc could do, regardless of how these organs performed.

That notion suddenly changed as recently as 1977. By that year, as a result of earlier federal legislation providing funds to pay for lifesaving dialysis for kidney patients, doctors already knew that in the process of having their blood artificially cleansed, these kidney patients developed various side effects. One of the side effects experienced by some dialysis patients is impotence. The cause for this wasn't known, but it was assumed that it was psychological in nature. At the same time, it was known that many dialysis patients are deficient in zinc. But the connection between zinc deficiency and impotence went unappreciated until a team of doctors at the Veterans Administration Hospital in Washington, D.C., began to put supplemental zinc in the dialysis "bath" which treats the blood of kidney patients. They discovered that the sexual functioning of patients who had been impotent improved dramatically—in a matter of a few weeks.

When they *stopped* putting extra zinc into the blood of these patients, their sexual functioning withered, only to return once more when zinc was again provided.

In further work, subsequently reported in *Lancet* (October, 1977), Lucy Antoniou, M.D., and her colleagues at the Veterans Administration Hospital found that just over half of all the dialysis patients with impotence they treated responded well to zinc therapy.

Now, here's where zinc really makes you think. To begin with, Dr. Antoniou has now found that even some dialysis patients who have relatively *normal* levels of zinc in their blood plasma *still* respond favorably to zinc therapy. Second, while most people think of testosterone as being the chief hormone involved in male potency, it now seems that the biologically active metabolite of testosterone, called dihydrotestosterone (DHT), is the critical factor so far as zinc is concerned. Dr. Antoniou found that only patients with low levels of DHT responded to zinc therapy.

Further, in every case where there was a low level of this "active" form of testosterone, zinc did the trick.

But when you get right down to it, says Dr. Antoniou, "The real sign of zinc deficiency is a response to supplementation" (*Sexual Medicine Today,* November, 1978). In other words, in purely practical terms, the only way to discover if someone needs more zinc is to give it to him or her and see what happens.

A similar study was conducted recently at the Veterans Administration Hospital in Allen Park, Michigan.

"It's a well-known fact that 70 percent of renal patients do have some degree of impotence," says Sudesh Mahajan, M.D., chief of nephrology at the Hospital and kidney specialist at Wayne State University School of Medicine.

But the bright side is that zinc supplementation has dramatically reversed these sexual woes in a group of kidney dialysis patients. The 20 subjects, aged 28 to 65, require machines—artificial replacements for their disabled kidneys—to filter impurities from the blood. All initially had low sperm counts and testosterone levels. During the double-blind study, no one knew which 10 men received the placebo or which 10 men got 50 milligrams of zinc a day.

After a year, every zinc-treated man showed biochemical improvements and reported restored potency. "In some cases," Dr. Mahajan told us, "changes occurred in just six weeks. Needless to say, their wives and girlfriends were happy."

The placebo-fed group, in contrast, could hardly boast of a new boost in their life. Their sex drives never accelerated, and impotency remained a problem. Furthermore, their low sperm counts and testosterone levels never perked up.

Can Zinc Help "Ordinary" Impotence?

While all this is most hopeful for kidney patients with a sexual problem, the big question is whether or not zinc therapy can do anything for men who are impotent, or partially so, and who are otherwise in reasonably good health. To put it another way, after physical disease has been ruled out, is it necessary to assume that the impotent man must be suffering from a psychological problem—or perhaps just "age"? Is it possible that nutrition could be involved?

Strangely, the answer is that no one seems to know. Not yet, anyway. But one person willing to speculate on the question is Ananda S. Prasad, M.D., Ph.D., professor of medicine and chief of hematology at the Wayne State University School of Medicine in Detroit. Dr. Prasad, a longtime pioneer in zinc research, suggests that it is probably worthwhile for physicians to try zinc therapy in cases where other causes of impotence have been ruled out, and where low levels of zinc are found in the patient. He mentions 20 milligrams or 30 milligrams of zinc a day as a reasonable and perfectly safe level.

Add Zing to Your Love Life with Zinc

It doesn't require a *severe* zinc deficiency to play havoc with sexual vigor. Even men who are only *slightly* zinc deficient are asking for trouble.

"Sexual dysfunction could be present in the marginal cases because the testes seem to be very sensitive to zinc," notes Dr. Prasad.

To test this hypothesis, Dr. Prasad and his colleagues induced mild zinc deficiencies through dietary manipulations in five healthy men aged 51 to 65. By eating controlled meals, the subjects actually lost about one milligram of zinc a day from their bodies. During a six-month period, sperm counts dropped in four out of five men. Testosterone levels dropped in all five men.

In three men, the sperm counts plummeted below the point of technical sterility, says Ali A. Abbasi, M.D., an endocrinologist at the Veterans Administration Medical Center in Allen Park, Michigan. And while admittedly "very subjective," the subjects complained of diminished sexual desire when fed the zinc-restricted diet, according to Parviz Rabbani, Ph.D., a nutritional biochemist working with Dr. Prasad.

After the volunteers resumed standard meals and were fortified with 30 milligrams of zinc a day, they returned to normal within 16 to 20 weeks.

However, a question every man might be wondering is: Could I be even moderately zinc deficient? Because smoking, alcohol, infections and medications can winnow away zinc reserves, Dr. Rabbani suspects marginal zinc insufficiencies may be commonplace.

Zinc-Blocking Factors

"Heavy smokers in particular might need more zinc," he told us. "The cadmium (a toxic heavy metal) in smoke interferes with zinc metabolism and can accumulate in the testicles. Therefore one might suspect there is an increased demand for zinc."

So, too, he denounces alcohol as one of the "most dangerous ingredients" we consume. Not only does abuse cause the body to excrete too much zinc, but it invites tippling a few too many at the expense of good eating habits.

Anxiety, maintains Dr. Rabbani, may also upset sound nutritional regimens. And if too much zinc is subtracted from your diet, that could mean a big minus in your sex life. "Eating badly," cautions Dr. Rabbani, "could very well be the reason for impotence."

Other Glands Need Zinc

According to Carl C. Pfeiffer, M.D., Ph.D., head of the Brain Bio Center in Princeton, New Jersey, insufficient zinc can lead to a greatly reduced sperm count, improper development of the penis and testes in young males, and prostate problems. (The prostate supplies the launching fluid for sperm during orgasm.)

Along the same lines, Dr. Pfeiffer has found zinc may contribute to the "glint in the eye of the more aggressive male" because both the retina and the prostate are exceedingly high in zinc content. He's also discovered large amounts of zinc in the pineal and hippocampus glands in the brain. The pineal gland is directly linked to sex drive, while the hippocampus controls emotions.

"With this knowledge," he contends, "we still can't say that anyone's sex life would be better with excess zinc." Still, he suggests *adequate* zinc levels are needed for normal sexual activity and reproduction.

Dr. Prasad recommends that once the physician has ruled out most organic and psychological causes of impotence, plasma zinc levels should be checked. If a zinc deficiency *does* exist, the doctor can begin treating it with 20 to 30 milligrams of zinc daily for six months to a year.

"One nice thing about this deficiency," he says, "is that it is correctable."

No need to overdo it, though. And certainly don't start by gorging yourself on oysters. Like other shellfish, oysters have the ability to concentrate dangerous levels of toxic microorganisms and other pollutants if they are harvested in polluted waters. But other good (and safe) zinc sources to rely on include liver and other meats, eggs, nuts, beans and zinc supplements.

CHAPTER

57

Kidney Stones

Recurrent calcium oxalate stones are the most common kidney stones plaguing the Western world. They represent about 70 percent of all kidney stones and may cause pain, fever, obstruction of the urinary passageway, infection and bloody urine.

In people who tend to develop that type of kidney stone, calcium and oxalic acid (both normal substances in urine) combine to form relatively insoluble crystals called oxalate. Although most stones are as hard as rocks and round, some are soft, white, chalky and many-pointed in shape. They may be the size of a grain of sand, small enough to be passed out in the urine, or the size of a walnut, large enough to obstruct the urinary passages. The pain they may cause is beyond description—severe enough to leave you doubled over in agony.

More Magnesium, Less Sugar
to Help Prevent Kidney Stones

Now, new evidence supports earlier findings that magnesium helps prevent the formation of certain kidney stones. When 67 patients who were stone formers were given 500 milligrams of magnesium hydroxide daily, they had a reduced rate of stone recurrence, Sverker Ljunghall and colleagues at the University Hospital in Uppsala, Sweden, found. (Five hundred milligrams of magnesium hydroxide equals approximately 200 milligrams of magnesium.) These findings suggest that magnesium lessens the chance of stone formation, the scientists reported during a conference of the American College of Nutrition in St. Louis, in June, 1979.

Actually, the new findings simply confirm clinical work with magnesium by Stanley N. Gershoff, Ph.D., director of the Nutrition Institute, Tufts University, Medford, Massachusetts, and Edwin L. Prien, Sr., M.D., urologist and emeritus member of the Newton-Wellesley Hospital, Newton, Massachusetts. Over a period of more than 15 years, these researchers, in cooperation with 64 other doctors from different regions of the United States, studied several groups of patients.

One group consisted of 149 patients who had at least 1 stone per year for the 5 years prior to time of treatment. Together, they had more than 871 stones during those preceding 4 or 5 years. However, in the next 4½ to 6 years, only 17 of the 149 patients developed stones while taking magnesium and vitamin B₆ supplements. In those 17, just 71 stones formed. That means 89 percent of the stone formers were symptom-free while taking magnesium, which appears to keep oxalic acid dissolved in urine, according to Drs. Gershoff and Prien (*Journal of Urology,* October, 1974).

It's also interesting to note that English researchers recently found that diets high in refined carbohydrates may actually *encourage* the formation of kidney stones. During a period of one month, the researchers fed a diet of low, normal or high levels of carbohydrates to 19 healthy young males. Reporting their findings in the *British Journal of Urology* (vol. 50, 1978), the researchers concluded, "There is the likelihood that a dietary structure which includes significant amounts of sugar or sugar products will increase the risk of calcium stone formation."

CHAPTER

58

Migraine Headache

Migraine headache. Not the garden-variety throbber, but the kind where the side of your head feels as if someone is walloping you with an iron skillet. Or a red-hot poker. Tears run down your cheek. You feel sick, helpless—and secretly wish a neurosurgeon would walk in and do an instant lobotomy.

Vasodilation—sudden widening of blood vessels—in the head are behind it all. Certain factors, ranging from stress to food chemicals to a change in the weather, seem to cause cerebral blood arteries to sometimes constrict and then immediately expand. Painful and distended blood vessels pressing against the nerves of the brain are what make migraine headaches the scourge they are. Sometimes you can actually feel the rush of blood into the cerebral arteries that tells you a migraine is on the way.

Precipitating factors are many. Certain foods are known migraine triggers in many people—cheese and chocolate are among the worst.

Alcohol (especially red wine) can do it. So can too much caffeine. (Or too little, as in the case of caffeine withdrawal headaches.) Or food additives, such as nitrites and nitrates (in ham, hot dogs and bacon) or MSG (monosodium glutamate, used widely in Chinese restaurants). Then there are everyday stresses and annoyances. A missed meal. A parking ticket. Cigarette smoke. Even the hormonal changes behind menstruation in some women.

For many poor souls, migraine attacks are a way of life, at times making them so ill they can't eat, sleep or work. And the triggering factors vary from one person to another. For relief, aspirin is the old standby. So are beta-blocking drugs, which prevent expansion of blood vessels. Relaxation, exercise, biofeedback, massage and acupuncture may be just as helpful, without the questionable or unpleasant side effects of drugs. And— needless to say—removing the noxious factor, whenever possible, is the best route. For some people, a low-salt diet may be the answer.

Salty Foods Vanish, Migraines Disappear

Few people are aware of it, but plain old salt—especially on an empty stomach—can trigger a migraine, according to a report by John B. Brainard, M.D., a surgeon from St. Paul, Minnesota. And avoiding a barrage of salt, it seems, removes a potent cause of migraine for some. Twelve of Dr. Brainard's patients—all of whom had suffered migraine attacks for years—were asked to avoid all other known precipitating factors and to record their incidence of migraine headaches before and after salt restriction. That went on for six months.

Specifically, salt restriction in this case meant avoiding all salted snack foods, such as pretzels, salted nuts and potato chips. Results were considered excellent if the patient was then free of migraine, good if he or she suffered fewer attacks than before, and poor if there was no change.

Most (10 out of 12) responded favorably. A few found glorious and dramatic relief, stating the migraine was wiped out of their lives—forever, presumably. For the 2 who responded poorly, Dr. Brainard suggests that sudden salt load was probably not a triggering device after all. Or that they had unknowingly run up against another migraine-provoking substance.

"The ubiquity of highly salted snack foods in our society may contribute to the presence of migraine," says Dr. Brainard. He explains, "The patients in this study had typical migraine, often being awakened by headaches in the night. The relief obtained suggests that sodium load requires several hours to precipitate a migraine. It has not been appreciated that the sudden salt load of a handful of salted nuts or potato chips, particularly if taken on an empty stomach, can cause severe migraine 6 to 12 hours later. The reason for the lag period is unknown" (*Minnesota Medicine,* April, 1976).

Salt-free snacking is not as impossible as it may sound. Unsalted nuts, crackers—and even potato chips, if you *must* have them—aren't as hard to find as they used to be. Better yet, try unsalted sunflower seeds. Or roast your own pumpkin seeds.

Try Herbs Instead of Salt

Can you get rid of your migraine and still enjoy your meals? How do you make your food tasty without adding salt? By substitution. Cultivate the use of herbs and enjoy a real taste adventure. Are you accustomed to salting your eggs? Try a light sprinkling of dill or chopped chives. You'll enjoy the zesty flavor. Have you been putting salt on sliced tomatoes? Try basil. Celery, spinach, beets, kale and Swiss chard have their own built-in sodium content; they don't need any more.

Experiment with a few herbs, and after a while you'll probably forget you ever needed salt. Try allspice, caraway, chili powder, curry, ginger, mustard seed, peppermint, coriander, tarragon, and lemon or lime juice. For a new taste in asparagus, sprinkle the stalks and tips with nutmeg before serving. Cucumbers take on a new flavor dimension when sliced very thin and marinated in tarragon vinegar before serving. For an exciting and exotic dish, try eggplant baked with tomatoes, and seasoned with a bay leaf and oregano. It's low-calorie and satisfying, too. Try green beans seasoned with nutmeg or savory; onions boiled with cloves and thyme, or unsalted veal with chopped or powdered mint.

59

Tics, Tremors and Twitches

The small muscles under your eye jump and quiver—a tic. An old man's hand shakes as he picks up a glass of water—a tremor. You begin to fall asleep, but your thigh jerks and jolts you awake—a twitch.

Tic, tremor or twitch. In each case, the muscles receive a garbled message about how to perform. Many diseases and conditions can send such a message. But one very common cause of these muscular mistakes is nutritional—a deficiency of potassium or magnesium. Why those minerals?

The answer is found at the neuromuscular junction, the meeting place between nervous system and muscle. At that junction, electrical impulses pass from the nerves into a muscle and control its movement. The impulses are conducted by minerals, but if those minerals are out of balance—if there's too little potassium, for instance—then too much electricity gets through. Your muscle is zapped.

"Potassium lack is a common nutritional deficiency," said Richard Kunin, M.D., a psychiatrist from San Francisco and author of *Mega-Nutrition* (McGraw-Hill, 1980).

And, said George Mitchell, M.D., from Washington, D.C., "Giving potassium is one part of a nutritional approach to solve a muscular disorder such as a tic or twitch.

"Potassium deficiency is a particularly big problem among people who regularly drink cola, tea or coffee," Dr. Mitchell told us. "Those liquids work like a diuretic and wash potassium out of the body."

And Dr. Kunin told us how a potassium deficiency can also be caused by a sugary diet. "When you ingest too much sugar, the body has to convert it into a chemical called glycogen and store it, and this process uses up a great deal of potassium," he said. "The end result may be a twitch or tic."

Magnesium and Potassium Calm Stuttering Muscles

If you have a potassium deficiency, you're probably low on magnesium, too.

"People are commonly deficient in both potassium and magnesium," said Dr. Kunin. "I find that a tremor in the tongue or the arms or legs often clears up when I give a person magnesium."

"Magnesium deficiency is a cause of a lot of muscular problems because one of its functions is to relax muscles," said Dr. Mitchell.

"Muscle jerks are often very easily helped with something as simple as dolomite," said Donald Thompson, M.D., from Morristown, Tennessee. "Our society tends toward a deficiency in magnesium—it's the magnesium in dolomite that makes it such a valuable substance."

"I've treated several patients who had tics or tremors with dolomite, and their symptoms cleared up," said Arnold Brenner, M.D., from Randallstown, Maryland.

"In each case I used one to two teaspoons a day. Analysis of their hair showed low magnesium levels, so it is apparently the magnesium portion of the dolomite that was effective in these individuals," he said.

"Tremors sometimes respond to magnesium and high levels of B complex vitamins," said Warren M. Levin, M.D., from New York City.

B Complex Vitamins Work with Minerals

Dr. Levin—and many of the other physicians we talked to—uses B complex vitamins because some tremors are caused by a disorder in the central nervous system. For the health of the central nervous system, B complex vitamins are a must.

"The B complex vitamins work on the central nervous system," said Dr. Kunin. "B$_6$, for example, is a natural tranquilizer. Niacin inhibits chemical activity in the brain that may cause tremors."

"I get some results clearing up tremors using vitamin B$_{12}$," said John Siegel, M.D., from Virginia, Minnesota.

Dr. Mitchell also treats tremors with B complex. "B$_6$ is especially important," he said, "because it plays a role in the body's utilization of magnesium." But, he points out, "a person with a tremor is usually deficient in several of the B vitamins."

Too much lead

A tremor isn't always caused by what's lacking. It can also be caused by an excess—of lead.

"A number of patients with tremors have higher than average lead levels—levels close to the toxic range," said Howard Lutz, M.D., of the Institute of Preventive Medicine in Washington, D.C.

"But if we give those people calcium or zinc, the minerals force much of the lead out of the body, and the tremor is cleared up."

Dr. Lutz also believes that many tremors are caused by foods or chemicals to which a person is allergic.

"If we relieve the allergic stress, tremors will go away in 50 percent of the cases," he said. "The other 50 percent will have a less marked tremor or a tremor that occurs less frequently."

Drugs Can Cause Tremors

To avoid chemical stress that may cause a tic, tremor or twitch, stay away from unnecessary drugs.

"When I see an elderly person who has a tremor, the first thing I do is check his medication," said Frederick Klenner, M.D., of Reidsville, North Carolina. "Many tranquilizers can cause tremors. If the medication is discontinued, the tremor clears up. And very few of these people really need tranquilizers, anyway."

A tranquilizerlike ingredient in antihistamines may also cause a tic, tremor or twitch. An article in a medical journal describes a woman who used antihistamines regularly and developed twitches and tremors in her face. When she stopped using the medication, her condition improved (*New England Journal of Medicine,* September 4, 1975).

And another medical journal reports a case of 20 hyperactive children who developed tics from their medication (*Journal of the American Medical Association,* March 29, 1976).

But, as we said earlier, tics, tremors and twitches can have many causes—not all of them treatable by nutritional supplements and a more natural lifestyle.

"If you don't get rid of the problem with your own treatment, then consult a doctor and have him check you out for further disturbances," said Dr. Kunin.

Better yet, prevent the problem.

"Nutritional supplements and a natural diet work together to chemically balance the body," said Dr. Mitchell. "A balanced body is a healthy body."

And that means a body free of tics, tremors and twitches.

PART
VI

MEETING YOUR PERSONAL MINERAL NEEDS

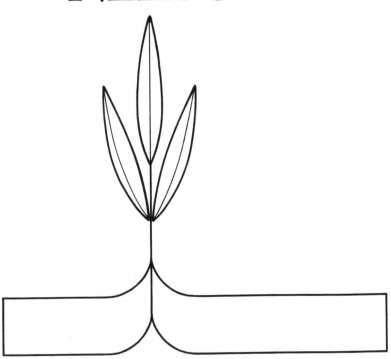

CHAPTER

60

The RDAs: What the Recommended Dietary Allowances Mean to You

Our bodies are amazingly adaptive. Unlike an electrical appliance, which refuses to run at all if its plug is pulled, the body can continue functioning on stored nutrients during times of short supply. In an earlier chapter, we explained how our bodies break down food and store energy for day-long use, so we don't have to eat round the clock. When it comes to minerals, the body is comparably adaptive—to a point. We automatically excrete less according to our intake and needs. At the same time, we can use some of what's been held in storage.

The book *Recommended Dietary Allowances* (9th Edition, National Academy of Sciences, 1980) gives an unabridged discussion of dietary requirements for minerals as well as protein, vitamins and other nutrients. For further reading, check your local or school library for a copy, or write to: Office of Publications, National Academy of Sciences, 2101 Constitution Avenue, N.W., Washington, D.C. 20418.

TABLE 41 ## Recommended Dietary Allowances for Minerals

Recommended Daily Dietary Allowances

	Age (years)	Weight (pounds)	Height (inches)	Calcium (milligrams)	
Infants	0-6 months	13	24	360	
	6 months- 1 year	20	28	540	
Children	1-3	29	35	800	
	4-6	44	44	800	
	7-10	62	52	800	
Males	11-14	99	5' 2''	1,200	
	15-18	145	5' 9''	1,200	
	19-22	154	5'10''	800	
	23-50	154	5'10''	800	
	51+	154	5'10''	800	
Females	11-14	101	5' 2''	1,200	
	15-18	120	5' 4''	1,200	
	19-22	120	5' 4''	800	
	23-50	120	5' 4''	800	
	51+	120	5' 4''	800	
Pregnant				+400	
Lactating				+400	

Estimated Safe and Adequate Daily Dietary Intakes

	Age (years)	Sodium (milligrams)	Potassium (milligrams)	Chloride (milligrams)	
Infants	0-6 months	115- 350	350- 925	275- 700	
	6 months- 1 year	250- 750	425-1,275	400-1,200	
Children and Adolescents	1-3	325- 975	550-1,650	500-1,500	
	4-6	450-1,350	775-2,325	700-2,100	
	7-10	600-1,800	1,000-3,000	925-2,775	
	11+	900-2,700	1,525-4,575	1,400-1,200	
Adults		1,100-3,300	1,875-5,625	1,700-5,100	

SOURCE: Reprinted from *Recommended Dietary Allowances*, 9th ed., 1980, with the permission of the National Academy of Sciences, Washington, D.C.

Phosphorus (milligrams)	Magnesium (milligrams)	Iron (milligrams)	Zinc (milligrams)	Iodine (micrograms)
240	50	10	3	40
360	70	15	5	50
800	150	15	10	70
800	200	10	10	90
800	250	10	10	120
1,200	350	18	15	150
1,200	400	18	15	150
800	350	10	15	150
800	350	10	15	150
800	350	10	15	150
1,200	300	18	15	150
1,200	300	18	15	150
800	300	18	15	150
800	300	18	15	150
800	300	10	15	150
+400	+150	30-60	+5	+25
+400	+150	30-60	+10	+50

Copper (milligrams)	Manganese (milligrams)	Fluoride (milligrams)	Chromium (milligrams)	Selenium (milligrams)	Molybdenum (milligrams)
0.5-0.7	0.5-0.7	.01-.05	0.01-0.04	0.01-0.04	0.03-0.06
0.7-1.0	0.7-1.0	0.2-1.0	0.02-0.06	0.02-0.06	0.04-0.08
1.0-1.5	1.0-1.5	0.5-1.5	0.02-0.08	0.02-0.08	0.05-0.10
1.5-2.0	1.5-2.0	1.0-2.5	0.03-0.12	0.03-0.12	0.06-0.15
2.0-2.5	2.0-3.0	1.5-2.5	0.05-0.2	0.05-0.2	0.15-0.30
2.0-3.0	2.5-5.0	1.5-2.5	0.05-0.2	0.05-0.2	0.15-0.50
2.0-3.0	2.5-5.0	1.5-4.0	0.05-0.2	0.05-0.2	0.15-0.50

But our bodies prefer that we replenish minerals daily. Over the course of a week or so, there's an optimum daily amount we should get to remain in good health. If not, we make it hard for our bodies to defend themselves against infection, injury or surgical trauma. And aside from outright deficiency diseases like iron deficiency anemia and goiter, other disorders—like poor vision and bone problems—are less likely to plague a body well supplied with minerals and other nutrients.

The Recommended Dietary Allowances for minerals, given in table 41, are values estimated to be high enough to cover basic needs of most healthy people. First established in 1943 by the Food and Nutrition Board of the National Research Council, the RDAs for minerals and other nutrients were originally developed to help the government decide how to adequately feed defense troops and manage domestic food supplies during World War II. Since then, the RDAs have been reviewed every five years, based on research in nutritional science, and have been used as guidelines for nutrition education programs, school lunch programs, nursing homes, public assistance programs, and, most recently, for nutritional labeling of food.

Not all vitamins and minerals are included in the RDAs—only those for which there is the most information. Those on which the Committee on Dietary Allowances feels there is enough data to make a reasonably sound estimate are calcium, phosphorus, magnesium, iron, zinc and iodine. For the first time, in 1980, the Committee recognized minerals for which there isn't quite enough data to go on to set a definite RDA, yet there is too much good data to ignore altogether. A new category—"safe and adequate intakes"—gives ranges of intake for sodium, potassium, chloride, copper, manganese, fluoride, chromium, selenium and molybdenum. Those are more tentative. For simplicity's sake, though, we'll refer to all the dietary allowances as RDAs.

The RDAs are really *dietary* allowances rather than true *daily* allowances, reflecting the body's adaptive nature. That is, if we're short on, say, magnesium one day, we can make it up the next.

And eventually, the list will probably be expanded to include many more trace minerals—like nickel and vanadium—which we know are essential but for which data on body functions and food sources are now scanty.

Guide, Not Gospel

Many people are surprised to learn that few of the RDA values are based on actual balance studies on people. For the most part, instead, the RDAs are simply extrapolated from population and dietary data. That is, they are nutrient amounts eaten by people who don't seem to run a deficiency—with an added amount as a margin of safety. Suggested values are passed around among Committee members—all nutrition scientists who sometimes act as consultants to the food industry—and submitted to the Food and Nutrition Board, which makes the final decisions.

To get a clearer idea of just how allowances are calculated, let's look at the RDA for calcium, the body's main mineral. The calcium content of a newborn baby is about 27 grams (approximately one ounce). Except for a few milligrams of calcium floating around in body fluids, most of the calcium we accumulate during our lifetime ends up in teeth and bones. We stop growing somewhere between age 20 and 30.

A tall man could accumulate 1,290 grams (nearly 3 pounds) of calcium by adulthood. That amounts to 141 milligrams of calcium a day needed to build teeth and bones. At age 25, a woman's body might contain 770 grams (about 1½ pounds) of calcium. So she'd theoretically need 84 milligrams of calcium a day.

But the RDA for adults is 800 milligrams—and 1,200 milligrams for teenagers. Why the big difference?

We absorb only about 20 to 30 percent of the calcium we eat—less if we eat a lot of meat or too much phosphorus, or get too little vitamin D. The rest is passed out, mainly in the urine and feces, plus a little in sweat. So to pluck 84 or 141 milligrams of calcium out of our food, for example, we have to eat three to five times as much—up to 420 for our hypothetical woman and over 700 for our hypothetical man. Add to that a few more milligrams of calcium for body fluids and to compensate for individual differences, and, in the Committee's judgment, 800 milligrams should do it for most healthy people. During pregnancy and lactation, women need 1,200 milligrams to insure the fetus and newborn ample calcium. That higher amount also applies during early adolescence, when growth is most rapid.

How the other RDAs are determined varies from one mineral to the next. For iron, the RDA is based on fairly well-established estimates of daily iron losses. In adults, that means about 1 milligram a day from miscellaneous cells that die and are sloughed off. For women of childbearing age, another ½ milligram or so is lost through menstrual flow. But because we absorb only 10 percent of the iron we eat, the RDA for adults is 10 milligrams, raised to 18 milligrams for menstruating women. In that way, the Committee feels, iron losses for most people will be covered.

For zinc, there have been some balance studies indicating that 8 to 10 milligrams are required to maintain good balance in adult men. Most people absorb about 40 percent, says the Committee, so the RDA is set at 15 milligrams, with an extra 5 milligrams during pregnancy and an extra 10 milligrams for breastfeeding mothers.

For iodine, the deficiency disease goiter seems to be prevented at an intake of about 1 microgram a day per pound of body weight. That's averaged at 150 micrograms of daily iodine across the board.

For copper, some balance studies indicate that young adults require about two to three milligrams a day. From those studies, values are adjusted for children.

Are the RDAs Too Low?

For most other minerals, there is often less to go on. Some critics say that, because of lack of firsthand studies, the values may not be appropriate for some minerals. For instance, women past menopause may require more calcium to forestall the weak and brittle bones of osteoporosis. Calcium absorption seems to decline with age, for one thing. And there is evidence that calcium balance in women may be better maintained by an intake above 800 milligrams a day. Some studies indicate that amounts as high as 1,500 or 1,600 milligrams a day are protective. The RDA committee acknowledges that evidence, especially in light of the negative effect of too much protein or phosphorus, but thinks that 1,000 milligrams a day is about as high as intake need go. At the same time, it concedes that there seems to be no actual danger from eating the larger amount.

Before menopause, iron is a woman's most critical mineral. One out of 20 menstruating women has heavier-than-usual monthly periods and loses up to three times as much iron as her moderately flowing sisters. For women with long or heavy periods, the RDA for iron may not replace all that's lost.

The evidence doesn't stop with calcium and iron. Nor are women's needs the only ones called into question. When protein intake was boosted in a study of older adults (both men and women), calcium, magnesium and phosphorus losses increased significantly *even though the RDAs for all three were met.* The protein intake was about equal to the average protein intake of many people in the United States—112 grams a day. One of the implications of the study, conducted by nutrition scientists at the University of Wisconsin, is that the typical American diet may demand more than the present RDAs for at least those particular minerals, if not others. In the words of the researchers who conducted the study, "It is possible, therefore, that the RDAs for calcium, magnesium and phosphorus may be too low for older adults" (*Journal of Nutrition,* February, 1980).

There's a good chance the RDA for zinc may also be too low. For one thing, the amount needed to maintain balance may be higher than previously thought. And absorption from even a healthy diet may be only 15 percent, in some cases, not the 30 or 40 percent formerly assumed.

The reason for that is fiber. Fiber is the indigestible part of food, present in whole grains and other plant foods, which is essential to a healthful diet. But because of the binding effect of plant fiber and substances called phytates in complex carbohydrates like grains, beans and legumes, eating a high-fiber diet may call for a trace mineral intake higher than is now judged adequate. As fiber content of the diet goes up, trace mineral absorption gradually goes down. Besides zinc, calcium, magnesium and iron are also affected.

That doesn't mean adding bran to your cereal is going to give you a mineral deficiency. What it probably *does* mean is that since we evolved on a high-fiber diet, RDAs for minerals based on assumed availability from a diet made up of low-residue foods, like white flour, meat and dairy products, aren't necessarily appropriate for a diet rich in whole grains, legumes, fruits and vegetables. Yet that's the kind of diet we do best on.

Evidence like that seems to call for more solid research to determine more precise—and in some cases, higher—RDAs. Unfortunately, we're told, that kind of research isn't likely to be forthcoming for a long time. The people who make up the RDAs explain that even if the money was there, nutrition is complicated. You can't always measure what goes in, subtract what comes out, and come up with an appropriate value for what's needed to keep all systems running smoothly. It's just not that simple. Besides, even if it was, what applies to some people doesn't necessarily apply to others. People's biochemical needs differ widely—by as much as 10 to 100 times, according to one researcher. And much depends on total diet of the individual. For instance, vitamin C increases iron absorption. Too much protein causes calcium losses. All that must be figured in.

The RDA committee is the first to admit that the allowances are incomplete and far from ideal—best guesses, really. (In their own words, based "on available scientific knowledge.") But they're the best they can offer, we're told.

How Our Needs Differ

The RDAs weren't intended to fit people individually. The allowances are broken down into age, sex and sometimes body weight, but beyond that, there are too many of us, with too many variables. And on top of that, our needs change from time to time.

It's like shopping for clothes and picking up one of those dresses marked One Size Fits All. There's no such thing. The dress will be too small for some people and too large for others. And with sheer luck, it may fit you at the moment. But if you go on a crash diet, it won't fit for much longer.

The RDAs will fit some people, but not others. And then only part of the time. The individual factors that determine whether or not you need more than the RDA aren't very hard to identify. Knowing about them can help you decide how the RDAs for particular minerals apply to you.

Stress

The RDAs take into account ordinary life stresses—little irritations we deal with daily. But severe physical and emotional stress—death of a spouse, money worries, infection, chronic disease, surgery, a heat wave or cold snap—can increase the need for not only minerals, but protein and vitamins as well. Calcium, zinc and iron are minerals most likely to suffer when stress becomes overwhelming, but all help to get us over the worst.

Environmental health hazards

Heavy metal pollution puts a special kind of stress on the body. Lead and strontium 90 compete with calcium for binding sites in the body. Cadmium accumulates quickly but takes a long time to leave. And people with low iron levels absorb more harmful minerals than those with adequate stores. Selenium and zinc, along with vitamins C and E, help combat harmful substances. So exposure to industrial fumes, auto exhaust, cigarette smoke, urban smog and radioactive leaks all boost requirements.

Alcohol and drugs

Alcohol flushes out so many minerals that even moderate, steady drinking can raise your requirements to compensate for those heavy urinary losses. The same goes for drugs like diuretics and steroids. Calcium, zinc, magnesium and potassium are the first to go. (For full discussion, see Alcohol, Drugs and Food Ingredients That Meddle with Health-Building Minerals, chapter 27.)

Fiber

While a diet rich in complex carbohydrates (fruits, vegetables, grains and legumes) is considered a definite bonus for health, it nonetheless calls for mineral intake at the higher end of the ranges given.

People Most Likely to Fall Below the RDAs

Mineral nutrition is a mystery to many people, including some of the best educated. Unless you're a dietitian, your total nutritional background probably consists of little more than a 20-minute pitch for the Basic Four Food Groups by the school nurse in the sixth grade. So a person can graduate summa cum laude in aerospace engineering, yet think of potassium only as that white powdery stuff he or she played with in high school chemistry class.

Coupled with a fuzzy grasp of where food minerals are to be found in food, certain people—the elderly, young adults and dieters, especially—fall into mineral-poor eating habits.

Elderly eat less

Our caloric needs go down as we age, because our metabolic rate—the speed at which we use up calories—decreases about 2 percent for every decade of adulthood. So older adults (age 51 to 75) need roughly 10 percent less food than they did when they were young in order to stay the same weight. After 75, we need up to 25 percent fewer calories. But mineral needs don't fall with that decline in calorie needs. If anything, they go up, because mineral absorption drops off with advancing age. Iron and calcium absorption decline, for example. And the chromium content of the body goes down. So the catch is, what older adults *do* eat must supply optimum amounts of each mineral.

Eating habits, though, may lean toward convenient but mineral-poor choices. Tea and toast. Rewarmed soup. Canned ravioli. Or just snacks. Living alone, as many elderly do, can take the fun out of preparing adequate meals. And fresh produce, fish and meat—prime sources of several key minerals—tend to be expensive. People on fixed incomes who try to save money at the supermarket may be shortchanging themselves of minerals and other nutrients.

Young singles commit nutritional sins

Young adults are at similar risk. Although digestive efficiency is at its peak during our late teens and early twenties, nutritional savvy may be quite low and eating habits erratic. Years ago, single people lived at home until they got married, feasting on mom's home-cooked meals until a spouse entered the picture. Meals retained their commonsense nutritional goodness without interruption. Now, young people are eager to move into their own apartment as soon as they land their first job. On their own, meals often become catch-as-catch-can. The nearest fast-food franchise becomes a surrogate mother to them, dishing out afternoon and evening meals. And mineral nutrition can suffer.

Dieting cuts minerals

Dieting is a national pastime in the United States. Yet as a people, Americans are as chubby as ever. And the startling fact is, it's not necessarily because we eat more than did our foreparents. We weigh more simply because we are sedentary. We sit most of the time, and lie down the rest of the time. Soon after we get up in the morning, we sit down to breakfast. Then ride to work in our cars—or a bus or train. Sit at a desk. Sit during coffee break. Ride home. Eat supper. Mow our lawns with lawn tractors. Sit and watch TV. Chat on the phone. Read, knit, play cards, go to night school. At the same time dieting feverishly to keep the pounds from ballooning around our waists and thighs. While cutting down on food in our struggle to stave off overweight, we cut mineral intake short.

What we need is *more* food, not less. If we simply *exercised* more, we could allow ourselves enough food to reach adequate mineral intake with no problem. But few of us exercise as much as we should. So we have to eat less, defaulting on mineral intake along the way.

CHAPTER

61

Supplements: How Much Should You Take?

The RDA committee of the Food and Nutrition Board says that all of our minerals should come from food. And that's certainly the *best* place to get them. They also say supplements aren't necessary for healthy people. But that's something only *you* can decide. The individual factors we mentioned in the preceding chapter may call for more minerals than diet alone can provide. Keeping certain factors in mind, we've broadened the standard Recommended Dietary Allowances for some major minerals to develop general guidelines for customizing mineral intake to your individual circumstances. These are the minerals for which the most research has been done. And like the standard RDAs, the guidelines here inevitably reflect a certain degree of opinion as well as current research.

For each nutrient, read the paragraph of descriptive statements accompanying the various amounts given. Find the paragraph that most sounds like you. It is not necessary, or in some cases even possible, for each sentence in the paragraph to describe you specifically. Go with the one that, *overall*, seems most applicable. Whether you need to supplement your basic eating plan depends on your own individual situation. (See Super-Mineral Foods, chapter 29, for information on beefing up your mineral intake from food.)

Don't try to use the information here to pinpoint nutritional causes of symptoms, though. Analyzing serious symptoms is your doctor's job.

Calcium

600 milligrams. Your diet normally includes substantial amounts of such calcium-rich foods as dairy products, tofu, salmon (with small, round, soft, cooked bones), and broccoli. You get a good bit of exercise out of doors and your health is excellent in almost every regard.

1,200 milligrams. Your diet is not especially high in the calcium-rich foods mentioned above. You eat a substantial amount of meat, which promotes excretion of calcium from the body. You sometimes have a tendency to develop muscle cramping, when you aren't performing exercise that might cause such a cramp.

Possibly, if you are a woman, you have begun to experience minor backaches. Or you've nursed several children. Your mother or your grandmother, when they were of advanced age, suffered from bone fractures or osteoporosis.

1,600 milligrams. You have aching bones, such as in the low back. You seem to be developing kyphosis (dowager's hump), and you are clearly not quite as tall as you once were. Recently you have suffered a broken bone. Perhaps you have been told by a doctor that you have osteoporosis or thinning of the bones. You may frequently suffer from cramps in the calf at night. It seems that your nerves are irritable, and you have pains for which your doctor has been able to find no obvious explanation. You may be taking steroid drugs, which cause your body to lose calcium.

Magnesium

250 milligrams. Your diet regularly includes generous amounts of soybeans, brown rice, peas, green leafy vegetables, nuts and whole grain products. Your nerves are steady and you have no particular reason to be concerned about the health of your heart. You do not engage in endurance sports such as cross-country running or Nordic skiing.

400 milligrams. Your nerves often seem to be on edge. You may even notice a certain amount of muscle tremor. You are concerned about doing everything possible that may help prevent a heart attack. Possibly you are a heavy drinker, which creates the need for extra magnesium.

Iron

10 milligrams. You are an energetic sort and have a hearty appetite as well. If you are a woman, you no longer have monthly periods. Or if you do, there is an extremely small amount of blood lost. Your diet regularly includes meat, liver, beans, green leafy vegetables, dried fruits and whole grain products.

20 milligrams. You are a woman in the menstruating years. Your appetite is not exactly ravenous, and there are many days when you eat no meat. Perhaps you drink tea, which interferes with the absorption of iron to some extent.

30 milligrams. Your periods are heavy. Or perhaps you have had surgery recently, or lost blood for some other reason. You have one or more of the many symptoms of iron deficiency anemia, which your doctor has told you are not caused by disease: weakness, easy fatigue, poor resistance, headaches and pale skin are among them. In which case, your doctor may recommend even higher amounts of iron for six weeks or more.

Zinc

10 milligrams. You are in excellent health and your diet includes such dependable zinc sources as meat, liver, oysters (from nonpolluted waters), fish, wheat germ and nuts. When you do injure yourself for some reason, the wound heals quickly. Your vision is excellent in dim light.

25 milligrams. You are concerned about the possibility of developing an enlarged prostate gland, and want to do everything possible to try to prevent it (although there is no black-and-white proof that zinc will do that). Your vision at night may not be all that it should be. You may have skin problems, or surgical incisions or injuries that have taken a long time to heal. Your resistance might need some beefing up.

50 milligrams. You may have any one of a number of problems that might possibly be helped by extra zinc, such as enlarged prostate, a variety of skin problems or a very poor sense of taste. Possibly you have had surgery recently and healing is proceeding very poorly. You may have acne, even though you are not an adolescent. There may be white spots on your fingernails, which may be signs of zinc deficiency.

Cobalamin (Vitamin B$_{12}$ with Cobalt)

5 micrograms. You are healthy, energetic, haven't yet reached retirement age, and you regularly eat animal foods such as meat, fish or chicken.

10 micrograms. You've passed your sixtieth birthday and your ability to absorb this vitamin in a useful form may be on the wane.

25 micrograms. Lately, your energy level and possibly your nerves just haven't been up to snuff. Possibly you've been ill or had surgery. You may be a strict vegan, one who avoids all animal-source foods. Those symptoms may well be serious enough to suggest a thorough medical evaluation.

Selenium

25 micrograms. You eat a lot of fish, liver and whole grain bread and cereal. You don't smoke, and never have breast lumps. You live in a high-selenium area of the country. Your blood pressure is normal and there's no history of heart disease in your family.

50 to 100 micrograms. You eat fish and liver only once in a while. You occasionally light up a cigarette at parties or under pressure. You live in an area of medium levels of selenium. High blood pressure and heart disease run in your family, but you show no symptoms so far.

250 to 400 micrograms. You eat very little fish, liver or whole grain foods, or a lot of fatty, refined foods. You smoke regularly. You get breast lumps every so often. You have high blood pressure or heart disease, or (if you're a woman) your mother or a sister has had breast cancer. You live in a low-selenium area.

Chromium

25 micrograms. You eat very little sugar, white flour or other refined carbohydrates. There is no diabetes or other blood sugar problems in your family. You exercise vigorously at least three times a week and eat high-fiber foods, liver and brewer's yeast.

50 to 100 micrograms. You're forty or older and a little overweight. Diabetes, heart disease or low blood sugar runs in your family. You frequently indulge in cravings for sweets. You have a sedentary job, but exercise on weekends.

250 micrograms. You have diabetes or low blood sugar. Your doctor says your cholesterol and triglycerides are higher than they should be. You get very little exercise. You're 65 or older.

That list is not complete. There are other minerals, as well as vitamins and foods, which may be advisable to eat regularly. For minerals not included, amounts are either so small or research so general that a more precise breakdown is not possible.

In general, if you find you need more of the above minerals, your need for other minerals may have increased also. In that case, it may be best to strive for a diet and supplement program that supply you with the higher range for each.

62

Is There a Hair Analysis in Your Future?

We are what we eat . . . and breathe and drink. Minerals in our food, water and air end up in our blood, skin, bones, spinal fluid, urine, hair—and even our fingernails. So samples of one or more of those tissues provide some clue as to whether or not we're overexposing ourselves to harmful minerals, like lead, cadmium and mercury. Or whether we're missing out on health-building minerals like zinc or chromium. In certain cases, specific mineral patterns may even point to specific diseases.

Tissue samples, however, can't always give a true picture of overall mineral status. Blood and urine—the body substances most commonly tested—may be relatively free of toxic metals, while at the same time other tissues, like bone, may harbor hidden deposits—caches of harmful minerals which may be mobilized at any time, at much peril to the brain and nervous system. Or they may register seemingly adequate—or even high— circulating levels of a nutrient, like calcium, when actual body levels are low. So blood and urine tests do not always assure us that all is well within.

What's more, viable substances such as blood and urine require careful handling—they deteriorate easily between the doctor's office and the lab, and are subject to contamination, which can skew the results.

Hair, a Running Ledger of Mineral Intake

A hair clipping serves as a nonperishable sample of minerals as they've accumulated over several months. That makes hair analysis potentially valuable as a retrospective recording of mineral status. For detecting chronic exposure to toxic metals like lead, high levels in hair generally mean high levels in the body—levels that must be brought down to avoid serious illness. In fact, hair analysis has its roots in criminal investigations of arsenic poisoning and other stealthy acts—a kind of medical snooping called forensic medicine. Today, hair analysis is being used more and more frequently in industry to monitor workers' exposure to lead, cadmium, mercury, nickel and other industrial pollutants.

Detection of harmful minerals doesn't stop with the crime lab or workplace, though. Because of everyday exposure to auto exhaust fumes, cigarette smoke and industrial emissions, hair analysis is beginning to catch on as a health check for the public at large. Amares Chattopadhyay, Ph.D., an eminent researcher in the area of hair analysis, and co-workers at the Institute of Environmental Studies at the University of Toronto, in Canada, found, for example, that the concentration of lead in hair paralleled exposure to environmental pollution: hair lead was lowest in rural population groups tested, higher in urban groups, and highest in individuals who lived close to lead smelters. The investigators also found the highest concentrations of mercury and cadmium in hair from individuals with known exposure to those minerals (*Archives of Environmental Health,* September/October, 1977). Similar results have been reported by others.

What Are the Shortcomings of Hair Testing?

Like blood and urine tests, however, hair tests, too, have their limits. While hair tests are just the ticket for detecting frank overexposure to such heavy metals as lead, they have real shortcomings as diagnostic tools or indicators of nutritional status. The drawbacks are chiefly due to inconsistent testing procedures.

Results Vary from Lab to Lab — and Person to Person

Actually, there are now a number of sensitive methods of analyzing hair, but the problem is, methods of collecting, preparing and analyzing hair samples vary from one lab to the next. Different labs use different washing procedures: distilled water, detergents, a combination of detergents and solvents, or chelating agents that trap minerals. And the different procedures produce different results. For instance, some washes remove iron and magnesium from the hair's inner structure, while others fail to remove those same minerals from the outer surface, as they should. Those differences represent the greatest source of inconsistencies among laboratories.

Haphazard sampling could also make a difference. Ideally, only hair clipped close to the skin—such as shaving stubble—would actually reflect mineral levels in the body. But that's not practical, so samples are taken from the first inch or two, usually from the base of the neck. Samples taken farther from the scalp may make it difficult to distinguish between, say, heavy metals contributed by the body itself, through sweat and scalp oil, or by air particles.

Then there are our zealous grooming habits. While tints, bleaches and dyes seem to have little effect on hair mineral levels, waving lotions add zinc and subtract calcium and magnesium. Hair sprays add manganese, and dandruff shampoos are likely to alter zinc and selenium.

In addition, dietary factors *other* than mineral intake, such as high levels of protein, as well as drug or alcohol use, can influence hair mineral levels. And believe it or not, even your age or the time of year you undergo a mineral test can leave a mark on the results.

Consequently, one of the stickiest areas is the problem of setting standard normal values for hair mineral analysis. There are none. Labs may use published data—what little there is—but are encouraged by federal and state licensing bureaus to establish their own set of norms, based on the many tests they run. (To qualify as an experienced hair testing lab, a lab should do a reasonable number of hair tests a year—about 100 annually. Some do thousands.) But regardless of how many they do, the norms will vary from one lab to the next, depending on sample preparation, equipment used—and expertise of the personnel.

Hair test results are also expressed in absolute values for each mineral (usually in parts per million or micrograms per gram). But those expressions, too, will vary with the lab.

All that explains why an individual (or his or her doctor) can send identical samples of hair out to three different labs and get back three different absolute values—and three different norms to compare them to. Each set of results could be correct *for that technique.*

Interpretation Is Tricky—Even for Doctors

Then there's the additional problem of interpretation. Given the most accurate test results possible, they're meaningless until they are correctly interpreted—preferably by a physician who has a lot of experience using hair analysis for his or her patients.

"I find hair tests valuable—but you have to know how to read them," said Jonathan V. Wright, M.D., a nutrition-oriented doctor and medical columnist for *Prevention* magazine. "If, for example, a person tests out low for several essential minerals but you know he's eating a high-mineral diet, it may be that the individual isn't absorbing them properly. That, in turn, may be a sign of a partial insufficiency of gastric acidity or pancreatic enzymes, which aid in digestion."

Also, after running hundreds of tests for patients, Dr. Wright and others have run into one of the most common problems of interpretation—false elevations. That is, minerals—most often calcium, magnesium and zinc—may appear high when in fact body levels are low. That's been confirmed with follow-up tests, usually blood and urine samples. Rarely would high levels of those minerals on a hair analysis truly reflect supernormal body levels, because excesses are excreted in the urine. What may be happening in such cases is, the patient isn't absorbing the minerals. Rather, they're being shuttled to the hair, squirreled away out of reach of the rest of the body. False elevations usually return to normal after the patient takes mineral supplements or enzyme digestive aids.

Along with that is the matter of ratios. False elevations of calcium could mask a low calcium-high phosphorus ratio in the body, increasing chances of developing osteoporosis.

"Those are only a few examples, but they show that even for a physician, hair analysis is tricky," said Dr. Wright. "Mineral analysis is an extremely valuable tool, but we are in the infancy of learning how to use it. Doctors are just beginning to learn what the results actually mean. For a person to go and have one done, to rely on the numbers alone to determine his or her mineral status and choice of supplements, is frequently not very useful."

As another example of the difficulties encountered in the interpretation of hair tests, consider this:

Nutritionists at the University of California at Berkeley, Virginia Polytechnic Institute and Johns Hopkins University School of Medicine took hair samples from two children with known copper deficiency due to severe malnutrition. Samples were meticulously collected and prepared—clipped from close to the scalp, thoroughly cleaned, washed with a proper detergent, rinsed in alcohol, dried and stabilized—then analyzed by atomic absorption spectroscopy. Even though the children were grossly copper deficient, hair copper levels registered normal when compared to controls. By way of explanation, the researchers took into consideration, among other things, the probability that changes in hair production itself during malnutrition altered hair copper values. But their report clearly illustrates that even for experienced nutritionists, the relationship between body stores and hair levels of a mineral is not always direct (*Lancet,* August 16, 1980).

How to Make the Most of Hair Tests

Taking those drawbacks into consideration, some people and their doctors nevertheless continue to seek out hair analysis, either to rule out toxic metal poisoning or to evaluate nutritional status. Many people feel more confident about supplementing their diet with mineral supplements based on a lab test than by hit or miss. How can one most effectively use a hair test?

Finding a Doctor Who Uses Hair Analysis Routinely

Beware of "interpretations" sent by labs for the layperson— especially those that include an exhaustive list of possible conditions that may explain the results. Not only can that raise concern where none is warranted, but unless the results are interpreted by someone who knows the nuances in hair test results as well as your medical history, it makes the interpretation only slightly more accurate than handwriting analysis.

Sample Hair Analysis

Out of curiosity, I had a hair sample tested by two different labs. The results, shown in tables 42 and 43, clearly demonstrate some of the limitations of trying to make heads or tails out of an analysis. They also show that two labs can come up with conflicting results.

Test No. 1 seems to indicate a deficiency in calcium, magnesium and potassium. That puzzled me, because I take dolomite nearly every day and eat plenty of cheese, nuts and fruit—good sources of one or more of those minerals. I do not drink a lot of alcohol, which is known to flush magnesium and potassium out of the system.

Some of the other results of Test No. 1 make sense, though. The sodium reading, for one, since I use no salt at the table or in cooking and rarely eat salty snacks. Cadmium and lead appear to be no problem, which is what I expected, since I neither smoke nor live in a highly industrialized area. Chromium and zinc seem on target, since I take zinc supplements and occasionally brewer's yeast.

Iron registers low on Test No. 1. At first I thought that was odd, because I take iron supplements off and on. But I have been very tired from time to time, and have been meaning to ask my doctor to check me out for iron deficiency anemia. While over-the-counter dosages of iron are fine for preventing anemia, you need much more—about 150 to 200 milligrams a day—if you've already got it. So in that way, the hair results may prompt one to seek medical help for a condition one already suspects.

TABLE 42   Hair Test No. 1

ELEMENTAL COMPOSITION OF HAIR EXPRESSED IN PARTS PER MILLION (PPM)

Sharon Faelten
Prevention
33 E. Minor St.
Emmaus, PA 18049

DATE: 9/30/80

30-F

ELEMENT	Major		PROVISIONAL STANDARDS	
			Female	Male
Calcium (Ca)	527	low	1500-5000	400-800
Magnesium (Mg)	70	low	120-600	100-300
Potassium (K)	167	low	300-1000	100-300
Sodium (Na)	63	low	4000-7000	1500-6500
	Minor			
Cadmium (Cd)	0.8	low	2	2
Cobalt (Co)	0.07	low	0.4	0.4
Copper (Cu)	45.0	normal	30-50	30-60
Iron (Fe)	23.0	low	40-60	50-70
Lead (Pb)	6.0	normal	6-12	6-12
Manganese (Mn)	0.5	low	2	2
Zinc (Zn)	173.0	normal	150-250	125-200

Special Determinations (< = less than)

Chromium (Cr)	0.8	high	0.11 - 0.33	
Mercury (Hg)	13.2	normal	11 - 25	

Comments: Values within 25% of the Provisional Standards are acceptable because there are
large seasonal variations in hair composition. Low levels of cadmium, lead, and mercury are
desirable because these are toxic elements. If the analysis indicates serious deficiencies,
review your diet with the aid of the many good books on nutrition, or help of your physician.
High levels of any element may indicate environmental contamination.

The major elements may have been washed out by shampooing and showering, as
well as swimming. More liver and liver products, frequent use of iron cooking
utensils, dietary mineral and vitamin B12 (low cobalt) supplements are
suggested to correct your deficiencies. High chromium probably originated
from the pipes supplying the water used in shampooing and showering.

Now, let's compare Test No. 1 to Test No. 2. The results for
calcium and magnesium are about the same in terms of absolute numbers,
but because the second lab used a different range for normal, they consider
my results normal, not low. So maybe my diet is providing enough of those
minerals, after all. Potassium here makes more sense, too. And the silicon
value (not tested by the first lab) seems right—I eat high-fiber foods, which
are high in silicon. Selenium is also high. My shampoo doesn't list any
selenium compounds on the label, but I eat a lot of fish and had been taking
selenium supplements a few weeks before the test. Chromium, cadmium,
lead and mercury all follow the same general pattern as in Test No. 1.

The most glaring inconsistency here is that Test No. 1 indicates my
iron is low and Test No. 2 shows it is high. Which is correct? That's where
a blood test might come in handy.

TABLE 43   Hair Test No. 2

```
                                    DATE TESTED:    OCT 10, 1980
                                    TIME TESTED:    10:24:55
        STATED DIAGNOSIS:           REF. NO:        253
                                    PATIENT NO.     253
                                    SEX:            FEMALE

ALL MINERALS ARE REPORTED IN P.P.M.
===================================================================================
NUTRIENT  USUAL    PATIENT  H/L :             :             :             :
MINERAL   RANGE    VALUE        :     LOW     :   NORMAL    :    HIGH     :
===================================================================================
   CA    200-600   539.          :*****************************
   MG     25-75     58.0         :************************
   NA     30-100    52.9         :*********************
   K      75-180   150.          :***************************
   P      50-100    59.7         :******************
   SI      5-22     21.3         :*****************************
   CR     0.5-1.5   .580         :******************
   MN      1-10     .306    LO   :*************
   MO     0.1-0.7   .273         :***************
   FE     20-50    102.    HI    :******************************************
   CU     12-35     34.4         :**************************
   ZN    160-240   157.    LO   :****************
   SE      5-15     22.1    HI   :*****************************************
===================================================================================
TOXIC     USUAL    PATIENT  H/L :             :             :             :
MINERAL   RANGE    VALUE        :             :   NORMAL    :   TOXIC     :
===================================================================================
   AL      2-10     16.3    HI   :****************************************
   CD     0-1.0     .530         :***********************
   PB     0-20      2.32         :*****************
   HG     0-2.5     .669         :*****************
   NI     0-1.0     2.08    HI   :*****************************************
```

** EXPLANATION OF SYMBOLS **

```
CA   CALCIUM      CR   CHROMIUM     SE   SELENIUM
MG   MAGNESIUM    MN   MANGANESE    AL   ALUMINUM
NA   SODIUM       MO   MOLYBDENUM   CD   CADMIUM
K    POTASSIUM    FE   IRON         PB   LEAD
P    PHOSPHORUS   CU   COPPER       HG   MERCURY
SI   SILICON      ZN   ZINC         NI   NICKEL
```

NOTE — CERTAIN SHAMPOOS CAN CAUSE EXCESSIVE LEVELS OF ZINC OR SELENIUM DUE TO
THOSE COMPOUNDS IN THE SHAMPOO. ALSO CERTAIN COLOR-BACK HAIR PREPARATIONS CAN
CAUSE ELEVATED LEAD VALUES.

YOUR ANALYSIS SHOWS THAT YOU ARE DEFICIENT IN THE FOLLOWING MINERALS:

MANGANESE
ZINC

YOUR ANALYSIS SHOWS THAT YOU HAVE HIGH LEVELS IN THE FOLLOWING MINERALS:

IRON
SELENIUM
ALUMINUM
NICKEL

NOTE: MINERALS IN EXCESSIVE LEVELS THAT CAN BE TOXIC INCLUDE:
      ALUMINUM, CADMIUM, COPPER, IRON, LEAD, MERCURY, NICKEL, SELENIUM, AND ZINC.

** SIGNIFICANT MINERAL RATIOS **

```
==========================================================================================
RATIO   USUAL    PATIENT  OBSERVATIONS
        RANGE    VALUE
==========================================================================================
CA/MG   7.5-11   9.34            WITHIN USUAL RANGE
CA/CU   20-60    15.7     LOW:   MAY BE ASSOCIATED WITH NERVOUS DISORDERS AND
                                 SOME DEGENERATIVE DISEASES
CA/FE   24-50    5.28     LOW:   IRON AT HIGH LEVELS IS TOXIC.
CA/PB   100-UP   232.            WITHIN USUAL RANGE
CA/ZN   1-6      3.43            WITHIN USUAL RANGE
ZN/CR   350-550  270.     LOW:   MAY BE ASSOCIATED WITH LUNG DISORDERS, ASTHMA
                                 OR OTHER ALLERGIES
ZN/CU   5-20     4.56     LOW:   MAY BE ASSOCIATED WITH DEGENERATIVE DISEASES,
                                 ARTERIOSCLEROSIS, HYPOGLYCEMIA, DIABETES, SLOW
                                 WOUND HEALING, MENTAL OR EMOTIONAL DISORDERS,
                                 INFERTILITY AND LOSS OF TASTE AND SMELL.
ZN/FE   7-11     1.54     LOW:  MAY BE ACCOMPANIED BY WHITE SPOTS ON FINGERNAILS
                                 AND SLOW WOUND HEALING.
ZN/MN   50-300   513.     HIGH:  MAY ACCOMPANY HYPOGLYCEMIA OR DIABETES.
ZN/CD   200-UP   296.     HIGH:  ASSOCIATED WITH GOOD HEALTH, NOT SMOKING, AND
                                 RELATIVELY FREE FROM POLLUTION EXPOSURE.
NA/K    1-6      0.35     LOW:   MAY BE ASSOCIATED WITH ADRENAL INSUFFICIENCY.
FE/CU   0.8-3    2.97            WITHIN USUAL RANGE
K/FE    1-5      1.47            WITHIN USUAL RANGE
ZN/MG   1-3      2.71            WITHIN USUAL RANGE
FE/MN   5-30     333.     HIGH:  MAY BE ASSOCIATED WITH DIABETES, HYPOGLYCEMIA AND
                                 IRON TOXICITY.
```

One thing that alarmed me about Test No. 2's results was the high aluminum and nickel values. According to the lab, those are high enough to warrant chelation therapy for immediate removal of those toxic metals. I stopped to consider possible sources. Although I've recently bought stainless steel cookware, I'd been using aluminum pots and pans for years. So it's remotely possible that I may have absorbed large amounts of aluminum from food. But I have none of the nausea, headaches, flushing or nerve problems associated with aluminum intoxication. Upon taking a closer look at the scissors I used to clip my hair sample, however, it looks as if they're not stainless steel — as recommended — but aluminum and nickel. Quite probably, the scissors contaminated the sample, producing the false elevations.

Another interesting observation is the apparent low zinc:copper ratio and high zinc:manganese ratio. According to the lab's interpretation, both may indicate hypoglycemia (low blood sugar). It just so happens that my doctor recently had me take a glucose tolerance test which indicated I am probably hypoglycemic. So there could be something to that.

So far, it would seem the test has some value — except for one thing. I use a creme rinse conditioner every time I shampoo. That could make both analyses invalid.

So you see, hair analysis can have real limitations. As it is, the results are difficult enough for a doctor to interpret — especially one who's not familiar with hair tests.

To locate a nutrition-oriented doctor in your area, who'd be more likely to use hair analysis, write to *Prevention* Readers' Service, 33 East Minor Street, Emmaus, PA 18049.

If you can't readily locate a doctor for guidance, you may want to know how to locate a lab on your own and how to send in your hair sample correctly.

Locating a Good Hair Test Lab

Out of 100,000 or so labs across the country, relatively few do hair analysis. Those that do may do hair analysis only, or hundreds of other tests — blood, urine, thyroid function, glucose tolerance, and so on. Magazines run ads for mail-order hair analysis. How do you know which are reliable?

There's really no way to tell for sure. But there are a few questions you can ask that may help rule out those that are least likely to give reliable results.

1. Is the lab either federally certified or state licensed?

Theoretically, regulations demand that a lab meet certain standards of quality control, procedures and personnel in order to be certified or licensed. Part of that includes general proficiency testing by the Centers for Disease Control, or CDC (a branch of the U.S. Public Health Service).

Certified labs send in random samples of various tissue test samples and results to see if their results jibe with those of CDC. The catch is, hair analysis is not one of the tests checked. "There are just too many different tests being done to check every single one in every single lab," explained a clinical chemist at CDC. A lab's general proficiency is judged by how well it conducts those tests that *are* checked. But just because they did it right once doesn't mean they do it right every time. So keep that in mind if your results come back way off base.

2. What kind of license?

If a lab claims it's certified or licensed, find out if it's licensed under Clinical Chemistry, Toxicology, or Special Chemistry.

Those are the general classifications for hair analysis. A lab certified for pathology or microbiology may be very good at detecting viruses, but it may not necessarily have the equipment, personnel or experience to do accurate hair analysis. It's like having your car fixed—you don't take it to a tractor repair shop.

3. Ask for the credentials of the director, supervisors and technicians.

Because a large percentage of lab mistakes are due to human error, asking about lab personnel's qualifications could possibly cut down on chances for error. Requirements vary from state to state, but in general the director should have a Ph.D. in chemistry, biology, microbiology, public health or pharmacy, or be a doctor of osteopathy, and have at least two years' lab experience. With a master's degree, he or she should have four years' experience, and with a bachelor's degree, five. Because the director is responsible for work of subordinates, ask how many hours a day he or she spends in the lab.

The requirements for supervisors are similar. As for technicians, they should have college experience in lab science at the very minimum.

4. Ask how many hair tests the lab does in a year.

It should be at least 100.

To offset variation between labs' norms, a good tactic is to go to the same lab every time. No need to have it done more frequently than every six months, though.

Slight deviations from the norm are the most difficult to interpret. They may mean very little in terms of health or diet. That's where acting as your own control—comparing tests before and after supplementation, for instance—may help give more meaningful results.

Snipping and Sending in Your Hair Sample

Scalp hair gives the best sampling of hair minerals simply because it grows the longest, in thick clusters. And because minerals from sweat, oil and the air around us also bind to the shaft along with body-borne minerals, the mineral concentration rises with the distance from the scalp. So the first inch or two of hair most closely reflects body levels. Consequently, most labs request that you clip a tablespoon or two of hair from the nape of the neck (or elsewhere if you are bald). Use a stainless steel scissors, to avoid contaminating the hair with metal. And wait at least three days after a shampoo.

Hair Test Costs and Coverage

The cost for a hair test runs from about $15 to $40, depending not only on the lab but the number of minerals you have analyzed. There's often a small discount for having three or more tests done at once—sort of a family plan.

Insurance may or may not pay

Blue Cross/Blue Shield told us they will only reimburse for a hair test if it's doctor-ordered. Medicare will not pay under any circumstances.

As for Health Maintenance Organization (HMO) plans, we checked with our regional representative. She told us that there is no blanket policy regarding hair analysis—claims are considered on an individual basis. In other words, maybe HMO will cover you, maybe they won't. The HMO representative also told us that such is likely to be the case for plans throughout the country, although it's actually decided at the regional level.

IRS picks up the tab

If your hair test costs aren't reimbursed by any of the above, you can deduct the costs from your federal income tax. We called the Internal Revenue Service in Washington, D.C., on this one. While there is no specific ruling on hair analysis tests per se, we were told that a hair test would be deductible as an expense incurred for a "cure, prevention, diagnosis or mitigation of disease," whether you had it done by a doctor or on your own.

Should you or your doctor then decide you need to take mineral supplements, though, that expense would not be deductible unless directly prescribed by your doctor. If so, get it in writing in case of a tax audit.

CHAPTER

63

Q and A

Answers to the Most Frequently Asked Questions about Minerals and Health

Q: What are the advantages, if any, of taking individual mineral supplements over a multiple tablet?

A: Each of us has different nutritional requirements. So the key advantage of taking individual supplements is that our daily mineral intake can be tailored to our personal needs. A multiple, on the other hand, may be more convenient, but it doesn't provide for individual differences.

Furthermore, only so much or so many minerals can be packed into a single tablet. So again, multiples rarely provide enough or the variety of minerals you may require. Trace minerals like chromium and selenium may be absent altogether.

If you rely on a multiple, you may want to boost it with certain individual minerals to help meet requirements raised by stress, disease, poor appetite or other conditions that may arise. A woman's need for calcium, for example, increases during pregnancy and breastfeeding. But as one nutrition text pointed out, "multi-vitamin-mineral pills seldom contain significant amounts of calcium. It is usually necessary to take a separate calcium supplement to obtain any appreciable amount" (*Introductory Nutrition,* C. V. Mosby, 1979).

In a similar way, zinc requirements rise to meet repair demands of wound healing after an injury or surgery. Women need extra iron during their menstrual years—often more than a multiple supplies. People with blood sugar problems may improve with extra chromium. Individual supplements are often the only way to meet those and other special situations.

Q: Do minerals lose their potency when stored for long periods of time?

A: No. They're tough as a rock. Even if the tablets crumble, the potency doesn't fade. However, when vitamins and minerals are together in one supplement, the storage rules are stiffer. Because minerals may cause a faster rate of breakdown, combination tablets should follow the rules for vitamin storage: keep in a cool, dry place in a tightly closed container. If you plan to store your supplements a long time, use single-mineral or all-mineral supplements. They have the longest shelf life.

Q: Every time I start a vitamin-mineral supplement program my appetite seems to increase. Is there anything to that? And if so, what can I do about it?

A: We spoke to a few nutritionists, among them Rebecca Riales, Ph.D., a clinical nutritionist in Parkersburg, West Virginia. She told us there is no scientific evidence that appetite increases when a person takes supplements unless you are correcting a very severe deficiency. For instance, zinc has been shown to renew lost sense of taste in many people. Or even sharpen it.

Beyond that, appetite is somewhat subjective. Perhaps your renewed interest in your diet has merely sharpened your appreciation of food. So eat less, but enjoy it more!

Q: What is chelation? Is it important to buy chelated minerals? For instance, is chelated zinc better absorbed than nonchelated zinc?

A: Minerals—like zinc or copper, for instance—are usually bound with some other substance or substances, even in nature. So mineral supplements consist of a mineral and a binder, or chelator. In other words, chelation simply refers to the binding of a mineral to another substance, natural or synthetic. Gluconate is a common chelator.

Chelation forms a weak bond, however, and once the mineral

supplement reaches the stomach, the mineral is quickly released from the chelator. So chelation usually makes little difference in how much we absorb.

More important are the conditions under which we take supplements. Eating them with meals enhances absorption because food components—protein and carbohydrates—carry minerals into the system.

Q: My neighbor told me not to eat a high-fiber diet because it makes minerals unavailable to the body. Is there any truth to that?

A: Your neighbor is probably referring to something she heard about phytic acid, a substance found in the husks of grains, legumes and some nuts. Phytic acid binds with calcium, zinc, magnesium and iron to form insoluble compounds called phytates, making a certain amount of those minerals unavailable.

If grains and legumes (peas and beans) make up such a large portion of the diet that those foods are the main sources of minerals, there could be a problem. But a high-fiber diet that balances grains and beans with other fibrous foods from the vegetable and fruit groups (apples, apricots, peaches, pears, broccoli, carrots, potatoes and so forth), as well as other good foods, will not lead to mineral deficiencies.

We asked Pericles Markakis, Ph.D., a food scientist from Michigan State University who specializes in fiber and mineral metabolism, about mineral deficiencies arising from phytic acid.

"People have been eating whole grains and beans for hundreds of years," he said. "Obviously, those foods don't cause mineral deficiencies. The only documented cases of mineral deficiencies (notably of zinc) caused by phytic acid in food were in small groups of Middle Eastern people. Eighty percent of their diet was unleavened bread. When added to bread, leavening agents such as yeast release enzymes which break down phytic acid as the bread rises so that it won't bind minerals. Without leavening of any kind, no breakdown takes place."

Phytic acid alone does not cause a mineral deficiency. Low mineral intake is a big factor. Dr. Markakis went on, "Because a diet of so much unleavened bread contains proportionately little dairy products, vegetables or other good food sources of calcium and other minerals, those people became deficient. Zinc deficiency was particularly common because zinc is not as abundant as calcium, magnesium and iron in food. However, it appears that the entire fiber complex of the food—bread in the case of the Middle East diet—is involved in the zinc deficiency cases studied.

"Those are extreme cases, though. We should all eat more whole grain products and less refined flour. While we don't know exactly how much whole grain or how many beans people have to eat before phytic acid levels become high enough to seriously interfere with mineral absorption, we do know that eating a variety of foods—vegetables, dairy products, fish, meat and so on—in addition to grains and beans will help outweigh the effects of phytic acid."

Q: There are so many different kinds of supplemental yeasts on the market—like brewer's, nutritional and primary— that I'm confused. What's the difference? And which yeast is the best source of chromium?

A: Brewer's yeast and primary yeast are the same type of organism (yeast is a super-tiny plant), but brewer's yeast is a *by-product* of beer-making, while primary yeast is a *product,* grown on molasses or grains for the express purpose of growing more yeast. Primary yeast may also be called "nutritional yeast."

The nutritional makeup of yeast—including its chromium content—depends in part on the medium in which it grows. But the chromium content is not required to be listed on the label. So while it's not always easy to choose a high-chromium yeast, you may contact the manufacturer of your brand of yeast for information on just how much chromium it supplies.

Q: Oysters have more zinc than any other food. Why don't you recommend eating oysters, clams or other shellfish? Because of the cholesterol?

A: Oysters are very rich in zinc. But oysters (along with their mollusk relatives, clams and mussels) tend to absorb contaminants from industrial waste and sewage dumped into the offshore waters where they live. People eating contaminated shellfish have suffered from paralysis and severe infection. A rich source of zinc, yes. A safe source, perhaps not.

Scientists also used to say that the amount of cholesterol in mollusks made them a less than ideal food. The reverse may be true. Recently, researchers lowered the cholesterol levels of laboratory animals by feeding them oysters or clams.

Q: What is the difference between zinc gluconate and zinc sulfate?

A: There is no difference nutritionally. Both are absorbed equally but the sulfate is more acidic and may irritate the stomach. You can avoid this by taking zinc sulfate with food or by switching to the gluconate.

Q: Which is the better calcium supplement, bone meal or dolomite?

A: Both are good sources of calcium. As to which is better, there's no clear-cut answer.

It just so happens that calcium and magnesium are well balanced in dolomite—in a ratio our body can use most efficiently. But none of the nutritionists we called could say what happens to that "perfect" balance when dolomite is eaten along with total nutritional intake for the day. So a balanced supplement may not necessarily guarantee a perfectly balanced intake for the day. Nor may a perfect balance be necessary. The body's own homeostatic (regulating) mechanisms take care of such fluctuations.

That's where bone meal comes in. Bone meal has plenty of calcium, but small amounts of magnesium and other minerals. For people who need extra calcium—like women with osteoporosis—bone meal can add a bonus of the mineral, over and above the calcium in food or dolomite. Other people may get all the calcium they need from food or dolomite (or both) with no need for bone meal.

Q: Will taking calcium supplements increase the chances of developing kidney stones?

A: For some people, high dietary calcium may be one cause of kidney stones. But for most stone formers, it is not.

The most common form of kidney stones involves not only calcium, but oxalic acid (a normal substance in the urine) as well. For a variety of complex and not completely understood reasons, calcium and oxalic acid sometimes combine to form relatively insoluble crystals called calcium oxalate—or kidney stones. So it's not calcium that's to blame, but the way the body handles calcium and oxalic acid in stone formers.

Some people can reduce their tendency to form stones by reducing calcium intake. But if you have no history of kidney stone formation, high-calcium foods or calcium supplements probably won't cause kidney stones.

Q: Can calcium deposits be treated nutritionally? Can taking too much calcium cause deposits?

A: Calcium deposits in the joints are due to a problem with the parathyroid gland rather than too much calcium in the diet.

Q: Is sea salt better than regular salt?

A: Sea salt is no better for you than regular salt. The only big difference between them is the price. Sea salt can cost up to four times as much as regular table salt. So why do people use it?

Many people believe that sea salt is rich in minerals. That would be true if sea salt were just evaporated sea water, because sea water contains substantial amounts of magnesium, calcium and potassium. But that isn't the case.

Sea salt is purified in order to meet government standards. Those standards specify that food-grade sea salt, whether taken from sea water or salt mines, must be at least 97.5 percent sodium chloride (salt). That doesn't leave much room for other minerals or for variation. Sea salt and regular salt are essentially the same.

In fact, that's just what the state of Oregon decided recently when it adopted a regulation that prohibits the use of the term "sea salt" in response to consumer complaints that the term was used as an excuse to charge higher prices for regular salt.

Besides that, all salt is really sea salt anyway. The deposits found in salt mines were left behind by sea water that evaporated millions of years ago.

So the next time someone tells you that sea salt is better for you than regular salt, take it with a grain of salt.

Q: I'm on a low-salt diet. Should I avoid taking vitamin C in the form of sodium ascorbate?

A: Vitamin C (or, as a chemist would say, ascorbic acid) comes in many forms. One of them is sodium ascorbate. When you take sodium ascorbate, the vitamin C and the sodium split apart in your body. The vitamin C is good for you. The sodium may not be.

Since you're on a low-salt diet, you probably know that too much sodium in the diet may cause or aggravate high blood pressure. So be cautious about the amount of sodium ascorbate you take. You get almost as much sodium from 1 gram (1,000 milligrams) of sodium ascorbate as you would from ½ cup of canned tomatoes. That's not a whole lot. But if you take large quantities of sodium ascorbate—10 grams, for instance—you'll get over a gram of sodium, a large chunk of the daily intake of salt for someone on a low-salt diet. If you want to take that much vitamin C, we suggest you stick with forms other than sodium ascorbate. A few people find that high doses of vitamin C in the form of ascorbic acid upset their stomach, and that's why they use sodium ascorbate. If you have that problem, try using calcium ascorbate, or an ascorbate-type vitamin C supplement that also contains calcium, magnesium or potassium. Those preparations don't aggravate the stomach.

Q: Since I no longer use salt in cooking meals, I'm concerned that my family may not be getting enough iodine (I used iodized salt). What do you suggest?

A: There's no need for concern. A lack of iodine in the diet (and the result of this deficiency, goiter) was only a problem in the days when people ate fruits and vegetables grown in iodine-poor soil and couldn't get produce from anywhere else. Health officials introduced iodized salt during the 1920s as a way of dealing with this problem. Today, however, produce grown in iodine-rich soils is available all over the country (and so is fish, which supplies lots of iodine), and goiter is very rare.

If you want to be extra sure about getting enough iodine, use kelp.

A teaspoon of kelp contains over 20 times the Recommended Dietary Allowance for iodine.

Q: A friend of mine told me that potassium chloride is a good salt substitute. Are there any dangers from using potassium chloride on food?

A: For most people, no.

Because too much sodium in the diet seems to encourage high blood pressure in many people, any means of cutting down on table salt (sodium chloride) is welcomed. For people who feel that food tastes bland without salt, potassium chloride provides the taste and texture of salt without the unwanted sodium. Check the label, though. Some brands are part potassium chloride and part sodium chloride. Others contain ammonium chloride, which may irritate the stomach and affect the bronchial tract.

For most people, up to a teaspoon or so of potassium chloride a day is no problem. Don't overdo it, though. Overuse can lead to hyperkalemia—dangerously high levels of potassium in the blood. That can lead to a heart attack. Also, people with kidney problems or diabetes are at special risk. If you have either of those conditions, or if you take a potassium-sparing drug (one that hoards potassium in the blood), you should check with your doctor before considering the switch to a salt substitute.

Q: When I put salt in my water softener, is that the same kind of salt that people use on their food, and if so, is there enough of it to give me high blood pressure?

A: Water is hard because it contains calcium and magnesium. Adding sodium chloride—table salt—to the water chemically pushes out those minerals and makes hard water soft. The harder the water to start with, the saltier the softened water will be. But is there enough salt in softened water to *give* you high blood pressure? Highly unlikely. Even in a city with very hard water, you'd need to drink two quarts of softened water a day to get 250 milligrams of sodium, a reasonably small amount (a safe level of daily sodium intake is 1,000 to 3,000 milligrams). But most doctors tell their patients who already have high blood pressure to avoid softened water, and we think that's good advice.

Q: I work in a hot, busy restaurant kitchen. Am I in danger of losing too much salt through sweat? Should I take salt tablets?

A: No, on both counts.

For one thing, our bodies can acclimate to heat—that is, adjust gradually to the heat and cut down the amount of salt lost in sweat.

Besides that, taking salt tablets freely can be dangerous. Concentrated doses of salt not only irritate the stomach lining, but can even be fatal.

Of course, some people need salt tablets for medical problems that cause heavy salt losses—in which case your doctor would recommend them. Only rarely will a healthy person need salt tablets—like an athlete competing in a hot climate to which he or she is unaccustomed—and then only under medical supervision.

The replacement of body fluids is more important than salt replacement. However, if you want to compensate for moderate salt loss, your best bet would be to drink tomato juice or eat foods that are naturally high in sodium.

Q: What exactly is mineral water? Does it have any nutritional benefits?

A: So far, no one has been able to define clearly what mineral water is.

Some mineral water may be spring water that flows naturally from an underground source. So spring water may contain insignificant or large amounts of minerals, depending on the source. Spring water may or may not include an undesirable amount of sodium. The Food and Drug Administration loosely regulates spring water standards, but information on mineral content is still hard to come by. Label information is often too general or unreliable.

Mineral water might also be distilled water to which minerals are added by the manufacturer.

The FDA does not regulate water labeled as "mineral water." So there is really no telling for sure what's in a bottle with that label.

So while mineral water is a good alternative to sugary soft drinks and alcohol, we wouldn't suggest you count on it to satisfy your body's mineral requirements. Foods and food supplements are much more reliable.

Q: What is mineral oil? Does it have any nutritional value? Is it safe to use?

A: Mineral oil is a chemical byproduct from the manufacture of petroleum. Sound unappetizing? Good. You should *never* ingest mineral oil—either as a laxative or by cooking with it. Granted, it's still on the market as an ingredient in some laxatives. But many doctors and nutritionists condemn its use. And well they should. It works by coating food particles and the intestinal walls so that food literally slides out of the system—without much nutrition being absorbed. Also, mineral oil dissolves vitamins A, D, E, and K, as well as some essential fatty acids. And, in spite of its name, it provides no minerals—or any other nutrient.

However, the oil isn't totally "good for nothing." As an ingredient in many cosmetics and skin lotions it helps preserve moisture and keeps your skin fresh.

Q: Does iron interfere with the absorption of vitamin E? Or is it the other way around?

A: Vitamin E does not seriously affect iron absorption one way or the other. As for the effect of iron on vitamin E absorption, it depends on the form.

Ferrous iron (present in food) has little if any interaction with vitamin E. It's the other form, *ferric,* not usually found in supplements or food, which blocks the vitamin. And as long as the iron in the supplements you take is combined with an organic compound such as gluconate or fumarate, you should have no problem. Avoid the inorganic forms, such as sulfate or phosphate, which seem to interfere with vitamin E absorption.

So look for organic ferrous iron supplements and get the most from your vitamin E capsules too.

Q: I read in a magazine article recently that eggs block iron absorption. Is that true?

A: Yes. Eggs contain a compound that interferes with iron absorption. That not only makes the iron in eggs relatively unavailable but will affect the absorption of iron from foods eaten with the eggs. So when eaten as part of a meal, eggs will sharply reduce iron absorption.

No need to give up eggs, though. If you're concerned about your iron status, taking an iron supplement is better than omitting eggs.

Q: What other substances interfere with iron absorption? Does milk or milk products? If so, how long after eating them should I wait to take an iron pill?

A: A number of substances are known to interfere with iron absorption, notably the tannic acid in tea, and, to a lesser extent, coffee, eggs, antacids and the antibiotic tetracycline.

Foods containing large amounts of phosphates, phosphate additives or the preservative EDTA also seem to inhibit iron absorption.

The possible interference of milk and milk products is controversial. In a study led by James D. Cook, M.D., professor of medicine and director of hematology at the Kansas University Medical Center, milk and cheese appeared to reduce iron absorption (*American Journal of Clinical Nutrition,* August, 1976). But it's not yet clear what the interaction is. "Iron absorption is very complex and more information is needed before a change in diet is recommended," Dr. Cook told us. "If you are concerned about your iron intake, it's a good idea to take iron supplements to be sure you are getting your requirements."

Iron supplements are best absorbed on an empty stomach. You should take them either before or three hours after the meal. If you experience stomach problems, take them with the meal.

Q: I'm considering donating blood. Will I need to take extra iron because of the blood loss?

A: The donor who gives a pint of blood once a year probably doesn't need to take extra iron. But, "for the person who donates blood three or four times a year, taking iron supplements may be a good idea," says Robert H. Kough, M.D., director of hematology/oncology at Geisinger Medical Center in Danville, Pennsylvania.

Each time blood is drawn, the body needs to replenish the iron that was lost. If the diet is not sufficient in iron, then the body will have to draw on stores of iron in bone marrow and the spleen. Besides robbing those sources of a vital mineral, blood hemoglobin suffers as well, since iron is its key ingredient. On top of that, women lose iron regularly in the menstrual flow. Those with heavy periods lose even more.

Unless the diet consists of many sources of iron-rich foods, food alone may not be able to compensate for the iron lost with frequent blood donations. Supplements help insure against serious iron losses. Taking iron supplements may be the best way to prevent serious loss of this vital mineral.

Q: A friend told me that baking powder isn't good for you. If that's so, what should be used?

A: You should avoid any baking powder that contains aluminum salts. Several studies show that aluminum can accumulate in the brain over time, causing loss of memory and brain deterioration.

You can find baking powder without aluminum salts in health food stores. However, you can make your own using this recipe from our Rodale Test Kitchen.

Baking Powder

2 tablespoons cream of tartar
2 tablespoons arrowroot
1 tablespoon baking soda

Mix the ingredients together in a small bowl with a wooden spoon, crushing any lumps. Store in a tightly covered jar in a cool, dry place.
Makes ¼ cup.

Q: I read somewhere that soaking eggshells in water or adding them to soups is a good way of adding extra calcium to the diet. Is that true?

A: Not really. An eggshell has about two grams of calcium. And, chances are, plain water won't coax it out. Only in a soup made with an acid, like tomato broth, lemon juice or vinegar—some calcium will leach out. Just how much calcium dissolves depends on how much acid you add and how long you cook the soup. So the exact amount of calcium gained would be hard to predict.

Besides, it may be next to impossible to strain out the bits of shell that are bound to break off.

Q: Recently I read that foods prepared in an iron skillet have a high iron content. Is that true? How *much* more do they have?

A: Yes, it's true. Foods cooked in iron pots may have a higher iron content. Exactly how *much* more iron depends on the kind of food, how long it cooks and even on the condition of the pan you're using.

The amount of iron that makes its way into food varies greatly. In some rare cases, iron reaches toxic levels, as is the case for the South African Bantus who brew their beer in iron pots. As a result, their daily iron intake has neared the 200-milligram mark compared to Americans, whose daily intake hovers around 15.

For the average American, however, the use of iron cookware for food preparation may boost the already low dietary iron intake. Foods cooked in iron pots can have on the average three to four times more iron than the same foods cooked in glass, for example. A 3½-ounce serving of macaroni-beef stew cooked 2½ hours in aluminum had 1.03 milligrams. But the iron content jumped to 4.7—more than four times as much—when the stew was cooked in an iron skillet.

The key to this iron bonus rests with the partnership between foods' acidity and length of cooking time. Many studies have shown that the more acid a food and the longer it's cooked, the more iron will be dissolved from the pot. Spaghetti sauce, for example, cooked for 3 hours in an iron pot contained 87.5 milligrams of iron per 3½ ounces. But the iron levels in that same sauce prepared in a glass pot yielded only 3 milligrams.

Seasoning—the process of sealing off the pores of a pan with oil—is usually recommended not only to keep foods from sticking but to prevent rust (a buildup of iron salts). Therefore, the better seasoned your pan, the less you may be able to count on that iron bonus.

Q: Do copper cooking utensils add copper to food? Is that good or bad?

A: Yes, you can get copper from copper cookware if your food comes in direct contact with the metal itself. Today, however, most copper pots sold in the marketplace are lined with either tin or stainless steel. So there's no problem unless the tin lining wears away with use, exposing the copper. If that happens, the pot should be relined, for although copper is needed by the human body in very small amounts, too much can be toxic. The amount of copper you're exposed to from worn pots will, of course, depend on how frequently you use your copper pots. Exactly how much copper will dissolve from a worn copper pot depends additionally on how highly acid the food is and how long it's cooked.

As might be expected, foods cooked in copper pans with worn tinning show higher levels of copper than foods from pans with intact plating or from aluminum pots. In one study, a four-ounce serving of fish prepared in an old copper pot contained about 0.65 milligram, a value which dropped to 0.26 in an unused pot with the lining intact. But in no case did the level of copper exceed the recommended limit.

Another big reason why you probably wouldn't want to cook in direct contact with copper is that it's destructive to vitamin C and possibly vitamins A and E.

The best way, then, to safely take advantage of copper's even heating properties, is to make sure it has a nontoxic liner.

Remember, also, to keep your pots clean. That greenish-blue film that forms when copper is exposed to the air—called tarnish—is actually a buildup of copper salts. This "verdigris," as it is sometimes called, can be poisonous and should never be in contact with food you're eating.

Aside from the potential health hazards from dissolved copper, foods cooked in contact with copper can have an off color and taste.

Q: I enjoy collecting handmade pottery, but hesitate to use mugs and pitchers for food and beverages because of lead poisoning. How do I know if handcrafted pottery is safe for food?

A: It isn't easy to determine if pottery is safe for food. Not all pieces are fired with lead glazes. Even so, glazes that don't contain lead must be properly formulated, applied, and fired so that acidic foods and beverages cannot penetrate.

Handmade stoneware—like the dishes you buy in a store—is safe for food. Fired over 2,100°F, it isn't porous, so any lead that may have been used cannot leach into the food. At this temperature, any lead volatilizes, or burns away.

Earthenware, however, is fired at low temperatures, usually under 2,100°F. Any lead in the glaze generally doesn't burn away. That may not have a chance to leach into foods briefly served in the earthenware—like a mug of soup or tea. But if acid drinks—like juice, soft drinks, wine, or vinegar-containing foods—are stored in earthenware, significant amounts of lead can leach into the foods.

The best advice we know of comes from some potters and pottery teachers we spoke to. If your pottery is very old or from a foreign country, have the piece checked for lead before you use it for food. This pottery is more likely to have been fired in an older, inefficient kiln or with lead glazes. If you're buying pottery from a craftsman, ask if the glaze is lead-free and whether the pottery was low-fired or high-fired. Some pieces of pottery are tagged, stating that the piece is safe for food.

Q: I've heard that canned tuna is loaded with lead and is unsafe to eat. Is that true?

A: We recently asked ourselves the same question and had an independent laboratory test the lead content of seven samples of well-known brands of canned fish we purchased at a local market. The lab, of course, did not know which brands were which.

The average amount of lead found in the canned fish was 21 micrograms per 100 grams (about 3½ ounces). These levels are extremely low and pose no danger, according to the Food and Drug Administration. The World Health Organization's recommended allowable intake of lead for adults is about 430 micrograms per day.

Kathryn Mahaffey, Ph.D., a leading researcher in the area of nutrition and lead metabolism, told us that a study conducted by E. J. Stuik in Holland showed that adult women, who are affected more easily by lead intake than men, have noticeable changes in their blood components when about 1,000 micrograms of lead are consumed per day for about 21 days. Rapid lead poisoning has been seen in adults after taking in 5,000 micrograms per day for under a month. So to develop even mild symptoms of lead poisoning from the fish samples, you'd have to eat a minimum of 24 cans a day for four weeks.

If you're interested in avoiding lead from canned foods, Clair C. Patterson, Ph.D., from the California Institute of Technology, suggests staying away from any food packaged in cans soldered with lead.

Soldering involves pouring hot molten lead solder on the outside of the can's seam and then brushing it into the seam as it cools and solidifies. This process makes an airtight seal, but it also transfers tiny amounts of lead into the food.

How do you identify a soldered can? According to Dr. Patterson, if the sides of the can flow continuously without a break around the bottom edge, so that it looks like one continuous piece of metal, it's probably lead-free. The kind to avoid has a break in the metal where the side joins the bottom. This kind also has a vertical seam running up and down the side from top to bottom, which is where the can may be soldered. Those that are not soldered may have a label which rolls smoothly and continuously over the seam. But if you can't tell, you can check by pulling the label about ¼ inch away from the seam. If it's soldered, there will be a rough patch of silvery, grayish metal of different color and texture from the smooth, shiny tinned surface of the can.

Q: Do copper IUDs add copper to the body? Is this good or bad?

A: Copper IUDs dissolve slowly in the uterus. As much as 20 to 50 milligrams of copper can dissolve in one year. Some of that copper will be lost through menstrual flow. Some copper, however, will remain in the uterus and be carried through the body by the blood system. That presence of copper in the uterus does cause uterine tissue damage and other changes which persist after the IUD is removed. As of yet there are no reliable tests to determine if copper also accumulates in the liver and other organs and causes damage in those tissues. There is concern that women using an IUD for several years may be subject to copper toxicity. You're probably better off with a less questionable form of birth control until more conclusive studies are done.

APPENDIX

MINERAL
CONTENT
OF FOODS

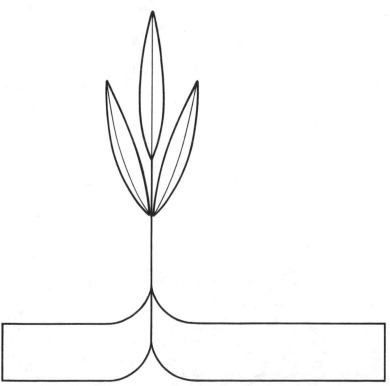

Mineral Content of Foods

We list here over 200 foods graded for the amount of minerals they contribute to the diet. Values are weighted on a scale of Excellent, Good, Fair or Poor, rather than expressed in absolute amounts, to enable you to choose foods more quickly and easily, rather than get bogged down in columns of numbers.

Values have been calculated for portions of foods as they're eaten—½ cup in the case of fruits and vegetables, 4 ounces of meat, poultry and fish, and 1 cup of juices and beverages. And, of course, when foods must be cooked before eating, that's considered in.

Remember, too, that using nutrient-saving cooking techniques such as steaming rather than boiling your vegetables will maximize the mineral content of your diet.

Food (average portion)	Calcium	Magnesium	Potassium	Zinc	
Dairy Products					
Buttermilk	●	—	⊕	○	
Cheese					
blue	⊕	—	—	—	
Cheddar	⊕	—	—	○	
Colby	⊕	—	—	○	
cottage	○	—	—	—	
Edam	⊕	—	—	○	
Gouda	⊕	—	—	○	
Monterey Jack	⊕	—	—	○	
mozzarella	⊕	—	—	—	
Muenster	⊕	—	—	○	
Parmesan	○	—	—	—	
provolone	⊕	—	—	○	
ricotta	⊕	—	○	○	
Swiss	⊕	—	—	○	

Key:

●	Excellent
⊕	Good
○	Fair
—	Poor
(NA)	Information not available

Copper	Iron	Selenium	Chromium	Manganese	Iodine	Cobalamin (Vitamin B₁₂)	Fluorine
—	—	—	—	—	—	⊕	○
—	—	—	⊕	—	—	○	—
—	—	—	⊕	—	—	○	—
—	—	—	⊕	—	—	○	—
—	—	—	○	—	—	○	—
—	—	—	⊕	—	—	○	—
—	—	—	⊕	—	—	(NA)	—
—	—	—	⊕	—	—	(NA)	—
—	—	—	⊕	—	—	○	—
—	—	—	⊕	—	—	○	—
—	—	—	○	—	—	(NA)	—
—	—	—	⊕	—	—	○	—
—	—	—	⊕	—	—	○	—
—	—	—	⊕	—	—	⊕	—

Mineral Content of Foods (continued)

Food (average portion)	Calcium	Magnesium	Potassium	Zinc	
Cream	—	—	—	—	
Ice cream	⊕	—	O	O	
Milk					
fresh	●	O	⊕	O	
dried	●	—	⊕	O	
Yogurt	●	—	⊕	O	
Fruit					
Apple	—	—	O	—	
Apple juice	—	—	O	—	
Apricots					
fresh	—	—	⊕	—	
dried	—	—	⊕	—	
Avocado	—	⊕	●	—	
Banana	—	⊕	⊕	—	
Blackberries	—	—	O	—	
Blueberries	—	—	—	—	
Cantaloupe	—	—	⊕	—	
Cherries	—	—	O	—	
Cranberries	—	—	—	—	
Dates	—	—	O	—	
Figs, fresh	O	—	O	—	
Grapefruit	—	—	O	—	
Grapefruit juice	—	—	⊕	—	

Key: ● Excellent   ⊕ Good   O Fair   — Poor   (NA) Not available

Copper	Iron	Selenium	Chromium	Manganese	Iodine	Cobalamin (Vitamin B$_{12}$)	Fluorine
−	−	−	−	−	−	−	−
−	−	−	−	−	−	⊕	O
−	−	−	−	−	−	⊕	O
−	−	−	−	−	−	⊕	O
−	−	−	−	−	−	⊕	O
O	−	−	O	O	−	−	O
O	O	−	O	O	−	−	O
O	−	−	O	O	−	−	−
O	O	−	O	O	−	−	−
⊕	−	−	O	O	−	−	(NA)
⊕	−	−	O	●	−	−	−
O	−	−	O	O	−	−	(NA)
O	−	−	O	O	−	−	(NA)
O	−	−	O	O	−	−	−
O	−	−	O	O	−	−	−
−	−	−	O	O	−	−	(NA)
O	O	−	O	O	−	−	(NA)
O	−	−	O	O	−	−	−
−	−	−	O	O	−	−	−
−	−	−	O	O	−	−	−

Mineral Content of Foods (continued)

Food (average portion)	Calcium	Magnesium	Potassium	Zinc	
Grapes	—	—	—	—	
Honeydew melon	—	O	⊕	—	
Lemon	—	—	—	—	
Lemonade	—	—	—	—	
Mango	—	—	O	—	
Orange	O	—	O	—	
Orange juice	—	—	⊕	—	
Papaya	—	(NA)	⊕	—	
Peach	—	—	⊕	—	
Pear	—	—	O	—	
Pineapple	—	—	O	—	
Plums	—	—	—	—	
Prunes	—	—	⊕	—	
Raisins	—	—	●	—	
Raspberries	—	—	—	—	
Rhubarb	O	—	O	—	
Strawberries	—	—	O	—	
Tangerine	—	—	O	—	
Watermelon	—	—	—	—	
Vegetables					
Amaranth	—	(NA)	(NA)	(NA)	
Artichoke	O	(NA)	⊕	O	
Asparagus	—	—	O	—	

Key: ● Excellent ⊕ Good O Fair — Poor (NA) Not available

Copper	Iron	Selenium	Chromium	Manganese	Iodine	Cobalamin (Vitamin B$_{12}$)	Fluorine
—	—	—	O	O	—	—	—
O	—	—	O	O	—	—	—
—	—	—	O	O	—	—	—
—	—	—	O	O	—	—	—
O	—	—	O	O	—	—	(NA)
O	—	—	O	O	—	—	—
O	—	—	O	O	—	—	—
O	—	—	O	O	—	—	(NA)
O	—	—	O	O	—	—	(NA)
O	—	—	O	O	—	—	—
—	—	—	O	O	—	—	—
—	—	—	O	O	—	—	—
O	O	—	O	O	—	—	—
O	O	—	O	O	—	—	—
O	—	—	O	O	—	—	(NA)
(NA)	—	—	O	O	—	—	—
—	—	—	O	O	—	—	(NA)
O	—	—	O	O	—	—	—
—	—	—	O	O	—	—	(NA)
(NA)	—	—	⊕	O	—	—	(NA)
(NA)	O	—	⊕	O	—	—	(NA)
—	—	—	⊕	O	—	—	(NA)

Mineral Content of Foods (continued)

Food (average portion)	Calcium	Magnesium	Potassium	Zinc	
Beans					
garbanzo (chick-peas)	O	(NA)	⊕	O	
lima	—	⊕	⊕	O	
navy	—	●	⊕	O	
red kidney	—	●	⊕	O	
snap	—	—	⊕	—	
soybeans	O	●	⊕	●	
soybean curd, see Tofu					
soybean paste, see Miso					
Beet greens	O	O	O	—	
Beets	—	—	O	—	
Black-eyed peas	—	⊕	⊕	O	
Broccoli	O	—	O	—	
Brussels sprouts	—	—	O	—	
Cabbage	—	—	O	—	
Carrots	—	—	O	—	
Cauliflower	—	—	O	—	
Celery	—	—	O	—	
Chick-peas, see Beans, garbanzo					
Chicory, see Endive					
Coleslaw	—	—	O	—	
Collards	O	O	O	—	
Corn	—	O	O	—	

Key: ● Excellent   ⊕ Good   O Fair   — Poor   (NA) Not available

Copper	Iron	Selenium	Chromium	Manganese	Iodine	Cobalamin (Vitamin B₁₂)	Fluorine
O	⊕	—	⊕	⊕	—	—	(NA)
O	O	—	⊕	⊕	—	—	(NA)
⊕	O	—	⊕	⊕	—	—	(NA)
⊕	O	—	⊕	⊕	—	—	(NA)
—	—	—	⊕	O	—	—	—
⊕	O	—	⊕	⊕	—	—	O
O	O	—	⊕	O	—	—	(NA)
O	—	—	⊕	O	—	—	—
⊕	O	—	⊕	⊕	—	—	(NA)
—	—	—	⊕	O	—	—	(NA)
—	—	—	⊕	O	—	—	(NA)
—	—	—	⊕	O	—	—	—
—	—	—	⊕	O	—	—	—
—	—	—	⊕	O	—	—	(NA)
—	—	—	⊕	O	—	—	—
—	—	—	⊕	O	—	—	—
O	—	—	⊕	O	—	—	(NA)
—	—	O	⊕	⊕	—	—	—

Mineral Content of Foods (continued)

Food (average portion)	Calcium	Magnesium	Potassium	Zinc
Corn grits	—	—	—	—
Cucumber	—	—	—	—
Dandelion greens	⊕	—	O	—
Eggplant	—	—	O	—
Endive (chicory)	—	—	O	—
Kale	O	—	O	—
Kohlrabi	—	—	O	—
Lentils	—	O	O	O
Lettuce				
iceberg	—	—	O	—
romaine	—	—	O	—
Miso (soybean paste)	—	●	⊕	●
Mushrooms	—	—	O	—
Mustard greens	O	—	O	—
Okra	O	O	O	—
Onions	—	—	—	—
Parsley	—	—	—	—
Sprouts, mung bean	—	(NA)	O	—
Squash				
acorn	—	—	⊕	—
butternut	—	—	●	—
yellow	—	—	O	—
zucchini	—	—	O	—

Key: ● Excellent ⊕ Good O Fair — Poor (NA) Not available

Copper	Iron	Selenium	Chromium	Manganese	Iodine	Cobalamin (Vitamin B$_{12}$)	Fluorine
—	—	O	⊕	⊕	—	—	—
—	—	—	⊕	O	—	—	—
O	O	—	⊕	O	—	—	(NA)
O	—	—	⊕	O	—	—	—
O	O	—	⊕	O	—	—	(NA)
O	—	—	⊕	O	—	—	O
—	—	—	⊕	O	—	—	(NA)
O	O	—	⊕	⊕	—	—	(NA)
—	—	—	⊕	⊕	—	—	(NA)
—	—	—	⊕	⊕	—	—	(NA)
⊕	O	—	⊕	⊕	—	—	O
⊕	—	—	⊕	O	—	—	(NA)
O	O	—	⊕	O	—	—	(NA)
—	—	—	⊕	O	—	—	(NA)
—	—	—	⊕	O	—	—	—
—	—	—	O	O	—	—	—
—	—	—	⊕	O	—	—	(NA)
O	O	—	⊕	O	—	—	(NA)
O	O	—	⊕	O	—	—	(NA)
O	—	—	⊕	O	—	—	(NA)
O	—	—	⊕	O	—	—	(NA)

Mineral Content of Foods (continued)

Food (average portion)	Calcium	Magnesium	Potassium	Zinc	
Sweet potato	—	O	⊕	—	
Swiss chard	O	O	O	—	
Tofu (soybean curd)	⊕	●	O	●	
Parsnips	—	—	O	—	
Peas	—	—	O	O	
Peppers, green	—	—	O	—	
Potato	—	⊕	●	—	
Pumpkin	—	—	O	—	
Radishes	—	—	—	—	
Spinach	O	⊕	O	—	
Tomato	—	—	O	—	
Tomato juice	—	—	●	—	
Turnip greens	O	O	(NA)	—	
Turnips	—	—	O	—	
Yams	—	(NA)	●	—	
Water chestnuts	—	—	O	—	
Watercress	O	—	O	—	
Grains and Grain Products					
Barley	—	—	O	(NA)	
Bread					
cracked wheat	—	⊕	—	—	
pumpernickel	—	—	O	—	
rye	—	—	—	—	

Key: ● Excellent ⊕ Good O Fair — Poor (NA) Not available

Copper	Iron	Selenium	Chromium	Manganese	Iodine	Cobalamin (Vitamin B$_{12}$)	Fluorine
O	O	—	⊕	⊕	—	—	(NA)
O	O	—	⊕	O	—	—	(NA)
⊕	O	—	⊕	⊕	—	—	O
—	—	—	⊕	O	—	—	(NA)
O	O	—	⊕	O	—	—	—
O	—	—	⊕	O	—	—	(NA)
⊕	O	—	⊕	O	—	—	O
O	—	—	⊕	O	—	—	(NA)
—	—	—	⊕	O	—	—	—
O	O	—	⊕	⊕	—	—	O
O	—	—	⊕	O	—	—	—
⊕	O	—	⊕	O	—	—	—
O	—	—	⊕	O	—	—	—
—	—	—	⊕	O	—	—	—
O	—	—	⊕	O			(NA)
—	—	—	O	O	—	—	(NA)
—	O	—	⊕	O	—	—	—
⊕	O	O	⊕	⊕	—	—	(NA)
O	—	⊕	⊕	O	—	—	—
—	—	O	O	—	—	—	—
—	—	O	O	—	—	—	—

Mineral Content of Foods (continued)

Food (average portion)	Calcium	Magnesium	Potassium	Zinc	
Bread (continued)					
white	—	—	—	—	
whole wheat	—	—	—	—	
Bulgur (cracked wheat)	—	(NA)	—	O	
Cereal					
corn flakes	—	—	—	—	
puffed rice	—	—	—	—	
shredded wheat	—	⊕	O	O	
Corn bread	O	(NA)	O	—	
Cornmeal	—	⊕	O	O	
Cracked wheat, see Bulgur					
Flour					
buckwheat	—	●	(NA)	(NA)	
rye	—	O	—	—	
white	—	—	—	—	
whole wheat	—	⊕	O	O	
Gingerbread	—	(NA)	O	—	
Macaroni	—	—	—	—	
Millet	—	O	⊕	(NA)	
Noodles, egg	—	—	—	—	
Oats, rolled (oatmeal)	—	⊕	O	O	
Pancakes, whole wheat	⊕	(NA)	O	O	

Key: ● Excellent   ⊕ Good   O Fair   — Poor   (NA) Not available

Copper	Iron	Selenium	Chromium	Manganese	Iodine	Cobalamin (Vitamin B_{12})	Fluorine
—	—	—	—	—	—	—	—
O	—	⊕	⊕	O	—	—	—
⊕	O	⊕	⊕	●	—	—	—
—	—	—	—	(NA)	—	—	—
—	—	—	—	(NA)	—	—	—
O	O	⊕	⊕	O	—	—	—
—	—	O	⊕	O	—	—	—
—	O	O	⊕	⊕	—	—	—
⊕	O	O	⊕	⊕	—	—	—
O	O	O	⊕	●	—	—	—
O	O	O	O	O	—	—	—
⊕	O	⊕	⊕	●	—	—	—
—	O	—	—	—	—	—	—
—	—	—	—	—	—	—	—
⊕	O	O	⊕	⊕	—	—	(NA)
—	—	—	—	—	—	—	—
O	O	O	⊕	●	—	—	—
⊕	O	⊕	⊕	●	—	(NA)	—

Mineral Content of Foods (continued)

Food (average portion)	Calcium	Magnesium	Potassium	Zinc	
Spaghetti					
white	—	—	—	—	
whole wheat	—	⊕	○	○	
Rice					
brown	—	○	—	○	
white	—	○	—	—	
Tapioca	—	—	—	(NA)	
Wheat germ	—	○	—	○	
Nuts and Seeds					
Almonds	○	⊕	○	—	
Brazil nuts	○	⊕	○	⊕	
Cashews	—	⊕	○	⊕	
Chestnuts	—	○	○	(NA)	
Coconut, flaked	—	—	—	—	
Filberts (hazelnuts)	○	⊕	○	○	
Peanut butter	—	⊕	○	○	
Peanuts	—	⊕	○	○	
Pecans	—	⊕	○	(NA)	
Pine nuts	—	(NA)	(NA)	(NA)	
Pumpkin seeds	—	(NA)	—	⊕	
Sesame seeds	○	—	—	(NA)	
Sunflower seeds	—	—	⊕	⊕	
Tahini (sesame seed butter)	⊕	○	—	(NA)	

Key: ● Excellent ⊕ Good ○ Fair — Poor (NA) Not available

Copper	Iron	Selenium	Chromium	Manganese	Iodine	Cobalamin (Vitamin B$_{12}$)	Fluorine
—	—	—	—	—	—	—	—
⊕	O	⊕	⊕	●	—	(NA)	—
O	—	O	⊕	●	—	—	—
—	—	—	O	O	—	—	—
—	—	—	(NA)	(NA)	—	—	(NA)
O	—	⊕	⊕	⊕	—	—	—
⊕	O	(NA)	(NA)	⊕	—	—	—
⊕	O	(NA)	(NA)	⊕	—	—	—
⊕	O	(NA)	(NA)	⊕	—	—	(NA)
O	—	(NA)	(NA)	⊕	—	—	(NA)
O		(NA)	(NA)	⊕	—	—	(NA)
⊕	⊕	(NA)	(NA)	⊕	—	—	—
O	—	(NA)	(NA)	⊕	—	—	(NA)
O	—	(NA)	(NA)	⊕	—	—	(NA)
⊕	—	(NA)	(NA)	⊕	—	—	(NA)
⊕	O	(NA)	(NA)	⊕	—	—	(NA)
⊕	O	(NA)	(NA)	⊕	—	—	(NA)
O	—	(NA)	(NA)	⊕	—	—	(NA)
⊕	O	(NA)	(NA)	⊕	—	—	(NA)
O	O	(NA)	(NA)	⊕	—	—	(NA)

Mineral Content of Foods (continued)

Food (average portion)	Calcium	Magnesium	Potassium	Zinc	
Walnuts	—	⊕	O	O	
Poultry and Eggs					
Chicken					
dark meat	—	—	O	⊕	
light meat	—	O	O	O	
livers	—	—	O	●	
Duck	—	—	O	O	
Goose	—	—	⊕	(NA)	
Turkey					
dark meat	—	—	O	●	
light meat	—	O	O	⊕	
Egg	O	—	—	—	
Fish and Seafood					
Bluefish	—	(NA)	(NA)	(NA)	
Clams	—	(NA)	O	O	
Cod	—	O	⊕	O	
Crab	—	O	(NA)	●	
Flounder	—	O	●	O	
Haddock	—	—	⊕	O	
Halibut	—	(NA)	●	O	
Herring, canned	(NA)	(NA)	(NA)	(NA)	
Lobster	O	—	O	⊕	
Mackerel	—	O	(NA)	O	

Key: ● Excellent ⊕ Good O Fair — Poor (NA) Not available

Copper	Iron	Selenium	Chromium	Manganese	Iodine	Cobalamin (Vitamin B$_{12}$)	Fluorine
⊕	○	(NA)	(NA)	⊕	—	—	(NA)
○	⊕	—	⊕	—	—	○	○
—	⊕	—	○	—	—	○	○
⊕	●	●	●	○	—	●	○
⊕	●	—	⊕	(NA)	—	⊕	○
○	⊕	—	⊕	(NA)		(NA)	○
○	⊕	—	⊕	—	—	○	○
○	⊕	—	○	—	—	○	○
—	○	—	(NA)	—	—	⊕	—
○	—	●	○	—	○	(NA)	⊕
—	⊕	●	○	—	⊕	●	⊕
○	⊕	●	○	—	●	⊕	●
⊕	—	●	○	—	○	●	●
○	⊕	●	○	—	(NA)	⊕	⊕
○	⊕	●	○	—	●	⊕	⊕
○	—	●	○	—	⊕	⊕	⊕
○	(NA)	●	○	—	⊕	●	⊕
⊕	—	●	○	—	●	⊕	⊕
○	⊕	●	○	—	⊕	●	●

Mineral Content of Foods (continued)

Food (average portion)	Calcium	Magnesium	Potassium	Zinc	
Oysters	O	O	O	●	
Salmon	●	O	●	(NA)	
Sardines	●	—	●	(NA)	
Scallops	O	(NA)	●	(NA)	
Sea bass	(NA)	(NA)	(NA)	(NA)	
Sea perch	—	(NA)	O	(NA)	
Shrimp	O	⊕	O	⊕	
Sole	—	O	⊕	O	
Sturgeon	—	(NA)	O	(NA)	
Swordfish	—	(NA)	(NA)	O	
Trout	(NA)	(NA)	(NA)	O	
Tuna	—	(NA)	⊕	O	
Whitefish	(NA)	(NA)	⊕	O	
Meat					
Bacon	—	—	—	(NA)	
Beef					
ground	—	O	⊕	●	
liver	—	—	⊕	●	
roast	—	O	⊕	●	
steak	—	O	O	●	
Calf liver	—	O	●	●	
Frankfurters	—	(NA)	(NA)	⊕	
Lamb	—	—	⊕	●	

Key: ● Excellent   ⊕ Good   O Fair   — Poor   (NA) Not available

Copper	Iron	Selenium	Chromium	Manganese	Iodine	Cobalamin (Vitamin B_{12})	Fluorine
●	●	●	○	—	⊕	●	⊕
○	⊕	●	○	—	○	○	●
—	⊕	●	○	—	○	●	●
○	⊕	●	○	—	⊕	⊕	⊕
○	(NA)	●	○	—	○	(NA)	⊕
○	⊕	●	○	—	●	⊕	⊕
⊕	⊕	●	○	—	●	⊕	●
—	—	●	○	—	—	⊕	⊕
○	⊕	●	○	—	(NA)	(NA)	⊕
○	⊕	●	○	—	(NA)	⊕	⊕
○	—	●	○	—	—	●	⊕
○	⊕	●	○	—	(NA)	●	⊕
○	—	●	○	—	—	(NA)	⊕
—	—	—	—	—	—	—	—
—	●	—	⊕	—	—	●	○
●	●	●	●	○	—	●	○
○	●	—	⊕	—	—	●	○
—	●	—	⊕	—	—	●	○
●	●	●	●	○	—	●	○
○	⊕	—	○	—	—	⊕	○
—	⊕	—	(NA)	—	—	●	(NA)

Mineral Content of Foods (continued)

Food (average portion)	Calcium	Magnesium	Potassium	Zinc	
Pork	—	—	⊕	●	
Rabbit	—	(NA)	⊕	●	
Veal	—	—	O	●	
Venison	—	O	(NA)	●	
Soups					
Chicken	—	(NA)	O	—	
Cream of mushroom	⊕	(NA)	O	O	
Split pea	O	(NA)	●	—	
Tomato	⊕	—	⊕	O	
Vegetable	—	—	⊕	⊕	
Snacks					
Crackers, saltines	—	—	—	—	
Popcorn	—	(NA)	(NA)	—	
Soy nuts	O	⊕	(NA)	⊕	
Miscellaneous					
Blackstrap molasses	O	⊕	●	(NA)	
Brewer's yeast	—	—	O	(NA)	
Kelp	O	(NA)	(NA)	(NA)	

Key: ● Excellent   ⊕ Good   O Fair   — Poor   (NA) Not available

SOURCES: Most values were adapted from
   Nutritive Value of American Foods in Common Units, Agriculture Handbook No. 456, by Catherine F. Adams (Washington, D.C.: Agricultural Research Service, U.S. Department of Agriculture, 1975).
   Composition of Foods, Agriculture Handbook No. 8, rev. ed., by Bernice K. Watt and Annabel L. Merrill (Washington, D.C.: Agricultural Research Service, U.S. Department of Agriculture, 1975).
   Composition of Foods: Dairy and Egg Products, Agriculture Handbook No. 8-1, rev. ed., by Consumer and Food Economics Institute (Washington, D.C.: Agricultural Research Service, U.S. Department of Agriculture, 1976).

Copper	Iron	Selenium	Chromium	Manganese	Iodine	Cobalamin (Vitamin B₁₂)	Fluorine
⊕	●	—	(NA)	—	—	⊕	(NA)
O	O	—	(NA)	—	—	(NA)	(NA)
O	⊕	—	⊕	—	—	⊕	O
O	(NA)	—	(NA)	—	—	(NA)	(NA)
—	O	—	O	—	—	—	(NA)
—	—	—	(NA)	—	—	(NA)	(NA)
O	⊕	—	O	⊕	—	(NA)	(NA)
O	—	—	O	O	—	—	(NA)
⊕	O	—	O	O	—	—	(NA)
—	—	—	—	—	—	—	—
—	—	O	O	—	—	—	(NA)
O	O	(NA)	(NA)	⊕	—	—	(NA)
⊕	⊕	—	(NA)	(NA)	—	—	(NA)
O	O	—	●	(NA)	—	—	(NA)
(NA)	—	(NA)	(NA)	(NA)	●	(NA)	(NA)

Composition of Foods: Poultry Products, Agriculture Handbook No. 8-5, rev. ed., by Consumer and Food Economics Institute (Washington, D.C.: Agricultural Research Service, U.S. Department of Agriculture, 1979).

"Provisional Tables on the Zinc Content of Foods," by Elizabeth W. Murphy, Barbara Wells W... and Bernice K. Watt, *Journal of the American Dietetic Association,* April 1975.

Introductory Nutrition, 4th ed., by Helen Andrews Guthrie (St. Louis: C. V. Mosby, 1979).

NOTE: This table was compiled by Takla Gardey and Carol Matthews.

INDEX

Rodale Press, Inc., publishes PREVENTION®, the better health magazine.
For information on how to order your subscription,
write to PREVENTION®, Emmaus, PA 18049.